PRAI~~SE FOR THE~~ *WAHLS* PROTOCOL

"There are very few books that have had the impact of *The Wahls Protocol*—for the first time, autoimmune conditions such as multiple sclerosis could be treated causally instead of reactively, supportively instead of suppressively. Now Dr. Wahls has written a revised and updated edition of her classic book, which includes new research, new testimonials of success, further clarification and simplification of her protocol, and most important, preventive treatment for autoimmune and other chronic conditions. This book is a must-read for all of us who want to see the end of the threats of multiple sclerosis and other chronic illnesses."

—Prof. Dale Bredesen, author of the *New York Times* bestseller *The End of Alzheimer's*

"Terry Wahls, MD, is one of the rare health experts and bestselling authors who not only walks the talk but actually *researches* the talk. Her rigorous clinical trials address diet quality, track microbiome and gene expression changes over time, and answer lingering questions that we all have about multiple sclerosis and other autoimmune conditions. Her newly revised book, *The Wahls Protocol*, is a classic in the emerging field of personalized lifestyle medicine and should be required reading for every medical student, practitioner, and patient who cares about their health."

—Sara Gottfried, MD, *New York Times* bestselling author of *Younger*

"In *The Wahls Protocol*, Dr. Wahls provides elegant firsthand validation that diet truly represents the most powerful medicine. This book is totally supported by the most leading-edge research and provides a beacon of hope when compared to the ever-changing landscape of pharmaceutical recommendations for multiple sclerosis."

—David Perlmutter, MD, #1 *New York Times*–bestselling author of *Grain Brain*

"Groundbreaking! Once you understand why you need to eat for health, Dr. Wahls delivers a detailed road map, guiding you step by step. This will be life changing for many."

—Robb Wolf, *New York Times*–bestselling author of *The Paleo Solution*

"Whether or not you struggle with autoimmune diseases, I can't recommend *The Wahls Protocol* highly enough. Dr. Wahls provides a clear, in-depth, copiously researched dietary and lifestyle protocol to help you take charge of your health and your life. An absolute must-read book."

—JJ Virgin, CNS, CHFS, *New York Times*–bestselling author of *The Virgin Diet*

"Dr. Terry Wahls is an incredible teacher, researcher, and physician who has turned her healing success into the Wahls Protocol, which can benefit many people. I've supported her work through the years because she is evidence-based, encourages colorful eating with copious plant foods, and recognizes the need to incorporate high-quality, nutrient-dense foods that will help prevent disease. In this new book, she addresses some of the more current topics in nutrition such as ketosis, fasting, the impact of the microbiome, as well as epigenetics. She is always on the pulse of what is new and provides a balanced perspective."

—DEANNA MINICH, PhD, CNS, IFMCP, RESEARCHER, EDUCATOR, AND AUTHOR OF *Whole Detox*

"In *The Wahls Protocol*, Dr. Terry Wahls offers a revolutionary way of reversing multiple sclerosis: nutrient-dense food. She does this artfully, combining scientific evidence with her own exceptional story of personal triumph over severe MS. You'll find many tools for healing in this accessible book, from detailed recommendations and recipes to much-needed hope and encouragement. It is a must-read!"

—MAYA SHETREAT, MD, INTEGRATIVE PEDIATRIC NEUROLOGIST AND AUTHOR OF *The Dirt Cure: Growing Healthy Kids with Food Straight from the Soil*

"Terry Wahls is a hero to many for her discovery that a nourishing ancestral diet can heal multiple sclerosis. In *The Wahls Protocol*, Terry sets forth a straightforward plan for achieving good health through good food. Not just for MS patients, *The Wahls Protocol* is a fascinating tale that proves the wisdom of Hippocrates: 'Let food be thy medicine.' Try it, it works!"

—PAUL JAMINET, PhD, AUTHOR OF *Perfect Health Diet* AND EDITOR IN CHIEF OF THE *Journal of Evolution and Health*

"I've long recommended that *anyone* diagnosed with MS who is also interested in health and healing research the work of Dr. Wahls online, but the game has now changed. *The Wahls Protocol* will be the go-to resource for anyone suffering from MS or another autoimmune condition who is ready to fight back. Dr. Wahls outlines a clear-cut, stepped approach to dietary and lifestyle changes—supported by her extensive research and testing of the plans—that will put *anyone* on a path to better health. Whether you have MS or not, *The Wahls Protocol* is a gold mine of easy-to-follow, real-food nutritional guidelines that will leave you feeling so amazing it'll make you wonder how you ever ate any other way."

—DIANE SANFILIPPO, BS, NC, *New York Times*–BESTSELLING AUTHOR OF *Practical Paleo*

"*The Wahls Protocol* is one aha after another of how Terry Wahls's realizations may help you in your health journey. Not only will you be captivated by what you read, you'll also learn how to be healthier. Highly recommended."

—DR. TOM O'BRYAN, CREATOR OF A GRAIN OF TRUTH: THE GLUTEN SUMMIT

"Terry Wahls's new book is one of the most important books on health ever written. That's not a hyperbolic statement, just plain fact. If doctors would take this incredible information to heart (and into their practices), the health crisis in this world would be over—the cancer industry crushed and the rise in autoimmune conditions would fall.

True health reform is contained within these pages. I cannot recommend a book any more highly. Bravo, Dr. Wahls!"

—LEANNE ELY, CNC, *New York Times*–BESTSELLING AUTHOR OF *Saving Dinner*

"Terry Wahls does an amazing job at highlighting the importance of micronutrients (vitamins, minerals, and essential fats) as an integral part in preventing and reversing disease. Her story is incredible and brings hope to millions needlessly suffering. *The Wahls Protocol* is a must-read for anyone looking to reverse autoimmune conditions naturally."

—MIRA CALTON, CN, AND JAYSON CALTON, PhD, AUTHORS OF *Rich Food, Poor Food*

"The best treatment for multiple sclerosis, autoimmunity, and chronic disease is teaching people how and why to eat and live for optimal health. By combining the latest science with the all-important factors of nutrition, exercise, and healthy lifestyle, *The Wahls Protocol* goes beyond conventional treatments and empowers you with real solutions."

—ANN BOROCH, CNC, AUTHOR OF *Healing Multiple Sclerosis: Diet, Detox & Nutritional Makeover for Total Recovery*

"Dr. Wahls engages us with her personal story of triumph over multiple sclerosis while educating us on the importance of a nutrient-dense diet for our cellular health. You will find yourself drawn in and inspired to take control of your own health as Dr. Wahls shares her experiences, knowledge, and compassion. The three levels of *The Wahls Protocol* provide a concrete plan—including both feasible diet and lifestyle changes—to help you on your road to recovery." —SARAH BALLANTYNE, PhD, AUTHOR OF *The Paleo Approach*

"*The Wahls Protocol* is essential reading for anyone suffering from a chronic disease and wanting to regain their health. All the therapies which restored Dr. Wahls to well-being are described in detail and are succinctly summarized in the appendices. The huge amount of scientific information, clear explanations, and practical advice make this book an invaluable resource and indispensable reference."

—ASHTON EMBRY, PhD, PRESIDENT OF DIRECT-MS

"Only Terry Wahls, MD, could have written a book as important as *The Wahls Protocol*. Her discovery of a path to recovery from disabling multiple sclerosis after failing to respond to the traditional medical approach is not only a story of great personal triumph but a manifesto of hope for many others with various chronic illnesses for which drug therapy has not worked. This is a book that provides a program that can be applied by anyone who is searching for solutions to health challenges."

—JEFFREY BLAND, PhD, PRESIDENT AND FOUNDER OF THE PERSONALIZED LIFESTYLE MEDICINE INSTITUTE

The
WAHLS
PROTOCOL

*A Radical New Way to Treat All Chronic
Autoimmune Conditions Using Paleo Principles*

Revised and Expanded

TERRY WAHLS, MD

with Eve Adamson

AVERY

an imprint of Penguin Random House

New York

AVERY

an imprint of Penguin Random House LLC
penguinrandomhouse.com

First Avery trade paperback edition 2014
Revised and updated 2020

Most Avery books are available at special quantity discounts for bulk purchase for sales
promotions, premiums, fund-raising, and educational needs. Special books or book excerpts also
can be created to fit specific needs. For details, write SpecialMarkets@penguinrandomhouse.com.

The Library of Congress has catalogued the hardcover edition as follows:

Wahls, Terry L.
The Wahls protocol : how I beat progressive ms using Paleo principles and functional
medicine / by Terry Wahls, M.D., with Eve Adamson.
p.   cm.
ISBN 978-1-58333-521-5
1. Wahls, Terry L.—Health.   2. Multiple sclerosis—Patients—Rehabilitation.
3. Physicians—Diseases—Biography.   4. Multiple sclerosis—Exercise therapy.
5. Multiple sclerosis—Diet therapy.   I. Adamson, Eve.   II. Title.
RC377.W34   2014   2013043692
616.8.'34—dc23
ISBN 978-1-58333-554-3 (paperback)

Printed in the United States of America
19   20

BOOK DESIGN BY TANYA MAIBORODA

To Jackie,
who has sustained me
through the challenges and joys of this life

A NOTE TO THE READER

Many of the Wahls Warriors who generously contributed their stories and are quoted in this book have included their actual names and locations, but a few prefer to remain anonymous, so some names and locations have been changed to protect the privacy of those who desire it.

Nutrient composition of recipes and menus were calculated with Nutrition Data System for Research (NDSR) Database Version 2012 © Regents of the University of Minnesota, at ncc.umn.edu/. Nutrient totals include all ingredients except those listed as optional. When a choice of ingredients is presented, the nutrient composition for the first item was used in the calculations. Reasonable effort has been made to check the accuracy of this data; however, variations in natural and manufactured foods as well as deviations from the stated recipe or menu ingredients, amounts, and preparation methods will impact the nutrient composition. All nutritional values should be considered approximate. Conclusions regarding the nutritional adequacy of the diets are based on the sample menus shown and the current nutritional recommendations for women in my age group (51 to 70 years), who have higher calcium intake requirements than premenopausal women, or men under the age of 71. Note that nutritional recommendations are otherwise relatively similar between age groups. Always consult your health care provider to discuss your personal diet and nutritional needs and have these concepts adapted and personalized to your circumstances.

Disclaimer

Medicine and nutrition are ever-changing sciences. As new research and clinical experience broaden our knowledge, changes in nutrition recommendations, treatment, and drug therapy are required. The authors have checked with sources believed to be reliable in their efforts to provide information that is complete and generally in accord with the standards accepted at the time of publication. However, in view of the possibility of human error or changes in medical sciences, neither the authors nor the publisher nor any other party who has been involved in the preparation or publication of this work warrants that the information contained herein is in every respect accurate or complete, and they are not responsible for any errors or omissions or for the results obtained from the use of such information. Readers are encouraged to confirm the information contained herein with other sources.

The Food and Drug Administration has not evaluated any of the statements made on my websites, in my lectures, or in my books. This is education and not intended to diagnose, treat, cure, or prevent any disease. This book is based upon my review of hundreds of basic science studies and animal model studies, hundreds of human clinical trials, my experience in my primary care clinics and traumatic brain injury clinics, my own self-experimentation over the last ten years, and our clinical trial.

Trademark Notice

The terms Wahls Protocol™ program, Wahls™ diet, Wahls Paleo™ diet, and Wahls Paleo Plus™ diet and Wahls Warriors™ are the trademarks of Dr. Terry Wahls LLC. Whenever the terms Wahls Protocol, Wahls Diet, Wahls Paleo, or Wahls Paleo Plus or Wahls Warrior are used in this book, they are referring to the Wahls Protocol™ program, the Wahls™ diet, the Wahls Paleo™ diet, and the Wahls Paleo Plus™ diet and Wahls Warrior™ individuals.

CONTENTS

PREFACE TO THE REVISED EDITION

MUCH HAS HAPPENED since the first edition of *The Wahls Protocol* was published in 2014. When I first found myself in the spotlight and under the scrutiny of my professional colleagues, I received a lot of pushback about the contents of this book (and my TEDx talk). Since then the world and the priorities of science and medicine have changed dramatically. Today there is a huge amount of research published about the influence of diet and lifestyle on human health. This is no longer a new or controversial topic. We have gone mainstream. Other concepts have become popular topics of research as well, such as the microbiome and the gut-brain axis, which directly influence human health, and which are largely shaped, fueled, and influenced by both food and lifestyle.

What has driven this change? To a large extent, you have. It was difficult to get our first paper published, which described the preliminary data on the first ten subjects in our trial who had secondary progressive MS and who, with the implementation of the Wahls Protocol, experienced a statistically (and more important, clinically) significant reduction in fatigue. Now, research like this is hardly unusual, and that is because you wanted to know. You demanded answers. You knew, instinctively, that food and lifestyle influence health. You wanted options beyond the latest disease-modifying drugs. You wanted to take control of your own health. That has led doctors, scientists, the media, and those who fund research to sit up and pay attention. The National MS Society (NMSS) monitors social media to understand the interests and needs of their constituency—people with MS. When *The Wahls Protocol* was first published, there was a dramatic uptick in the mentions about diet, exercise, lifestyle, and the Wahls Protocol, which eclipsed all the mentions about all the drug disease-modifying therapies! This ultimately led the NMSS to have a wellness conference, and they invited me to attend. They had 45 scientists and 45 patients with MS (I was a twofer). I urged the NMSS to create a new peer review process for dietary intervention studies, since it is a very different science from drug development. I also urged the NMSS to create resources so patients would know about the Wahls diet, the Swank diet, the Mediterranean diet, and gluten-free diets, including the limited research behind each diet and the potential benefits and risks of each diet.

The NMSS[1] did create those educational resources and did make diet and lifestyle interventions for wellness a research priority. They also funded our research lab to conduct a study comparing the Swank diet to the Wahls diet, with a million-dollar four-year grant.[2] We will be analyzing the data in 2020 and presenting our results once the analyses are completed. That is because of you.

Since 2014, we have been busy. We have had all of our subjects complete twelve months of the protocol. The second paper was published, which also showed significant reduction in fatigue and improvement in quality of life. The third paper showed reduction in anxiety and depression scores, and improved verbal and nonverbal reasoning.[3] All this is remarkable.

Next we completed a randomized controlled trial, but this time, our subjects had relapsing-remitting multiple sclerosis only. People were randomized to receive diet instruction right away, or at 12 weeks. We measured clinical outcomes at baseline and 12 weeks, and demonstrated that our diet was associated with significantly less fatigue, improved quality of life, and improved motor function.[4]

We recently published another paper that showed our diet increased HDL ("good") cholesterol and that this was associated with less fatigue in MS patients. Further dietary analysis will becoming in a future paper.[5]

After that, we did a randomized controlled trial comparing the original Wahls Diet to the Wahls Paleo Plus ketogenic diet, to investigate whether the ketogenic version was more beneficial than the original Wahls Diet. The results of this study will be forthcoming in a future publication.

I cannot overstate the significant ways our research has changed research into this area.[6] Other investigators are now talking about our work. Since *The Wahls Protocol* was published, there have been hundreds of scientific papers about diet and MS published and available on PubMed. Only a few involve actual clinical trials, and most of these came from our lab.

I also have collaborations with other scientists here at the University of Iowa to investigate how our protocol impacts the microbiome and vision function. We are also developing collaborations with MS researchers at other universities who have expertise in lipids, metabolomics, vitamin K and vitamin A, and brain structure analyses. We have more data to analyze and more papers to write.

In addition to my research, I remain committed to public education. I have created a website and newsletters, recorded my lectures, and given lectures around the country. I do webinars, interviews, radio shows, and talk shows. One of the highlights of my career was when I was awarded the 2018 Linus Pauling Award, presented to me by the Institute for Functional Medicine, for my contributions as a researcher, teacher, clinician, and patient advocate. (You can read more about this at terrywahls.com/i-did-all-that-i-could/.)

I have joined the faculty of the Institute for Functional Medicine, teaching dietary approaches to reduce neuroinflammation and neurodegeneration for the IFM advanced practice module on energy. I lecture for the American Academy of Anti-Aging Medicine. I also work with philanthropists who believe in our mission of testing how therapeutic diet and lifestyle interventions create health and control neuroinflammation and neurodegeneration. I travel across the country and around the world, teaching the public, clinicians, and research scientists about the use of therapeutic diets and lifestyle to create a more healing environment for our cells.

Many health professionals who had been forced to stop working because of their health challenges discovered my work and restored their health. During that journey, they too have found new purposes. They have often transformed their clinical practices and have become certified Wahls Protocol Health Professionals. They have shifted the focus of their clinical work toward using therapeutic diet and lifestyle within the realm of their clinical expertise. We have in-person and virtual health professional training programs, which you can also learn about at terrywahls.com.

I also have a small private practice where I complete comprehensive assessments and provide six months of support to help people implement the recommendations. Details of the types of programs I offer can be found on my website.

And now I can offer you a revised, updated version of *The Wahls Protocol*. This edition is full of new information, including new scientific developments, furthered understanding of old concepts, more references to more new research, and more things you can add to your Wahls Protocol arsenal. I've also included some new recipes, new testimonials, and my assessment of what is new and important in the world of health and wellness. I've also expanded many of the discussions in this book to apply to people with chronic diseases other than MS, as I meet and learn about people using the Wahls Protocol to resolve a wide variety of health challenges. Even if you read this book before, it's worth another look now so you can keep up on the latest developments and tools available for you.

We are very optimistic about the future. We have just recently published four papers with one more under review.[7] All are about the role of diet in multiple sclerosis. Three analyze data from our previous studies. The others look at how diet composition may influence MS-related symptoms and disease activity. And other scientists are now also making the case that diet and lifestyle factors impact the risk of developing autoimmune issues, including MS.

I could not have done any of this without my Wahls Warriors behind me. We will always have more to learn, but the more we learn, the more you can benefit, and the more you can benefit, the more the world changes. Our epidemic of health is spreading—it's contagious, indeed, and I can only hope that someday, the knowledge that food, movement, and lifestyle are the most important factors for health will be the standard of care in every doctor's office and every clinical trial the world over.

This revised edition is my thank-you. I want to take you along with me into the future. No matter what else is happening in the world, I have hope because I see how far you have come, how much more you demand, how dedicated you are to change—and how that has changed the world for the better.

INTRODUCTION

I USED TO RUN marathons and climb mountains in Nepal. I've competed multiple times in the American Birkebeiner 54-kilometer cross-country ski marathon (once while pregnant), earned a black belt in tae kwon do, and won a bronze medal in women's full contact free sparring at the trials for the 1978 Pan American Games in Washington, DC. I used to feel invincible.

Then I developed multiple sclerosis. After decades of troubling symptoms I tried to ignore, I was finally diagnosed in 2000. By that time, the disease had a good footing in my central nervous system. My health decline progressed rapidly. Within two years of my diagnosis, I could no longer play soccer with my kids in the backyard. By fall 2002, walking from room to room for my hospital rounds exhausted me, and by summer 2003, my back and stomach muscles had weakened so much that I needed a tilt/recline wheelchair. Within three years of initial diagnosis, my disease had transitioned from relapsing-remitting multiple sclerosis into secondary progressive multiple sclerosis. In that phase, disability slowly progresses despite increasingly aggressive therapy. By 2007, I spent most of my time lying in a zero-gravity chair. I was 52 years old.

Everyone with multiple sclerosis has a story—the years of clues and strange symptoms that finally, in retrospect, make sense. Those with other autoimmune diseases, as well as other chronic neurological, medical, and mental health issues, have their stories as well. It is in the nature of most chronic diseases and health conditions that symptoms accumulate slowly, bit by bit, over the course of decades. Long before there can be a diagnosis based on discernible damage to the organs and systems of the body, the disease is progressing. This is what happened to me. As a doctor, I was compelled to find answers: a diagnosis and a cure. As a patient, I was compelled to save my own life.

Like most physicians, I had always been focused on quickly diagnosing my patients, then using drugs and surgical procedures to treat them—that is, until I became a patient myself. This turned my whole understanding of health care on its head. Conventional medicine was failing me. I saw that. I was heading toward a bedridden life.

But I wasn't willing to give in or give up. Since the first doctor ever treated the first patient, physicians have used self-experimentation, either to prove a scientific point or to treat themselves when the conventional treatments of the day were not enough. In that tradition, and in the face of this chronic, progressive disease for which I knew there was no cure, I began to experiment on myself. What I didn't expect were the stunning results I got from my self-experimentation: I did much more than arrest my disease. I achieved a dramatic restoration of my health and function. What I learned changed forever how I saw the battling worlds of health and disease. It changed me as a doctor, and it saved me as a patient.

More than a hundred years ago, Thomas Edison said, "The doctor of the future will give no medicine, but will interest his [or her] patients in the care of the human frame, in a proper diet, and in the cause and prevention of disease." This became my new course, my passion, and my mission. I understood health and disease in an entirely new way. I became a new person, both physically and emotionally, both personally and professionally. I also became passionately committed to helping other people become new people, too.

My Diagnosis

The stress and pressure of medical school may have been what triggered my first symptoms in 1980, years before I had any idea what they were. I would eventually call them "zingers"—intense stabs of facial pain. They lasted just a moment and would come on randomly, sometimes in waves, the episodes building over a week or two and then gradually fading over the next several weeks. They were most likely to happen during my busiest and most brutal hospital rotations, with shifts lasting thirty-six hours and allowing for little sleep. Over the years they became steadily worse, resembling electrical pain that felt like a 10,000-volt cattle prod sticking me in the face.

At the time, I thought the episodes of face pain were an aggravation, nothing more. I thought it was an isolated, unexplained problem—one of those medical mysteries that don't really require solving. Even as a doctor, I didn't think much about it. I was too busy with my own patients to dedicate too much diagnostic thought to myself. I certainly never suspected an autoimmune problem.

The shocks of facial pain were my first symptom, but that first incident was not likely the moment when multiple sclerosis began its relentless march through my central nervous system. For at least a decade before that moment— probably two decades, in retrospect—my brain and spinal cord had been under siege from "friendly fire"—my own immune system attacking the myelin that insulated my nerves. I couldn't feel it at first. In many cases, autoimmune attacks are mostly asymptomatic for years. Nevertheless, I know now that it was already happening.

As the years passed, I became a mother, first to my son, Zach, then to my daughter, Zebby. The rigors of parenting and full-time work distracted me, but unbeknownst to me, my multiple sclerosis clock was ticking. This was a clock I did not hear, even though I developed other alarms, like visual dimming, along with more of those excruciating zingers to the face. I had no idea what was in store for me. I fully expected to be an active, adventurous, vibrant woman for at least forty more years. I imagined mountain climbing with my children, even as a white-haired old grandma. I never thought my unexplained symptoms would have anything to do with something as basic as my mobility or as crucial as my ability to think clearly.

One evening at a dinner party, I was talking to a neurologist and I happened to mention that I perceived the color blue somewhat differently in my right and left eyes. Blues were a bit brighter when I used my right eye than if I used the left. She seemed interested.

"You'll have multiple sclerosis someday," she said. It was the first time anyone had ever said those words to me. My father died the next morning, and so her words were forgotten in the chaos of grief. Years later, I recalled those prescient comments.

The day my wife, Jackie, noticed I seemed to be walking strangely, I didn't believe her. I didn't even notice until she insisted we go for a three-mile walk to the local dairy for ice cream. She wanted to prove her point, and she did. By the time we got back, I was dragging my left foot like a sandbag. I couldn't pick up my toes. I was exhausted, nauseated, and scared. I scheduled an appointment with my physician.

I spent the next few weeks going through test after test, dreading each result. Some tests involved flashing lights and buzzers. Others involved more electricity and more pain. There were more blood tests. I said little and feared much. Everything came back negative, which was a relief, but deep down I knew the truth: there was something wrong with me.

Finally, we were down to the last test: a spinal tap. If there were oligoclonal-band proteins (an indicator of excessive amounts of antibodies) present in the spinal fluid, then the diagnosis would be multiple sclerosis. But if this test was also negative, then I likely had what they call "idiopathic degeneration of the spinal cord" (meaning they don't know the cause). Considering the long list of potential diseases I had faced, this seemed like the best option. I was hopeful.

When I got up the next morning, I knew that the results should be in my chart. I could get into the clinic medical records from my home computer through remote access. I brought up my medical record on the screen and went to the laboratory section. Positive. I stood up. I paced. Two hours later, I logged onto the system and checked again. Five times I looked up my results, hoping they would somehow change. They never did.

It was official: I had multiple sclerosis.

My Decline

In summer 2000, I moved with Jackie and my children from Marshfield, Wisconsin, to Iowa City, Iowa, to accept a joint appointment as assistant professor at the University of Iowa and chief of primary care at the VA hospital. Because I was newly diagnosed with multiple sclerosis, I was taking Copaxone, which my physician had prescribed. Like most patients, I relied entirely on my physicians for treatment decisions. Even though I was a physician myself, I had been conditioned to believe that specialized physicians know best. I had to step back and be the patient now, at least in terms of my own care. Besides, what did I know about multiple sclerosis? It wasn't my area. I was seeing the very best people and getting the very best treatments available, so I assumed I was doing all that I could do.

I was also determined not to let my diagnosis influence my new job. I vowed not to let anyone know—not to show any weakness. I was in a leadership position with plenty of challenges, and I loved it. I enjoyed teaching the medical students, and my children were thriving in their new home. I thought I was doing pretty well, and so did my doctors. I even began to imagine I might never get much worse. I dreamed I might not even have to confess to my kids that I had multiple sclerosis. Nobody had to know!

But as is typical for MS, my disease progressed. When my right arm and hand became weak, my doctors gave me steroids to suppress my immune cells, and my strength slowly returned. But this was the beginning of a slow and steady decline. I could see it. Jackie could see it, and so could the kids. They've since admitted that sometimes it was embarrassing to have me around because I was less and less mobile. Sometimes they wished I wouldn't attend their activities, and that made me feel guilty for wanting to be there. It was a strain on the whole family, and I felt responsible. It was all my fault. I was supposed to be the provider, and I was slowly losing my ability to manage my own body. It had been only two years since my initial diagnosis, but the change in me was dramatic.

Then something happened that altered the entire course of my life. In 2002, my neurology doctor at the Cleveland Clinic noted that I was slowly getting worse and suggested I check out Ashton Embry's website, Direct-MS, at direct-ms.org. Dr. Embry is a geologist with a PhD whose son has MS. Dr. Embry's son improved dramatically by changing his diet, so Dr. Embry became an active and vocal proponent of the link between diet and multiple sclerosis. This was the first I'd heard of such an idea—or at least the first time I paid attention. Although it sounded suspiciously like "alternative care" to me—being a conventionally trained doctor, I didn't put much stock into what I saw as fringe medical practices—this was a suggestion from my *neurologist*, so I took her seriously. I decided to check it out.

Dr. Embry's website was full of scientific references, which I began to read one by one. The articles were from peer-reviewed journals, written by scientists from highly respected medical schools. This wasn't "soft science." This wasn't "fringe." This was legitimate research. It was difficult science, too. A lot of it was in fields outside my expertise, or it relied on basic science concepts that hadn't been part of my medical training. I had trouble absorbing everything, and the MS-related brain fog didn't help. There was so much new information—how did I not know about any of this? After a lot of intensive reading, I determined that Dr. Embry was not a charlatan and that maybe he was onto something. What if diet could have a major impact on MS? I had spent years leaving my health in the hands of doctors while continuing to decline, so this idea fascinated me. I could control what I ate. It seemed too easy and too good to be true. I had to know more.

Dr. Embry's website was the first place I heard about Dr. Loren Cordain. Dr. Cordain linked changes in the human diet to the development of chronic disease in Western society. He had published a number of articles and had also recently published a book for the public called *The Paleo Diet: Lose Weight and Get Healthy by Eating the Foods You Were Designed to Eat.* This level of reading, geared for the general public, was much easier reading than the technical scientific papers I'd been slogging through.[1] I began to absorb information more quickly: molecular mimicry, leaky gut, lectins, immune modulation (I'll talk about all these things later in this book). I began to see where Dr. Embry and Dr. Cordain were going with their theories. I began to consider that what we eat might actually have a major, rather than a minor, influence on how our bodies work.

I was particularly interested in the idea that excessive carbohydrates and sugars in our modern diet lead to excess insulin and inflammation. The evidence that the original human diet could possibly improve my MS was compelling, but switching to this kind of diet would be a major change for me. I had been a vegetarian since my college days and I loved my beans and rice. I loved making bread. Could I really cut out grain, dairy, and legumes, the current staples of my diet?

But I wanted to arrest my disease more than anything else. I wanted to keep walking, working, and playing with my kids. I decided to try it. Meat was back on the menu, and I gave up the now-forbidden foods I loved so much. At first the smell of meat was nauseating to me. I started slowly, adding meat to soup in small amounts. With time, it got easier.

I was hopeful about this change, but despite this switch to what Dr. Cordain called a Paleo diet, my decline continued. I was frustrated. It wasn't working! I couldn't play soccer in the backyard with my kids without falling. I couldn't take long (or even short) hikes with the Boy Scouts or Girl Scouts. Then it became harder to take even short walks with Jackie. Fatigue became more and more of a problem. I was disappointed, at times despondent, and tears came at inconvenient times. But I was also determined. I didn't want to give up on the idea that there were things I could do to help myself. Some of the entries on Embry's website said that recovery took five years. I realized I could not expect an overnight miracle, so I stuck with the changes. Even if progress would be slow, my new dietary regimen came with its own sense of empowerment.

Meanwhile, I rearranged my schedule to avoid walking. My doctor told me that it was time to get a scooter, and then changed his mind and suggested a tilt/recline wheelchair because of the worsening fatigue. He also suggested I try taking mitoxantrone, a form of chemotherapy. When that didn't help, I switched to a new, potent immune-suppressing medication called Tysabri; but before I went in for my third injection, Tysabri was pulled from the market because people were dying from the activation of a latent virus in their brains. After this, my doctor suggested that I take CellCept, a transplant medicine, which would suppress my immune cells. I often had mouth ulcers after that. My skin was grayish. I started every day tired, and despair gnawed at me each night as I lay in bed. Jackie, Zach, and Zebby were my lifelines. Jackie would hold me and tell me we'd get through everything together. We often discussed our kids and how they were absorbing the ways that we dealt with what was happening. For their sakes, I didn't want to let my discouragement and fatigue show.

Though I had resisted getting the tilt/recline wheelchair, it actually felt liberating once I had it. I was able to go outside and stroll (or rather, roll) with my family as we hiked around the county park or the neighborhood. It did make my life easier. It weakened my back muscles, however, and the more those muscles atrophied, the more time I spent in bed. I didn't talk about it much, but I thought it likely that eventually I would become bedridden.

Sitting at my desk at work was exhausting. Then I found a zero-gravity chair, designed like the NASA chairs used during space flights. When I was fully reclined, my knees were higher than my nose and gravity held me in the chair. I had one for my office and another for my home. That helped with the fatigue a great deal, but this wasn't how I wanted to live my life. I was getting through life day by day, but I couldn't accept that this would be my future.

Taking My Life Back

Getting into that wheelchair triggered something in me. I realized that conventional medicine was not likely to stop what was happening to me. I still hoped that the Paleo diet would make a difference, but I hadn't seen much of a change thus far. I decided to go back to reading the medical literature. I wanted to know if there was something I was missing—some other avenue, something the doctors had overlooked. I had come to accept that recovery was not possible, but maybe I could slow things down. I was through ceding my power to doctors and not seeing results. I needed to be more forward thinking. I vowed to research and study and exhaust every possibility, just in case there was some other answer for me out there, something that would delay a little longer the inevitable life as a bedridden invalid.

At first I began to read all about the latest clinical drug trials going on, but then I realized that those all involved medications that I'd be unable to get. This kind of knowledge would be only theoretical. So I started to think outside the box. I knew how science worked—I knew that studies on mice and rats are always the source of tomorrow's treatments, but that it's typically years, often decades, before anything becomes a matter for a clinical trial, let alone a standard of care. This was the cutting edge of the cutting edge, so I began to look there. I wanted to know what the brightest minds were thinking and how they envisioned the future of diseases like mine.

Each night I spent a few minutes searching pubmed.gov for articles about the mouse model for MS. I knew that brains afflicted with MS shrink over time, so I also began reading about the animal models of other conditions with shrinking brains. I researched Parkinson's disease, Alzheimer's dementia, Lou Gehrig's disease (amyotrophic lateral sclerosis, or ALS), and Huntington's disease. I discovered that, in all four of those conditions, the mitochondria—small subunits within cells that manage the energy supply for that cell—stop working well and lead to early death of brain cells, causing shrinking of the brain. More searching led me to articles in which mouse brains and their mitochondria had been protected using vitamins[2] and supplements like coenzyme Q10, carnitine, and creatine.[3]

I didn't have anything to lose, so I decided to take action. I translated those mouse-size doses into human-size ones, then made an appointment with my primary care doctor. She looked over my list and decided the supplements were likely safe. She entered them all into my medication list, one at a time, to check for potential adverse interactions. There were none. I was excited about starting my new, experimental vitamin-and-supplement routine. I began to take them and was disappointed when nothing immediately happened. After a couple of months, I stopped taking them . . . and a few days later, I couldn't get out of bed! When I resumed the supplements, I could get up again. They were helping, after all! If nothing else, they seemed to be slowing my decline.

This was a ray of hope. Obviously, I thought, my body was getting something from those supplements that it wasn't getting without them—something it needed. This was a valuable clue.

Discovering E-Stim

My next discovery was in a completely different realm than food. I came upon a research protocol that used electrical stimulation of muscles to treat people who had become paralyzed due to an acute spinal injury. According to the research, the purpose of this therapy, known as e-stim, was to maintain bone health and quality of life for these patients. Reviewing that research protocol made me wonder if the electrical stimulation might slow down my disability. I talked to a physical therapist who used this technology, and he warned me that it was painful and exhausting for the athletes who did it. He wasn't sure if it would help me, but he finally said he was willing to give it a test session.

During my first session, the therapist had me lie on my belly and applied the electrodes to my left paraspinal back muscles. I lifted my left leg off the table and held it there as he dialed up the electrical current. If felt like bugs racing across my skin. He kept dialing up the current. The bugs raced faster. It became more and more electrical, and then painful. After a minute my therapist asked if he could turn up the current again. This is the typical procedure because the brain releases endorphins and nerve growth factors that make the e-stim more comfortable, so after a few minutes, the pain lessens and patients can typically tolerate a higher dose of electricity. When that was done, we did my quadriceps muscles on my left leg, where I suffered particular weakness. After it was over, I had completed thirty minutes of "exercise" that was more rigorous than what I had been able to do in years. It felt like progress, so I began doing e-stim therapy three times a week.

Discovering Functional Medicine

Every night, after everyone else was sleeping, I continued to search the Internet, looking for more information that might help me. I was relentless. One night I stumbled onto the web page for the Institute for Functional Medicine and was immediately intrigued. This organization's goal was to provide clinicians like myself with a better way to care for people with complex chronic disease by looking at how the interaction between genetics, diet, hormone balance, toxin exposures, infections, and psychological factors contributes to the development of disease or the improvement of health and vitality.

This was exactly what I had been searching for since I'd hit the wheelchair. The institute had textbooks, conferences, and continuing education courses for physicians and other health care professionals. One course captured my attention immediately: *Neuroprotection: A Functional Medicine Approach for Common and Uncommon Neurologic Syndromes*. I ordered it and began studying, night after night. Although it was difficult at first, that functional medicine course taught me more strategies to improve the condition of my mitochondria and my brain cells. It reinforced the importance of mitochondria and gave me more tools to help my mitochondria. I had a much deeper understanding of the significance to the brain of leaky gut, food allergies, toxins, and mitochondria that were not providing enough energy for the cells. I now understood neurotransmitter problems, and the impact of having inefficient enzymes for the metabolism of B vitamins and sulfur. I had a deeper understanding of why my brain was on fire, under attack by my immune cells, and what I could do. Based on all this new information, I created a much longer list of vitamins, minerals, amino acids, antioxidants, and essential fatty acids that I understood were helpful for mitochondrial and brain cell function.

But practical considerations imposed themselves on my big ideas. How would I do it? I had a long list of nutrients, but was I really going to take huge fistfuls of pills every day? And would that even work? The Paleo diet suggested that food was the best source, but many functional medicine concepts relied on supplements. Our Paleolithic ancestors didn't take supplements, obviously. The Paleo diet had taught me to eliminate certain foods but didn't necessarily tell me how to get the precise nutrients I now knew I needed. Functional medicine helped me to determine what nutrients I needed with their list of advised vitamins and supplements to take, but it didn't necessarily tell me how to get them. I could see two approaches that were each incomplete, and it was almost like they were reaching out toward each other and I could see it. I wanted to bring those two ideas together into something that would be even more powerful.

If I could get those same nutrients I was taking in pill form from the food I was eating, I reasoned, those nutrients might be more effective than the synthetic versions of the nutrients I was taking in supplements. In addition, I might also pick up many additional compounds—maybe thousands of compounds—occurring in the whole foods that had yet to be named. I reasoned that a whole food that contained a particular vitamin or supplement I was after might also contain compounds that contributed synergistically to the absorption of that nutrient, or other aspects that might make it more usable in the body. There was a reason why these nutrients existed together in the package that was a particular vegetable, for example. In nature, most vitamins are part of a family of related compounds that are all biologically active in our cells, so why wouldn't they work better together than in isolation?

To realize this new idea and incorporate it into my routine, I knew I would need a whole-food, nutrient-targeted eating plan specifically designed to maximize my mitochondrial and brain function—an eating plan that went beyond anything I'd already encountered. It would incorporate Paleo principles, functional medicine concepts, and my own extensive research. Maybe that would jump-start the changes in my body I desperately wanted to see and feel.

I stared at my new list of the nutrients my research and functional medicine suggested I needed for better brain health and wondered which foods contained these nutrients. I had no idea. I showed my list of nutrients to my registered dietitian friends, but they didn't know where to find those things in the food supply, either. This simply wasn't something people were thinking about. Next, I went to the health science library. I couldn't find any answers there, so I went back to the Internet and began searching once again. Answers began to emerge. With some more work, I finally developed a long list of foods, rather than relying only on the supplements, to add to my diet that seemed to match up with my list of nutrients. I began to add these to every meal, whenever I could.

That's when things really began to change in my brain and body. I didn't know it at the time, but I had also sown the seeds that would grow into the Wahls Protocol.

Generating the Proof

I was just about to start a new position as the primary care doctor for the polytrauma unit, treating veterans with head injuries. It was a job I wasn't sure I could do, and Jackie and I both wondered whether the hospital had assigned me the position in order to force me to face the fact that I could no longer work. But my new food regimen could not have been better timed. Instead of failing, I surprised everyone, including myself. After just three months of practicing the new diet, gradually increasing my e-stim exercises, and practicing daily meditation and a simple self-massage for stress management and muscle care, I said goodbye to that old tilt/recline wheelchair. I could walk between exam rooms using just one cane!

After six months I could walk throughout the entire hospital without a cane. My thinking was clearer and multitasking was easier. But it wasn't just my body that had changed. My whole outlook was transformed. I experienced and saw the world very differently than before. The old me—the conventional internal medicine physician—had been struck down like Paul on the road to Damascus. The old me, who had relied on drugs and procedures to make my patients well, who had been made progressively more feeble by my illness, had been replaced with someone who understood intellectually and physically that disease begins at the cellular level, when cells are starved of the building blocks they need to conduct the chemistry of life properly, and that the root of optimal health begins with taking away the things that harm and confuse our cells while providing the body with the right tools and the right environment in which to thrive. I finally understood what I had to do to provide my cells with all the building blocks of life they needed to heal. I was doing it, and it was working.

This completely altered how I practiced medicine. I began teaching residents and patients in our primary care clinics how to care for themselves in a way I had only just discovered as optimal, using diet and health behaviors for diabetes, high blood pressure, high cholesterol, mood disorders, post-traumatic stress disorder, and traumatic brain injury instead of relying only on drugs. The residents learned that diet and lifestyle are powerful treatments—often as effective, if not more so, than drugs. The patients in the traumatic brain injury clinic were also eager to learn what things they could do to speed the healing of their brains. In patient after patient, I watched symptoms and the need for drugs decrease as diet and lifestyles improved.

The many people I helped notwithstanding, however, anecdotal evidence wasn't good enough for me. There was no question that the medical establishment wouldn't believe, let alone endorse, my protocol without a clinical trial, and as a doctor, I understood that. I felt compelled to apply the same rigor to my own work that I had required when researching what to do for myself—because what if my success was just an isolated occurrence that happened only to me? What if my methods didn't apply to others? I knew intuitively that they did, but I needed definitive tests to prove it. My chief of medicine at the university and my chief of staff at the VA gave me the task of developing a proposal for a feasibility study. So I began the long, complex, and expensive process of doing a clinical trial to demonstrate that my new protocol didn't work just for me—that it would work for anyone with a similar affliction. That meant designing the trial, writing the grant, securing funding (in a world that funds fewer than 2 percent of grants), and getting my study approved by the institutional review board (the committee that oversees research at the VA and the university). In less than eighteen months, I achieved the seemingly impossible. On October 6, 2010, we enrolled our first patient.

In the fall of 2011, a group organizing a local TEDx talk asked me to submit a proposal to speak. For those not familiar with TEDx, it is an offshoot of TED, which stands for Technology, Entertainment, and Design. This is a set of nonprofit conferences on a variety of topics that are filmed and available for public viewing on the Internet. TEDx is similar, but conferences are organized locally. They are also available to view for free online, and speakers are not paid. Millions of people view the TED and TEDx talks, and many have gone viral. I would have eighteen minutes to tell my story and explain how I designed a diet specifically for my mitochondria and my brain. I agreed.

In my TEDx talk, I briefly related my story and explained the specifics of my intensive nutrition plan. I challenged people to become ambassadors for their mitochondria and to eat for health. At the end of November, that TEDx talk, "Minding Your Mitochondria," was placed on YouTube. It spread into the Paleo community, the MS community, and the functional medicine community. Within a year, that lecture had more than 1 million views, and as of 2018, was well past 3 million views. Unbelievably, I'd reached more people and touched more lives than most physicians or scientists could in a lifetime. I was exhilarated. It felt like I was doing something to change the world for the better. But this only made me want to do more.

My mission was never clearer. I needed to continue to do the research so I could reach my physician colleagues and eventually change the standard of care. I needed to continue to teach the public because I believe the public will soon be far ahead of the medical community when it comes to understanding the power of food to reclaim and maintain health.

The next step was to write this book.

Meanwhile, I've expanded the lab, we have additional studies under way, and our preliminary results continue to be very exciting. We have published several papers from our initial feasibility study in which we used the dietary and lifestyle interventions I used. We enrolled patients like me—they had either secondary or primary progressive multiple sclerosis and were expected only to decline. There would be no spontaneous remissions, no spontaneous improvements. Any improvements would be evidence that the protocol was in fact helpful for reducing MS-related symptoms. The goal of the study was to assess if people could implement the study diet, daily meditation, daily exercise, and electrical stimulation of muscles. I needed to show that people could adopt the same complicated regimen I had used, that it was safe (meaning no serious adverse events or patient injuries), and that there was a trend toward reduced fatigue and/or improved quality of life. With only 20 subjects the sample size was small, yet the changes observed were so great that we achieved both clinically and statistically significant change in the quality of life measures. The interventions were so radical (in research, the concept of doing a study not defined by a prior animal study is considered radical) that I was required to report the safety and outcomes data to the institutional review board for our first 10 subjects before enrolling the rest of the subjects. The pre-study analysis proved the diet was not nutritionally deficient, so we were allowed to proceed. The only side effect of any significance were that for those who were overweight or obese—they lost weight without being hungry! Patients had a marked and clinically statistically significant reduction in fatigue severity and improvement in quality of life. We published the results: "A Multimodal Intervention for Patients with Secondary Progressive Multiple Sclerosis: Feasibility and Effect on Fatigue,"[4] showing that the protocol can be implemented by others safely and can lead to a clinically and statistically significant reduction in fatigue.

Next, we added another 10 subjects and analyzed more data, showing clinically and statistically significant improvements in the quality of life, verbal and nonverbal thinking, and improved mood. We took videos of people doing the Timed Up and Go test (they stand up from a chair, walk eight feet, turn around, walk back to the chair, and sit down again). We analyzed the changes in gait over the study period. Again, with progressive MS, you would expect people to experience steady decline in walking speed over that time period. Instead, we observed that half of the subjects experienced improvement in their walking speed and endurance. That is remarkable.

CALL TO ACTION

If you want to see a link to all the papers I have written and published about my research, including the paper that has links to the video of the gait changes, find them at terrywahls.com/bonus.

It will take many years and millions of dollars for us to do clinical trials that can prove whether the Wahls Protocol is effective for multiple sclerosis and other chronic diseases. Our next big hairy audacious goal is to do a clinical trial that compares a therapeutic diet and lifestyle intervention (in those who have declined disease-modifying drug therapy) to newly diagnosed patients who are receiving usual care and likely receiving disease-modifying drug therapy. It would be quasi-experimental (that is, non-randomized), and so it would not be as good as a randomized trial that could result in a quality of evidence appropriate for creating a new standard of care. It is, however, a first step at prospectively examining what happens to people who decline drug therapy and choose a therapeutic diet and lifestyle instead. My neurologist co-investigators are very excited about this proposed study. They agree that it is vitally important to understand the clinical course for those people who use therapeutic diet and lifestyle and decline disease-modifying drug therapy—and it is a question that many of their patients (and you, my readers) are all asking. No one knows for sure as of yet, but it is my intent to do the research required to answer that question. This is the kind of study that will need philanthropic support, and we are well on our way toward meeting this funding goal.

Your Story

This is my story—and you have your own story. I still have multiple sclerosis, but now I also have my life back—and so do the many thousands of people who have implemented the Wahls Protocol. The word is out there—I have lectured to tens of thousands of clinicians, sold over 200,000 copies of *The Wahls Protocol*, and reached millions of people through my TEDx talk. The purpose of my years of self-experimentation was to determine exactly what my body needed to fight back against autoimmune disease. The result is the Wahls Protocol and a new updated edition of this book, which lays out a systematic and aggressive intervention to combat your body's downward spiral. It is a mending of your broken biochemistry that comes not from your doctor or your pharmacist but from you. I invite you to read my book, take my story to heart, and talk to your family and your physician about whether the Wahls Protocol might be something that could work for you.

But no matter what you decide and how you proceed, here's the most important thing I want you to realize: Your doctor cannot cure your autoimmune disease. Your medication can only ease your symptoms, sometimes with side effects that make you feel even worse. The power of healing is within you. All you need to do is give your body what it needs and remove what poisons it. You can restore your own health by what you do—not by the pills you take, but by *how you choose to live.* When you eat and live in accordance with the needs of your cells, your body can finally concentrate on healing, and that is when the dramatic changes will happen for you.

You don't have to wait until all the proof comes in for your specific condition and is vetted by the medical community. That could take another several decades to occur. You don't have to wait until a "food prescription" becomes part of the standard of care in your conventional doctor's office (which I believe someday will happen—it is the only rational course). You can have this information *right now.* Food is the bedrock of health. Our food choices can either lead to disease or create health and vitality.

As you implement the Wahls Protocol, you will likely begin noticing that your thinking is clearer, your moods are better, and your energy is coming back. Those over their ideal weight will find that their weight normalizes without hunger. In my clinics, when people come back in three months, everyone who has fully implemented the diet has begun noticing all these things. For the next three years, I typically see my patients "youthen"—they look younger and younger each time I see them as their cells revitalize and their bodies become healthy once more.

My story is not over yet, and yours isn't, either. If I can rise up from a tilt/recline wheelchair by changing the way I live my life, consider what the people you love, your community, your country, and the world would look like if everybody began eating and living to optimally fuel their cells. We could restore health and vitality to the world and dramatically lower the cost of health care, saving billions of dollars. What choice will you make? How will you choose to live the rest of *your* life? With disability? Or with vitality? Are you ready to take action to improve your quality of life? It's all up to you.

Part One

BEFORE YOU GET STARTED

Chapter 1

THE SCIENCE OF LIFE, DISEASE, AND YOU

YOU HEAR THE DOCTOR say those words—*multiple sclerosis*—and you wonder if your life will ever be the same. Maybe you aren't entirely sure what it means, but you've seen it—you've seen the people in wheelchairs who can't seem to remember things, who have a hard time even using their hands. Or maybe you are already there, your mobility declining or seemingly lost. Maybe you think that you are on the downhill slope and there is no climbing back up. Not in your condition.

Or perhaps you have a different kind of autoimmune disease, like rheumatoid arthritis or lupus. Maybe you are also saddled with obesity or severe allergies, food intolerances or celiac disease, diabetes or a heart condition. Perhaps you must endure depression or anxiety or attention deficit disorder along with your other limitations. Whatever you are facing, you may suspect or fear that the days of feeling good, feeling like yourself, are far behind you. Your body no longer works the way it should, and neither does your brain.

You have probably seen a doctor, and maybe you already have a diagnosis. Physicians treat your symptoms, but they cannot cure chronic diseases like multiple sclerosis, depression, high blood pressure, diabetes, or even obesity, for that matter. You may be prescribed a list of pharmaceutical interventions to ease your symptoms, but these may only exacerbate your problem long term because of medication side effects and the worsening nutrient depletion that may accompany long-term medication use. Medications for autoimmune disease *do not cure the disease*. Their only purpose is to make you feel a little better, which might work, and possibly slow the progression, which also might work. Or not. Meanwhile, the side effects may make you feel just as bad in different ways . . . or worse than you did before you started the medication.

Perhaps you are losing hope. I want to restore your hope.

This book is about hope. My overarching message couldn't be more straightforward: *You don't have to be a victim.* The disease or condition you have is already happening, but there are many significant things you can do to slow, halt, or even reverse your symptoms. Medication can't take away your autoimmune disease, *but your body can heal itself*—if you give it the tools.

Disease is not a simple cause-and-effect condition. It is a complex melding of forces, both genetic and environmental. Fortunately for all of us, the environmental aspect is of much greater significance than the genetic, and you can start doing something about your environment today. The lifestyle you choose can actually repair your broken biochemistry and restore your vitality. That's big, big news for anyone with an autoimmune or any other chronic disease. *You* can turn your life around. Not your doctor. Not your pharmacist. Not that bottle of pills. *You*. The power is in your hands.

When chronic disease is the result of a *deficiency*, drugs aren't going to solve the problem. As I'm sure you realize, multiple sclerosis is not a deficiency of the latest multiple-sclerosis-disease-modifying drug like Copaxone, just as fatigue is not a deficiency of wakefulness-promoting drugs like Provigil or even caffeine, and depression is not a deficiency of antidepressants like Prozac. No, these problems are not deficiencies of drugs, but they are triggered by deficiencies *in your cells* that lead to broken biochemistry and impaired signaling between your cells. When you look at chronic disease in this way, it's obvious that the most logical course of action is to treat the cellular deficiencies that cause diseases to develop in the first place, rather than focusing all your efforts on merely treating the symptoms. The latter is what most conventional pharmaceutical treatments do.

But unless you understand what your body actually needs to function and heal, you can't possibly make wise decisions about what you should do to keep your body going. You might decide to take someone else's advice about diet—advice that might be motivated by wanting to help you lose weight or gain strength but not necessarily fix the deficiency in your cells. That diet you want to follow might even be based on political, environmental, spiritual, or ethical concerns, all of which are valid considerations. However, unless you understand what your body actually needs, you won't know what advice to take and what advice to ignore in order to genuinely address your condition. You won't know what foods to choose. You won't know which diet is the right one for you. You won't know how to fuel your own cells for optimal health if the diet and lifestyle you follow is not designed for that purpose.

I challenge you to stop believing everything you read and everything everyone tells you, and to learn something about biology and biochemistry yourself so you can make your own decisions. When considering nutrition at the cellular level, we have plenty of scientific studies to guide us. We don't know everything there is to know about nutrition yet—not by a long shot—but we do know quite a bit about how to facilitate many of the biochemical repairs we need. Science has already demonstrated that when you give your cells more of what they need, your cells will thrive, even heal. If you deprive them of essential nutrients, they will deteriorate. They might not die—at least, not right away—but they'll soon begin to falter in their functionality, and that is exactly when problems start.

As a doctor and a scientist as well as a patient, I base the decisions I make for my own health and for the health of others on science. I would never ask anyone to just "believe me." I want you to understand *why* I designed the Wahls Protocol the way I did. If you don't understand why you must make the dietary and lifestyle changes I suggest, you might not be willing to stick to them. The results you'll experience by following the Wahls Protocol speak for themselves, of course, but an informed and proactive patient is an empowered patient. I want to empower you, so before we begin—before I give you even one bit of advice about what you should or shouldn't be eating, drinking, or doing—let's take a look at what's really going on in your body.

What Creates Health?

You are made of cells. A cell is the unit that is the basis for a living organism. Some organisms consist of only one cell, like an amoeba. Some, like human bodies, consist of trillions of cells. Cells come in different sizes and shapes, and they all do different things, but they are, essentially, the building blocks that make up our bodies.

Cells, however, don't work under just any conditions. They need certain nutrients in order to do the work of keeping you alive and healthy. Without those nutrients, the cells begin to malfunction, even die. Where do those nutrients come from? They come from the food you eat—nowhere else. If you aren't providing the right nutrients and environment for your cells, then they won't work as well as they could, and a malfunction at the cellular level could

WAHLS WARRIORS SPEAK

My first multiple-sclerosis-related episode at age 33 involved facial numbness and vertigo, and for the next seven years, I experienced increasing fatigue and heat intolerance. I used Copaxone for five years but went off it when I ran out of tolerable injectable space. Over the next eight years, I experienced a decline in energy, a massive decline in heat tolerance, and an increase in brain fog and fatigue, so much so that working two days a week was all I could muster.

I found the Wahls Diet completely by accident, when I ran across the TEDx talk online. I started the diet in July 2012 and called my son after two weeks to say I felt as if I had new eyeglasses—everything was sharper and clearer than it had been for years. I have had such an improvement in my mental clarity and fatigue that I feel like I should pinch myself! I really am still in shock that I have energy again and do not need a nap every day. The quality of my sleep has improved, and when I do nap, it is for 10 minutes. When I awaken, I am as energetic as I was in the morning. You can see why I think it is miraculous!

—Jan W., Steamboat Springs, Colorado

eventually impact any aspect of your health. Your genetics may determine *what* goes wrong, but when the cells aren't getting what they need, the body doesn't work right, and *something* (usually many somethings) will go wrong somewhere.

People often wonder whether health is mostly a matter of genetics. Do your cells work well or poorly depending on your DNA? If it were all up to your genes, then what you eat and how you live wouldn't matter very much. However, we know this is not the case.

Living in Iowa, we hear a lot about corn and see a lot of corn, and so I use this as an example reflecting my midwestern roots—an example of how important fuel is for your mitochondria (the energy-producing factories within each of your cells), and by extension, your cells, your organs, and your entire body, including your brain. A packet of seeds can all contain the same DNA, but if you plant a handful of corn seeds in rich black Iowa soil and you toss another handful onto a toxic trash heap topped with a thin layer of old, spent dirt, the seeds will grow into much different plants (if they grow at all). The seeds planted in the rich Iowa soil will be tall, sturdy, and lush, with healthy ears of corn. The seeds planted in the trash heap that do manage to sprout will be spindly and pale and probably won't produce much, if any, corn because there were not enough nutrients to nourish the plant. Same DNA, completely different result.

Your cells—and you—are like that corn. If your cells don't get the nutrients they require to function properly and aren't protected from harmful toxins, you will wilt. Your mitochondria won't produce enough energy (more about mitochondria in a moment) or won't produce energy efficiently, and that can trigger a cascade of dysfunctional biochemical reactions that can eventually launch a chronic disease process. (I will talk more about how the toxins trip up your chemistry in chapter 8, "Reducing Toxic Load.")

Don't get me wrong—genetics do play a role. Our cells rely on enzymes to facilitate the chemistry of life, and how we make those enzymes is determined by our genes—that is, our DNA. We know that there are hundreds of different genes, maybe more, that could each slightly increase the chance that someone will develop multiple sclerosis. A handful of the more than two hundred MS-related genes do increase the risk of getting MS more significantly, but if you have one, it does *not* mean you will *definitely* get MS. MS develops as a result of complex interactions between the genes you have and

THE ORIGIN OF MITOCHONDRIA

Long before animals evolved, when the earth was populated only by microbes, oxygen first appeared. It was toxic to most bacteria and killed off 90 percent of all the bacterial species. But some tiny bacteria were able to use oxygen for burning sugar in their environments. Those small oxygen-using, sugar-burning bacteria were eventually engulfed by larger bacteria and made the larger bacteria much more efficient organisms.

As life evolved, these tiny bacteria evolved, too—they were the precursors to the modern-day mitochondria living in each of our cells. They continue to make *us* far more efficient at extracting energy from our food than if we were still using the fermentation process bacteria uses. It is because of mitochondria that those ancient bacteria were able to evolve into multicellular organisms!

the lifetime of diet, physical activity, and environmental exposures that you have experienced.

These genes do affect a number of relevant factors, however, such as whether some enzyme doesn't work very well, some process interferes with inflammation control, toxins are managed sufficiently, nutrients are fully absorbed, hormones are working effectively, or neurotransmitters production is healthy.

Very few conditions, however, are caused solely by a single mutation in our DNA. The vast majority are caused by the interaction of multiple genes—sometimes as many as fifty or even a hundred—that shift the efficiency of our enzymes in response to our environments, including nutritional deprivation or toxic exposure. Environment largely determines which genes are silent, or "turned off," and which are active, or "turned on." For example, you may have a propensity to develop cancer, but if your body is fully nourished and not exposed to excessive toxins, you are far less likely to develop cancer, even with that propensity. Or if you do develop cancer, your white blood cells may be strong enough to kill the cancer cells as soon as they develop and you won't ever experience symptoms or be diagnosed. Or if you do get cancer that spreads or metastasizes, you will have a much better chance of beating it.

WAHLS WORDS

Epigenetics is the science of understanding how the environment determines which genes are active, or "turned on," and which genes are inactive, or "turned off." Currently, hundreds of millions of dollars are being poured into epigenetics research because epigenetics is thought to hold the answers to why we develop chronic diseases like cancer and diseases of aging. Much more information will be forthcoming in this field, but why wait for scientists to develop new, expensive drugs based upon epigenetics when you can learn how to optimize the environment for your genes right now, using the Wahls Protocol?

Through optimal lifestyle choices, you can keep the most harmful genes in the off position and the most health-promoting genes in the on position.

The bottom line is that your genetics alone will play a remarkably small role in whether you develop a particular disease like multiple sclerosis, even if it runs in your family. It's the epigenetics that determine which genes turn on, and that determines your risk.

Some 70 to 95 percent of the risk of developing autoimmune problems, obesity, heart disease, and mental health problems comes from the environment.[1] "Environment" means what you eat, what you drink, what you breathe in, what you bathe in, how you move, and even how you think and interact with people. What really matters is how your genes interact with the accumulation of your choices. This is what will determine whether you have good health or develop a chronic disease. The key is to know how to shift the odds toward achieving the most optimal health, given the genes that you were born with, by making your internal environment—your cellular environment—as favorable as possible.

We are still learning how lifestyle factors like prior infections, diet, environmental pollutants, amount and type of exercise, stress, vitamin D levels, hormone balance—even attitude and approach to life—can turn on harmful genes, interfere with our biochemical factories, and lead to harmful changes in nutrient absorption, hormone production, neurotransmitter function, and

WAHLS WORDS

The scientific term for a mutation in a DNA sequence is *single nucleotide polymorphism*, or *SNP*. We know that people with specific SNPs (pronounced "snips") that affect the production of enzymes for handling the B vitamins or sulfur are more likely to have heart disease, brain disease, mood problems, and/or autoimmune problems. It is often possible, however, to overcome problem enzymes by using a specific nutritional regimen once we know which enzymes are affected and which vitamins and which forms of the vitamins or foodstuffs can help the person bypass that particular SNP. If a disease or condition runs in your family, that's a sign that you and your relatives might have a particular SNP. A functional medicine doctor can make some predictions about the SNPs based on family history and genetic testing, and can recommend a personalized plan of action. (See chapter 12, "Recovery," for more information.)

more, but we do know that a genetic propensity may never come to anything if the body stays healthy and fully nourished. Cellular dysfunction caused by a lack of proper nutrients and/or the presence of toxins, however—including those the body generates during times of excessive stress—can be all it takes to flip the genetic switch.

In other words, genes are not your destiny. You get to decide how you live, and that means you have a lot of control over which genes will become active. Even if you already have a chronic disease like MS, it's not too late to intervene. Correcting your lifestyle now can do more than just arrest disease progression; in many instances, it may even reverse it. Healthier choices can turn off those harmful genes and turn on the most health-promoting ones.

Fueling Your Cells

This brings us back to the cell. Here is a simple fact: Cellular fuel comes from the food you eat. This is one of the most important things I want you to take away from this book: *What your cells use to fuel the chemistry of life comes directly from what you feed yourself.* The food you eat has everything to do with how well your body functions, how likely it will be that your genetic suscepti- bilities will be activated, and whether you develop a chronic disease—as well as how well you are able to come back from the disabilities that a chronic disease has inflicted on you.

If you put sugar into the gas tank of a car, the car isn't going to run right. If you are missing half of the parts in an "assembly required" toy, it's not going to work. This is not a new concept, but for some reason people tend not to apply it to our cells. They have some general concept that "you are what you eat" or that certain foods are "healthy" or "unhealthy," but really, it's more concrete than that. Your diet directly correlates to your cells' ability to function.

In other words, cellular nutrition is everything. It is the very basis of health. It all comes down to the cell, because when cells malfunction, eventu- ally organs malfunction. When organs malfunction, eventually *you* malfunc- tion. The disease you have today began in your cells, and while the susceptibility to that disease might have a genetic component, whether those genes get turned on or turned off has everything to do with what you are giving your cells and what you aren't giving them. It's never too late to turn your cellular dysfunction around, but unless you know how to do this, based on what cells actually require, you're just guessing about what you should or shouldn't do.

You're probably used to hearing about giving your body what it needs, but I believe a better question is: Are you giving your *mitochondria* what they need? This is where it all begins—with cellular health. If you want to be healthy, strong, and sharp, then your cells have to be healthy, and your cells won't be healthy unless their (that is, your) mitochondria are healthy. That is how you start at the very root, the very beginning of the dysfunction in your body. That is how you turn your health around.

Mitochondria aren't something you would typically read about in a diet book. They are more a subject for a medical text. The word isn't catchy; it doesn't roll off the tongue. Mitochondria aren't sexy. They are the cellular workhorses. Yet they are *incredibly important* for your life and health. Without mitochondria, a cell would be like the chassis of a car. It might look like a cell, but without an engine, it's not going to do anything. It won't keep you run- ning, and it won't shuttle the trash out the exhaust pipe. And as is true of any engine, mitochondria need fuel. Not just any fuel—high-quality fuel.

WAHLS WARRIORS SPEAK

My diagnosis with multiple sclerosis was a true wake-up call, but Dr. Wahls has created a wonderful road map for teaching the importance of nutrition. My improvements have been dramatic! Not only has my physical stamina improved greatly, to an extent I cannot overemphasize, but I have experienced drastic improvements with my balance, fatigue, mental clarity, and decreased neuropathy pain, and the list goes on and on. It is truly amazing. I have not used my cane since April 2011. I do still have MS issues. I still lose my balance and fall sometimes. I still have optic neuritis sometimes. I still get fatigued, but it is all 10,000 percent better than it was! Dr. Wahls has proven how profoundly food affects our physical bodies, our disease, and our mental outlook and clarity. The Wahls Diet really does prove the old adage "you are what you eat."

—*Pam J., Pecatonica, Illinois*

To fully understand how this works, I want you to understand what a cell is, exactly, and in particular how a cell is fueled by the organelles inside it called mitochondria.

Maybe you remember having to draw a cell on a high school biology test, but you may not remember what you drew. Generally, a cell contains a nucleus, which contains DNA, or the genetic instructions for the organism. The nucleus is the heart of the cell, where all the information lives. However, there are other things floating around in that cellular space, including the engines that power the cell. Those engines are called mitochondria. The singular term is *mitochondrion*.

Most cells in your body contain mitochondria. Some contain many more mitochondria than others. The more energy that a particular cell needs, the more mitochondria it requires to churn out that energy. For example, your brain, retina, heart, and liver cells contain a lot more mitochondria than most other cells in other parts of your body because thinking, seeing, pumping blood, and processing toxins are all high-energy activities.

Cells need fuel for multiple functions: building, maintaining, repairing,

THE EVOLUTION OF MITOCHONDRIA

About 1.5 billion years ago, when the only life-forms on Earth were bacteria, small bacteria invaded larger bacteria; but instead of harming their hosts, these smaller bacteria benefited them by generating energy more efficiently for the host.

The effect of these small "invader" bacteria was to open the door to specialization so that the larger bacteria were able to evolve into even larger, multicellular organisms that eventually became animals. The smaller bacteria evolved into mitochondria. Interestingly, a similar process seems to have happened with plants: Cyanobacteria engulfed smaller bacteria that were capable of photosynthesis, which evolved into plants having chloroplasts—organelles in which photosynthesis occurs. These potent nutrient-packed, energy-generating chloroplasts are one of the reasons why fresh leafy green vegetables are so good for us to eat.

and eliminating toxic waste. Toxins can come from medications, pesticides, herbicides, and pollution, as well as from the by-products of basic cell functioning (every engine has its waste products). Too much toxic waste can overwhelm cells and organs, but fortunately, your versatile and hardworking mitochondria are busy powering the cells that do the processing of fat-soluble toxins, converting them into a water-soluble form that can be eliminated by your equally hardworking liver and kidneys.

Mitochondria also orchestrate cell death. All cells die eventually, and timely cell death is crucial for health. When the mitochondrion gives the signal, the cell opens up to a flood of calcium, which kills it in a sort of cell "suicide" or preprogrammed cell death. (The technical name for this is *apoptosis*.) The cells that do not die when their time is up will continually grow at the expense of all other cells, becoming cancer cells.

You should also know a little bit about ATP. Mitochondria produce a compound called ATP (adenosine triphosphate), which stores energy in the bonds between its molecules. ATP helps your body create proteins and antibodies. It is the fuel that powers the chemistry used by our cells for all that

MITOCHONDRIA IN CELL LIFE AND DEATH

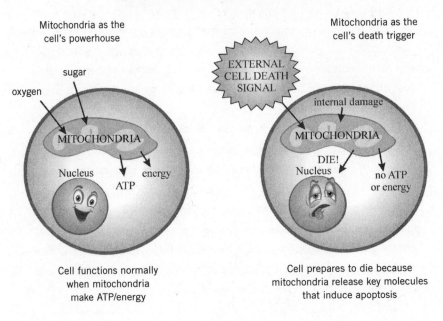

Mitochondria as the
cell's powerhouse

Mitochondria as the
cell's death trigger

Cell functions normally
when mitochondria
make ATP/energy

Cell prepares to die because
mitochondria release key molecules
that induce apoptosis

they do. Without it, your cells couldn't function as they should and could perish prematurely. Just like some cars need unleaded fuel and some cars need diesel fuel and other kinds of vehicles like jet airplanes need their own kind of fuel, cells need a particular kind of fuel to operate, and ATP provides it.

To produce ATP efficiently, the mitochondria need particular things: glucose, amino acids, or ketone bodies from fat (more about this in chapter 7) and oxygen are primary. Your mitochondria prefer to burn sugar and can limp along, producing a bit of ATP from only sugar and oxygen, but to really do the job right and produce the most ATP molecules, your mitochondria also need thiamine (vitamin B_1), riboflavin (vitamin B_2), niacinamide (vitamin B_3), pantothenic acid (vitamin B_5), minerals (especially sulfur, zinc, magnesium, iron, and manganese), and antioxidants. Mitochondria also need plenty of L-carnitine, alpha-lipoic acid, creatine, and ubiquinone (also called coenzyme Q10, coenzyme Q, CoQ, or CoQ10) for peak efficiency.[2] They also need to be protected from toxins like lead, mercury, and arsenic.

If you don't get all these nutrients or if you are exposed to too many toxins, your ATP production will become less efficient, which leads to two problems:

1. Your cells will have less energy to run on, so they may not be able to do everything they need to do.
2. Your cells will generate more waste than necessary, in the form of free radicals.

Without the complete spectrum of nutrients to fuel the ATP production in the mitochondria—which in turn produces energy for the cellular processes required to sustain life—your mitochondria can become starved. The cell then can't do its job very effectively. Furthermore, if the mitochondria are too strained, they will begin to disintegrate. With fewer mitochondria in a cell, there are greater demands from the existing mitochondria for the necessary energy. This strain on mitochondria can send a signal to the nucleus that it is time to die, and then the cell will die prematurely. That leads to more rapid aging in the organs and in the body as a whole, especially in the brain, where mitochondrial action is so important. This can eventually lead to brain fog (confusion, memory loss, feeling out of it) and even shrinking of the brain.

LET'S SUMMARIZE WHAT we've learned so far: When your mitochondria are working at peak performance, your cells have the energy they need to function so your body can work the way it's supposed to, without having to compensate for deficiencies in energy and nutrients. Your cells will produce fewer free radicals, minimizing cellular damage. The proper diet will facilitate this entire process. A deficient diet derails this process, leading to mitochondrial strain, rapid aging, and worsening chronic disease(s).

WAHLS WORDS

All chemical processes involve some waste, and free radicals are some of the trash your body produces in order to make the energy you need. Free radicals are molecules with an open place for an electron that creates a "dangling" bond, making them highly chemically reactive. Free radicals can cause problems in your cells because they scavenge for something to oxidize (in other words, destroy) to get rid of the dangling bond. The free radicals cause problems by stealing electrons, thereby changing the shape of a protein, a cell membrane, or your DNA and altering its function. If a cell gets too damaged by free radicals, it can stop working correctly and even die prematurely. Too much premature cell death eventually results in rapid aging of your internal organs and of you.

Antioxidants to the rescue! Antioxidant compounds from plants stimulate the production of enzymes in our cells that will neutralize those free radicals before they can damage our cells. They make the biochemical machinery much more efficient and effective at protecting the cell from the free radicals.

Imagine what your house would look like if you never cleaned it or threw away any trash. Eventually, trash and dirt would clog up your vents and plumbing, interfere with your electrical system, and cause rot and decay to the structure until your home is no longer livable. Antioxidants are your cleanup crew, your cellular housekeepers, and they keep the free radicals at bay. They sweep up the trash created by ATP production. (I'll talk later about the best dietary sources for antioxidants.)

Signs of Mitochondrial Starvation

Now, you may be realizing how important your mitochondria are to your health, and you are right! You may also be thinking that you need more nutrients so your mitochondria will have what they need to produce ATP—nutrients like B vitamins and minerals and coenzyme Q10 and antioxidants. You are probably correct about that, too: Most people don't get enough of the nutrients their cells need.

But how do you know whether your mitochondria are properly nourished? You can't look in the mirror and see your mitochondria or assess their health. There are, however, a few clues that I've discovered in my practice—signs and beacons to indicate that your mitochondria probably aren't getting what they need to keep your system up and running at peak capacity:

- **You experience fatigue.** If you always feel exhausted and low on energy, even when you've gotten enough sleep, your mitochondria may be starved for the vitamins, minerals, and antioxidants they need to produce energy at the cellular level. Low energy at the cellular level can translate to low energy you can actually feel.

- **You eat a high-sugar, high-starch diet.** Too much white flour, sugar, and high-fructose corn syrup can "gum up" your mitochondria, diminishing their efficiency. Sugars and refined starches affect your body detrimentally in two ways: (1) They are high in calories but low in nutritional quality, so you can fill up without getting the nutrients you need, starving your cells; and (2) they encourage the growth of unfavorable bacteria and yeasts in your gut, which can lead to a lot of other problems. (I'll talk more about this throughout the book.)

- **You are over 50 years old.** Your ability to manufacture coenzyme Q10, an important nutrient for healthy and efficient mitochondria, slowly declines with age. Your stomach may make less stomach acid and less intrinsic factor (a glycoprotein in the stomach that helps you to absorb certain vitamins) that together decrease your ability to digest protein, absorb minerals, and absorb cobalamin (vitamin B_{12}). As you pass 50 years, your mitochondrial efficiency also slowly declines, particularly if your nutrition is suboptimal.

- **You are on statin drugs.** Statin drugs help lower cholesterol, so many doctors recommend them for people at risk for heart disease or who have uncontrolled cholesterol. Some doctors even recommend them as preventive medicine. The problem with the statin class of drugs that are commonly prescribed to lower cholesterol is that they make it more difficult for cells to manufacture coenzyme Q10. Because cholesterol tends to be higher in older people, they are the ones most likely to be on statin drugs, and older people (over the age of 50) already often have problems manufacturing coenzyme Q10, further compounding the issue. Several studies have shown that improving the level of coenzyme Q10 reduces symptoms in patients with neurodegenerative brain disease.[3] If you have been prescribed statins, don't go off them without talking to your doctor first, but you might want to consider this information and increase your coenzyme Q10 intake to compensate.

- **You take prescription or over-the-counter medication regularly.** Many common prescription and over-the-counter medications can deplete your B vitamin, mineral, and coenzyme Q10 supplies. The longer you are on the medications, the more depleted these levels may become. Some of the medications that interfere with coenzyme Q10 include:

- tricyclic antidepressants
- benzodiazepines
- sulfonylureas
- thiazide diuretics
- beta-blockers
- acetaminophen (Tylenol)

- Medications that can interfere with B vitamin absorption and your metabolism include:

  - diuretics
  - metformin and other common diabetic medications
  - birth control pills
  - medications that lower stomach acid
  - certain antibiotics
  - benzodiazepines
  - tricyclic antidepressants
  - NSAIDs (nonsteroidal anti-inflammatory drugs, such as ibuprofen)
  - aspirin
  - proton pump inhibitors (like Prilosec and Prevacid)

- **Diuretics and medications that lower stomach acid may also interfere with the absorption of minerals.** The nutrient depletion associated with long-term medication use may be a factor in why so many diseases continue to progress when treated with medications.[4]

- **You have chronic migraine or tension headaches.** There is a correlation between chronic tension headaches and mitochondrial dysfunction.[5]

- **You have a chronic disease.** The list of health problems linked to mitochondria not working well is growing every day and now includes diabetes, high blood pressure, obesity, heart failure, hepatitis C, fibromyalgia, schizophrenia, mood disorders, epilepsy, strokes, neuropathy, memory problems, and autoimmune disease.[6] Even with cancer, the evidence is growing that dysfunctional mitochondria may be a factor.

Chronic disease is the most obvious manifestation of long-term mitochondrial dysfunction. When your mitochondria aren't powering your body correctly, everything begins to break down in a negative spiraling chain reaction that eventually contributes to cell aging, organ dysfunction, and chronic disease. Science increasingly shows that mitochondrial strain is at the root of most of the chronic diseases afflicting modern society. Want to grow healthier? Then restore your mitochondria to the healthiest function possible for you.

If any or all of these symptoms or categories apply to you, your mitochondria will benefit greatly from a tune-up. Every aspect of the Wahls Protocol

WAHLS WARRIORS SPEAK

I was diagnosed with relapsing-remitting MS in January 2003, when I was 46, although I had the disease many years earlier. I stuck with traditional medicine for years. I have been on Avonex, Tysabri, and Copaxone, but continued to decline. My neurologist suggested Gilenya, but I was reluctant to go on it because of recent deaths and dangerous side effects, so I started looking for another way. This led me to Dr. Terry Wahls.

I've been practicing the Wahls Diet for six months now, and also use the e-stim device. I am clearer mentally, my decline has stopped, and I have some strength returning. The color in my legs is better and I exercise 20 to 30 minutes a day, meditate, breathe deeply, and spend time outside. Dr. Wahls is my role model and heroine on several fronts. (I am also a gay mom with two young adult children of my own.) I had asked doctors for years about diet, exercise, and stress, and they blew my questions off. I so appreciate the depth of her research and her willingness to relate her personal experience. She is a lifesaver!

—Ann P., Houston, Texas

program will improve your mitochondrial function, either directly or indirectly, but none more so than the improvements you will make to your diet. You are going to start flooding your body with the B vitamins, minerals, antioxidants, and amino acids that your body needs to keep your mitochondria well fed so that every aspect of your health, from the cellular level on up, can begin to repair itself.

Your New Prescription: Food

Your cells have approximately 4,000 different enzyme systems with more than 1,000 different chemical signals, performing trillions of chemical reactions every second.[7] More than 250 different nutrients have been identified as impacting your health, and likely there are thousands more that scientists have not yet identified that are important to enjoying optimal health.[8] Are you getting them all? Probably not.

And is your gut capable of properly digesting the food you eat and absorbing the nutrients you need into your bloodstream, providing your cells with a sufficient supply of the vitamins, minerals, essential fatty acids, and antioxidants they need to thrive? This may also be a problem for you.

Biochemistry is complex, and the workings of the human body are unimaginably intricate and involved. Although we have some idea of the nutritional requirements of mitochondria, we don't yet fully understand every single mitochondrial requirement, nor do we fully understand all the nutritional needs of every cell type in our body. When I talk about "global nutrition," or what our bodies need overall, understand that while we know we have these nutritional needs for thousands of different functions, we still don't understand it all.

But nature does. This is why we can't have optimal health by relying only on vitamins and nutritional supplements on top of our usual diets. Real foods contain all the secrets we don't yet understand, and that is why the Wahls Protocol is specifically designed to use real foods in very particular ways in order to fulfill the vast nutritional requirements of your cells—even the thousands of requirements we don't yet understand.

What we do know is that when vitamin, mineral, and antioxidant levels in the body fall below optimum levels, we see a clear decline in health. This isn't just theory. Case in point: Dr. Bruce Ames, a biochemist who studies nutrition at the cellular level, provides evidence that illustrates how an individual is much more likely to have more rapid aging and the development of cancer with inadequate vitamin and mineral levels, even if she or he is okay short term.[9] For example, when the supply of vitamin K is limited, your body will prioritize how to use the limited supply. It will make proteins that will clot your blood if you are cut, but it will not make the proteins you need to maintain flexible blood vessels and heart valves. So although you won't bleed to death if you get an injury today, if your deficiency continues over the long term, you will develop stiffness in your heart valves and/or high blood pressure.[10] The result could be that in the future you may need heart surgery to replace your heart valves, or you may need to take blood pressure medication.

There was an interesting study that measured the blood levels in seniors of over thirty-one different vitamins, minerals, essential fats, and antioxidants that were thought to impact the health of the brain, in order to examine the impact of these nutrients on both brain size and thinking capacity. The Oregon Brain Aging Study looked at 104 adults (mean age 87). The researchers analyzed blood levels of various nutrients, brain size as measured by MRI, and thinking ability as measured by various neuropsychological tests, and then did regression analysis to measure the relationship between nutrient levels, brain size, and cognitive performance.[11] The results were illuminating. High levels of vitamins B_1, B_2, B_6, B_9, B_{12}, C, D, E, and fatty acids were the most powerful predictors of brain health. Additionally, high levels of vitamins A and K and antioxidants corresponded with increased brain volume and better thinking capacity.

The study also looked at detrimental substances, or "antinutrients." Notably, the more trans fat (hydrogenated vegetable oil) in the blood, the smaller the brain and the lower the thinking capacity, as determined by how well the subjects performed thinking tasks.[12] In other words, spending all of your calories on foods packed with the nutrition your brain needs is likely the most powerful thing you can do to protect your brain. If you want a smaller brain that thinks poorly, eat more antinutrients like trans-fat-laden processed foods. Eat fast food daily or even just three times a week and you are well on the way to early dementia!

Food can't do everything. I want you to understand that up front. I still have multiple sclerosis and I still have lesions in my cervical spinal cord. Some scarring and degeneration is permanent. But my (and your) brain and spinal cord can make new synapses (connections between brain cells) and repair the damaged myelin, restoring function. That is the key point. Quite a lot more degeneration may not be permanent, either. My lesions no longer keep me from walking. You can see them on an MRI, but they do not affect me the way they once did. Food can directly influence the firestorm of destruction inside your body. Will you continue to fuel the fire, or will you douse it by infusing your body with the particular nutrients it needs to best fight its way from the debilitating effects of an autoimmune or other chronic health condition, back toward steadily greater health and vitality?

Micronutrients Your Brain Needs Now

Cellular nutrition is crucial for overall health, but of particular interest to those with MS and other diseases that impact the brain is nutrition that specifically targets brain health. Your brain is an amazing and complex organ, and it needs a lot of resources in order to function properly. One of the most important structures to repair and maintain in your brain is myelin, and myelin is the very thing that the immune system attacks in people with MS.

Myelin is the fatty insulation around the nerve cells. There are 10 billion brain cells with 10 trillion connections. All that connective wiring must be insulated with myelin. However, your doctor probably didn't tell you which nutrients your brain cells need to function optimally, not to mention repair damage. Your doctor probably doesn't even know about this, as physicians receive very little nutrition training. However, I know. To make healthy myelin, you need to consume thiamine (vitamin B_1), folate (vitamin B_9), cobalamin (vitamin B_{12}), omega-3 fatty acids (in particular, docosahexaenoic acid, or DHA), vitamin K, and iodine. (Later in the book I'll tell you what foods you need to eat to be sure you have all these essential building blocks on hand.)

Your brain also depends on neurotransmitters. These are the molecules our brain cells use to talk to one another. When neurotransmitters malfunction, the result can be depression, anxiety, irritability, and increased pain. Many physicians give patients with mood problems drugs like Prozac to boost the production of particular neurotransmitters, but oftentimes patients don't get much relief, in part because they aren't eating the building blocks the brain cells need to make the neurotransmitters in the first place. The Prozac can't work as well if your brain doesn't have the building blocks it needs to run the chemistry of the brain. For proper neurotransmitter function, your brain cells need, in particular, certain amino acids, sulfur, and pyridoxine (vitamin B_6).[13]

When I first began researching the nutrients that fuel the proper biochemistry of cells, especially brain cells, I identified the micronutrients that scientists had said were important to either mitochondrial efficiency[14] or optimal function of brain cells.[15] I have listed the micronutrients and their main

BRAIN CELLS: WHERE THE BUILDING BLOCKS DO THE WORK

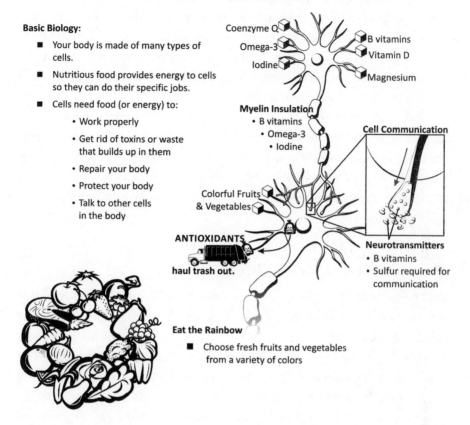

Basic Biology:

- Your body is made of many types of cells.
- Nutritious food provides energy to cells so they can do their specific jobs.
- Cells need food (or energy) to:
  - Work properly
  - Get rid of toxins or waste that builds up in them
  - Repair your body
  - Protect your body
  - Talk to other cells in the body

Coenzyme Q
Omega-3
Iodine

B vitamins
Vitamin D
Magnesium

Myelin Insulation
- B vitamins
- Omega-3
- Iodine

Cell Communication

Colorful Fruits & Vegetables

ANTIOXIDANTS haul trash out.

Neurotransmitters
- B vitamins
- Sulfur required for communication

Eat the Rainbow

- Choose fresh fruits and vegetables from a variety of colors

functions for you here. I have also listed food groups that are excellent sources for the calories consumed based upon the food itself (as opposed to those foods with vitamins added back after processing).[16] Keep in mind that synthetic vitamins do not have the same shape as naturally occurring vitamins, and they don't occur within the context of all the other elements in whole food. In addition, I have listed a key antinutrient that has been associated with worsening brain health.

Beyond Food: The Wahls Protocol

Food is the core component of the Wahls Protocol, and cellular as well as brain-targeted nutrition can determine what happens to your health for the rest of your life. It is not the entirety of the Wahls Protocol, however, and it is not the only thing I changed in my life in order to drastically reverse my symptoms. Many other factors led to my continuing recovery. These include targeted toxin reduction, electrical stimulation of muscles, a regular and appropriate exercise program, a few key supplements, and a commitment to a targeted program of stress reduction.

These round out the Wahls Protocol and are all things you can do for yourself. Combined with an improved diet, you can give your body the best possible shot at healing. Throughout this book, I will take you step by step through the various components of the Wahls Protocol that I developed to help myself and that I systemized to help others, but here's a preview of the basic elements:

The Wahls Diet, Levels 1, 2, and 3

This is the crux of biochemical restoration. I'll walk you through the steps that will take you from your current diet, which may be lacking in some of the potent nutrition your cells require for health, to eating the Wahls way. There are three levels, and you can start wherever you are most comfortable. The most basic level, the Wahls Diet, involves adding some things and taking some things away. The next level, Wahls Paleo, gets a little bit stricter. Finally, Wahls Paleo Plus is for those who want serious and rapid intervention. I'll also explain when you may want to try the Wahls Elimination Diet, a low-lectin version of my diet that is especially appropriate for those with inflammatory bowel disease, rheumatoid arthritis, other food-related symptoms that are difficult to pin down, and autoimmune conditions that are still symptomatic after doing the protocol for a few months.

The dietary steps may sound difficult at first, but you'll be eating great natural whole foods, including lots of vegetables, fruit, meat, poultry, seafood, nuts, seeds, and even some surprising foods you might never have considered trying before. You won't be hungry; in fact, you'll be required to eat a *lot* of food, and if you are overweight, you'll find those extra pounds melting away (a bonus of the Wahls Protocol!). Don't be nervous. You don't have to make the changes all at once. I'll talk you through them so you understand exactly what you are doing and why before you try anything radical.

Table 1 · List of Nutrients Critical to Brain Cell Health[17]		
Nutrient	Main Function	Top Food Sources for Nutrients
Vitamin A, retinol (animal form of vitamin A)	Involved in synthesis of visual pigments in the retina	Cod-liver oil, liver
Vitamin B_1 (thiamine)	Facilitates use of glucose, generation of myelin	Organ meat, seeds, nuts
Vitamin B_2 (riboflavin)	Helps produce mitochondrial energy	Liver, greens
Vitamin B_3 (niacin)	Helps produce mitochondrial energy	Liver, chicken
Vitamin B_6 (pyridoxine)	Aids in neurotransmitter production	Fish, greens
Vitamin B_9 (folic acid)	Facilitates myelin generation	Liver, greens, asparagus
Vitamin B_{12} (cobalamin)	Facilitates myelin generation	Liver, shellfish
Vitamin C	Fights infection, supplies intracellular antioxidants	Greens, citrus
Vitamin D	Aids in proper reading of the DNA, protects cells in the brain	Cod-liver oil, sunlight
Vitamin E	Promotes cell signaling; protects cholesterol-carrying molecules from oxidation; reduces brain cell death, which protects against aging	Nuts, seeds, avocado
Iron	Helps supply oxygen to the brain	Organ meat, greens, molasses
Copper	Promotes iron/copper balance involved in higher brain functions	Organ meat, shellfish, nuts, seeds
Zinc	Aids in perception	Liver, shellfish, nuts, seeds
Iodine	Involved with intelligence and myelin production	Seaweed, seafood, iodized sea salt
Magnesium	Stabilizes cells against excess glutamate (too much stimulation)	Greens, raw soaked nuts, seaweed
Selenium	Protects against oxidative stress	Brazil nuts, sunflower seeds, seafood, seaweed
Lycopene, lutein, zeaxanthin, alpha- and beta-carotene, beta-cryptoxanthin (carotenoids)	Antioxidants, which protect cell membranes and mitochondria and are key nutrients for a healthy retina and brain cells.	Brightly colored vegetables and berries
Carnitine	Assists with energy production in mitochondria	Heart, kidney, liver, beef, and all other meats, including poultry

Toxic Exposure

The modern world is chemically burdened and many of those chemicals interact with our cells, often thwarting the natural chemical processes. I'll explain how many of these chemicals are associated with the leading causes of disability and disease in America. I'll help you identify where your exposures to these chemicals lie and the specific steps you can take to reduce your exposure. I'll also explain how your body processes the toxic chemicals and eliminates them. Most important, I'll give you the specific steps to take to safely strengthen and optimize your body's toxin elimination systems so that you can slowly and safely reduce the body burden of toxins that are stored in your fat. I'll talk more about this in chapter 8.

Exercise and E-Stim

Your brain and your body need you to use your muscles and *move*, even if you have a degenerative disease. Exercise is important to maintaining the proper balance of hormones in the brain and in the body. Exercise is a critical part of rehabilitation for anyone who has had a stroke or traumatic brain injury. It is also a critical part of restoring health for anyone with a systematic autoimmune or chronic health problem. I encourage you to commit to an exercise program because exercise is the only way to prevent the decline of muscle mass. Muscle loss occurs during normal aging, and exercise slows the rate of age-related muscle loss. Being sedentary or in bed further accelerates muscle loss.[18] This is why it is critical to exercise and stay active—to maintain muscle mass and prevent accelerated muscle loss. Strength training in particular increases muscle mass.[19] When you have a chronic disease, it's also important to do enough, and not too much, and to do the right kinds of exercise for your needs. After I talk about exercise, I'll also tell you all about electrical stimulation, or e-stim, a process that has had a dramatic effect on my mobility as well as my mood. Athletes have been using e-stim to speed their recovery, and physical therapists are increasingly recommending that their patients use e-stim to speed their rehabilitation and recovery from a wide variety of injuries and illnesses. I encourage you to explore e-stim to aid your exercise program and rehabilitation as well. I'll talk more about this in chapter 9.

Supplements, Medications, and Alternative Medicine Treatments

I strongly believe that most nutrition should come from food, but depending on your particular needs, you could benefit from certain supplements; I'll tell you which ones I recommend and which ones I believe are contraindicated. I'll also talk about your medications and how physicians approach disease-modifying drug treatments, when drug treatment is beneficial, and what the research says about the risks of continuing and the risks of discontinuing disease-modifying drug therapy, so you know how to approach this as you begin the Wahls Protocol. Finally, I will give you my conventional-doctor-turned-functional-medicine-advocate perspective on alternative medicine treatments you might want to try and those I believe you should avoid. Learn what's proven and what's merely speculation, as well as what's safe and what might not be. I'll talk all about this in chapter 10.

Stress Reduction Techniques

Stress reduction is absolutely critical for optimizing your body's ability to heal. The stress response causes a cascade of changes in the body that can be highly beneficial in the short term and drastically destructive over the long term. I'll explain exactly why and how you can get yourself back out of fight-or-flight mode.

Looking Back over Your Life: The Prodromal State and the Power of Intervention

I hope you can still remember a time when you felt well. You could work or play all day and you felt happy, or at least normal, in your body. At some point, however, you probably noticed some subtle changes. Perhaps you noticed that you couldn't move as freely or think as clearly, or you began to experience pain. These very outward symptoms were a signal that your biochemistry was changing. The signaling between your cells was gradually becoming confused.

You could recognize that you didn't feel well, though you may not have been able to explain precisely what was amiss. You eventually saw your doctor, who performed an examination and conducted blood tests but found nothing wrong. Maybe a test showed that you have *some* autoantibodies (antibodies against one of the constituents of your cells) but your doctor told you the levels were not that high—that you did not have an autoimmune diagnosis. Perhaps you were told to come back in a year. When you did, you felt a little worse than you did the year before, but all your tests still looked okay and the doctor continued to say you were "fine." Perhaps this dance went on for years, perhaps decades, before your body finally suffered enough damage that a test or two began to come up abnormal. Finally, your doctor began to investigate more seriously. And perhaps, at long last, you were given a diagnosis. Your doctor had not been trained in functional medicine, and so opportunities to recover your vitality were missed, but the inexorable process of biochemical decline was happening all along, through all those years of negative test results and doctors reassuring you. Your body began to produce and accumulate incorrectly made molecules in your cells and your organs. To you, it probably felt like the music of your life slowly began to deteriorate, note by note, losing the melody and harmony, moving from a beautiful symphonic concert to chaotic noise. That's how it felt to me.

Why weren't you told, during those years and years of feeling bad but not meeting a specific diagnostic criteria, that there are things you could be doing to improve your health? Those years before diagnosis are critical—as the body experiences cross-reactivity between environmental antigens (proteins that elicit a response from our immune cells), food, and human tissue. This is also a period when molecular mimicry (molecules from one thing resembling another thing, such as human tissue and the gluten molecule) continues to confuse the immune system, triggering continued production of autoantibodies to even more cellular parts of you. This period before you are diagnosable is called the prodromal state, and it can last for two to fifteen years prior to full-blown autoimmune disease diagnoses of multiple sclerosis, rheumatoid arthritis, systemic lupus erythematosus, psoriasis, inflammatory bowel disease, or celiac disease (just to name a few autoimmune conditions). This prodromal state is precisely when diet and lifestyle changes can often completely normalize cellular function, reverse the damage, and lead to disappearance of the autoantibodies and resolution of symptoms, so disease diagnosis never happens. *This is huge.*

Likely, all autoimmune conditions, and likely even chronic conditions like high blood pressure, metabolic syndrome, fatty liver disease, anxiety, and depression, have this prodromal period. This is *exactly when a diet and lifestyle intervention will be very effective at stopping the damage and restoring health and vitality.*

What this means for you is that when you don't feel well but you aren't diagnosed, or your tests are just on the edge of normal, or just a little over, and nobody says anything to you about it, you may still be at risk for developing autoimmune disease or some other chronic disease. If the trajectory of your cellular health does not change, you will likely experience worsening symptoms, including progressive disability . . . unless you intervene. The prodromal state is the flashing yellow hazard light in your disease progression—the "caution" that comes before the light turns red and you are diagnosed with a full-blown disease and significant tissue damage. *Intervene now!*

The Wahls Protocol can be that intervention. If you have autoimmune disease or some other chronic health issue, you may still be able to restore significant function. And if you don't have it yet, you could head it off and never have to experience it! Believe me when I tell you that everyone who has MS or any other chronic disease would give almost anything to be able to go back in time and intervene during the prodromal state. It could prevent you from experiencing dim vision, difficulty walking, crushing fatigue, or relentless pain. It could save you from having to cut back on your work hours or stop working entirely because of worsening disability.

The most exciting thing about the Wahls Protocol is that no matter what stage you are in, the results of the protocol can reverse that state—whether you have received a diagnosis and are beginning to decline or whether you are just beginning to feel some bothersome symptoms. But in the early stages, it could prevent that dreaded diagnosis from happening at all. The Wahls Protocol puts your care back under your control. It's so easy to feel helpless, lost, and dependent on doctors and family members when your health declines. The Wahls Protocol offers you a chance to wean yourself off excessive dependence on others. If you are on medications, you will still need to take them, at least for now. You will still need to do as your doctor asks. If your health issues are already significant, you will likely still need help from your family—but who doesn't? However, if you are not there yet, you could avoid it, and if you are, the Wahls Protocol could restore your cellular function, which can then lead to a steadily healthier and more vital you. You have a future, and it can be one of steadily improving health or steadily declining health. It's up to you—your future doesn't have to be a dark one.

In Viktor Frankl's powerful and moving book *Man's Search for Meaning*,[20] he states that we all have a choice about how we will respond to the events in our lives. He says that between every event and our response is a space. In that space, we show the strength of our character. After I was diagnosed with MS, I resolved to get up every day, go to work, and do my job, however fatigued I was. I determined which things I could still do, rather than focusing on what I couldn't do. I decided I would do everything in my power to slow my descent. Remember, at that time, my doctors all told me that functions, once gone, were lost forever—that once you hit secondary progressive MS, it is a long, slow, steady, inevitable decline. When I started this journey, I was only hoping to slow the decline.

I couldn't have done what I did—get back out of my wheelchair, not to mention develop the Wahls Protocol and begin teaching it to others—if I hadn't made that initial decision not to give up but to keep pushing and living and being who I was, apart from my disease. This is what I want for you: to choose life rather than disability, and to choose your own well-being and health over sickness, even if it sounds difficult, even if you don't want to get out of bed.

The beauty of the Wahls Protocol is that no matter what deficiencies you might have or what faulty enzymes might be at work in your body—and no matter what you have been eating and drinking and doing and thinking up until now, even as recently as yesterday—you can still shore up your body and begin to replenish your cells. This is a new paradigm, and ironically it's exactly the way your body was originally intended to function. Your cells determine if you will continue to decline or begin to heal. With healthier cells, you become stronger, smarter, and younger. I see it in my primary care, therapeutic lifestyle, and traumatic brain injury clinics every week.

I call my patients and the many others who have written to me to tell me about their success Wahls Warriors, because they are fighters. They take action, one step at time, to begin changing their lives. You can be one of them. It's not too late for any of the good things you still want for your life. You can start over. This can be your new beginning. Will you join us?

Chapter 2

AUTOIMMUNITY, INFLAMMATION, AND CHRONIC DISEASE: CONVENTIONAL VERSUS FUNCTIONAL MEDICINE

W HAT IS IN a name? What *is* a disease, exactly? Diseases seem real and specific to those who have them or fear they have them because, as patients, we understand diseases according to what they do to us and how they make us feel. This is logical, after all: What we feel is all we know. In my body, multiple sclerosis was causing degeneration in my spinal cord, and I could feel the results: a slow loss of mobility, brain fog, and episodes of horrific pain.

Although MS looks like a particular condition on the outside, at the cellular level, MS is not so different from other autoimmune diseases like rheumatoid arthritis and systemic lupus; chronic diseases like diabetes and heart disease; and even from mood disorders like depression, autism, and schizophrenia. My biochemistry was malfunctioning, and in my case these dysfunctional processes began in the cells in my brain and spinal cord. But that root cause—cellular dysfunction—has everything in common with other diseases that have other names. How different are they, really? How different is multiple sclerosis from rheumatoid arthritis, or even from heart disease, obesity, diabetes, anxiety, or depression? Not that different, at the most basic biochemical level.

Scientists are discovering that nearly all of the chronic diseases that cause so much suffering and are steadily driving up the cost of health care share four things in common:

1. Mitochondrial dysfunction
2. Excessive and inappropriate inflammation
3. High cortisol levels
4. Absence of or insufficient health-promoting microbes living in and on us (together, these represent our microbiomes)

Yes, there are some other markers of broken biochemistry, but in the vast majority of chronic health issues, there is evidence of problems at the cellular level. That means, in a very real sense, *we all have the same disease.*

All disease begins with broken, malfunctioning biochemistry and disordered communication within and between our cells. For health to return, the chemistry must revert to normal, and communication within and between our cells must be restored. This is true for every disease.

Whether you are diagnosed with multiple sclerosis or rheumatoid arthritis or systemic lupus or inflammatory bowel disease or some other chronic disease that doesn't seem to have an autoimmune component—or whether you are told your symptoms are idiopathic (meaning we don't know what is causing them)—depends largely on how your disease looks on the outside. Inside, the distinction between these autoimmune diseases is, frankly, fairly arbitrary, although there are different ways to view, think about, and understand what is happening when cellular dysfunction gains a foothold. As a conventionally trained doctor, I learned one way; in my studies of functional medicine, I learned a different way. However, the fact remains that inside the body, health problems begin in the cells.

Enter the prodromal state, which I told you about in the first chapter— that pre-disease state where your cells are beginning to malfunction. Is that a disease? Or is that not a disease? You can see how the waters can get muddy. But I know my patients. They don't want muddy waters, and neither did I.

How Diagnosis Works

People who feel ill want a diagnosis. They want to know *what they have*. This is a very typical response, to which I am quite sympathetic. I wanted to know what I had, too. I wanted a name, something to blame, something to cure. It's part of how the human mind works. We want to separate out and define and categorize things, to better understand them.

Let's take a step back from all of that for a moment and try to think outside the box. To help you do this, I'm going to explain something that most doctors know but many patients don't totally understand. The truth is that diagnoses are simply names we put on conditions, based on the parts we can actually quantify, like symptoms, test results, and which medications improve or worsen symptoms, as well as through a process of elimination. If it's not *this* or *this* or *this*, then it must be *that*. This stems from the impulse to categorize and name, but it doesn't actually mean that one disease is something completely different from another disease.

What many people also don't know is that the names we put on chronic diseases are frequently the result of studies that look at what treatments—most often pharmaceutical or surgical, although it could be some other treatment or therapy—will make a difference in the symptoms. In other words, for example, when specific symptoms are relieved by a specific drug, then scientists often name the disease based on this information alone. Everyone who gets relief of symptom X by taking drug Y has disease Z. Disease isn't some inherent thing. It is just a label based on limited human knowledge of how to relieve symptoms that appear to be similar.

Whatever the treatment is, if it has an effect on symptoms, then that defined population gets a name for their particular type of illness, along with a specific treatment that eventually becomes what doctors call the standard of care, which means it is the generally accepted treatment for that condition. That is how, for many generations, physicians created diagnoses. They named conditions like multiple sclerosis, diabetes, congestive heart failure, asthma, depression, and inflammatory bowel disease based on what seemed to help those problems. They were not yet able to look into the biochemical workings of the cells to understand the root cause of these diseases or how similar, at the cellular level, all these diseases really are.

It's important to understand this so you don't give your diagnosis more power than it deserves. Diagnoses are often based on the external effects of treatments and historical observation rather than on the biochemical processes that cause the disease themselves. As our understanding deepens about disease processes and treatments, diseases are reclassified, treatments are adjusted, and diseases are renamed. Sometimes one disease is divided into several, or several diseases are merged into one.

This process also applies to scientific research. To study disease, scientists must follow a precise research protocol. We always have a tightly defined group of patients and a tightly controlled intervention (preferably a drug or a very specific procedure so it can be easily reproduced), so there are fewer variables to study. This makes the results seem more concrete and objective, but that approach isn't necessarily reflective of how our cells actually work when they function optimally or how they can deteriorate when they begin to malfunction. The research is easier to do and to analyze this way, making it easier to show if the study intervention works or not; but the effectiveness of any given drug to relieve symptoms may not have much if anything to do with what's really wrong with the broken biochemical pathways that are at the root of many of your symptoms.

Let me say this again in yet another way: *The names we first put on most chronic diseases—names we still use today, in many cases—are the result of observations made prior to the scientific understanding of the biochemical workings of individual cells.*

The National Institutes of Health and the pharmaceutical industry spend billions of dollars studying disease symptoms and developing drugs to control those symptoms. But what is spent on studying how to create optimal health and vitality through lifestyle choices that can lead to healthier biochemistry and, consequently, healthier people? Not much.

This may seem counterintuitive and counterproductive to you. It certainly does to me. Fortunately, this myopic view of health is changing. We are beginning to understand the disordered biochemical pathways that lead to the broken chemistry at the root of many chronic symptoms across many diagnoses. I believe that eventually this will transform the way all diseases are diagnosed.

But we aren't there yet. Although science is beginning to discover how those broken pathways disrupt the biochemistry of cells and disease, most conventional physicians are still using the traditional models of disease and diagnosis. The old ways still govern the standard of care. As a result, most conventional physicians focus on symptoms that can be improved by drugs or surgery instead of trying to create more health and vitality in their patients by improving the biochemistry of the cells through optimal lifestyle choices. They mostly patch rather than cure, and they rarely address prevention or intervention during the prodromal state of disease development.

But there is another, quiet revolution happening in health care today: functional medicine. This alternative method of health care focuses on discovering and treating the root causes of broken biochemistry by looking at the physiological systems for everything from the cells to the organs to the entire organism, and addressing the causes of the problems at their root. This is why I have embraced this form of medicine. I believe it is the only sensible way to correct biochemical dysfunction so you can return to health, rather than simply easing symptoms with drug therapy.

Conventional medicine still has its place. I still do conventional diagnosing in my clinic and still prescribe medication for my patients. This is useful to a point. However, I now add a second layer: I diagnose the person's health behaviors, exposure to toxins, stress level, nutrition quality, and exercise level. I try actively to create more health and vitality in my patients by increasing their knowledge about what they can do on their own. I try to help them intervene sooner and more aggressively, not with drugs, but with food, movement, stress management, deeper connections with others, awareness of their life purpose, and more.

This is where the Wahls Protocol differs from conventional treatment, more closely resembling the functional medicine model. I help my patients reset their broken biochemistry by teaching them to fix how they live, from multiple directions. I teach them how to eat, how to move, how to minimize their exposure to toxins, and how to improve their hormone balance and connect more deeply to their purpose in life. We untie the biochemical knots so the cells can work the way they were intended to. In turn, this allows the body to work the way it is meant to work: to maintain and optimize health.

This is what I want to do for you, but first I want you to understand what is going wrong in your body. Let's look first at autoimmune disease in general,

WAHLS WARRIORS SPEAK

I am a registered dietitian who understood cognitively the role of diet for health, but it wasn't until after my diagnosis with relapsing-remitting multiple sclerosis that I began experimenting with whole foods and specifically anti-inflammatory foods that I noticed a change in my body. My first symptom was optic neuritis (inflamed optic nerve). Subsequently, I experienced paresthesias (painful sensations due to diseased nerve transmission) in my legs and severe fatigue. Then I got numbness in my feet and I had difficulty remembering recent information. After seeing Dr. Terry Wahls speak via her TEDx video clip, I felt pushed to another level. I increased my intake of the foods she suggested, including fish (I was previously a vegetarian), and I eliminated gluten and dairy. I began to feel more energy and focus and noticed a distinct reduction in my symptoms. Then I went further, eating even more kale and other nervous system and mitochondrial substrates, as the Wahls Diet suggests.

I now feel even better than I did before. I am so grateful that a Western-trained physician is promoting what I have been trying to convey to doctors for years: that diet is more powerful than drugs in the long term. I am so grateful to see clinical research beginning to back this up so that others in the medical profession will begin to see credibility in what we already know in our bodies and minds.

—Marla B., RD, LD, CNSD, Chicago, Illinois

and then at multiple sclerosis in particular, through the lenses of both conventional and functional medicine.

What Is an Autoimmune Disease?

First, let's consider autoimmunity. In biology, *auto* means self, and autoimmunity is a condition in which the immune cells become confused and begin attacking the cellular structures of the person's own body. All of our cells have receptors on the cell membrane that allow the immune cells to recognize our cells as part of our own bodies. When the body doesn't see or sense these "self" receptors, it interprets a structure or substance as foreign and a possible threat. Is it a virus? Bacteria? An object that shouldn't be there? Your body doesn't know. It knows only "self" and "not self," and if the structure or substance is "not self," your body must then determine whether something is "not self but safe to ignore" or "not self and dangerous." Your immune cells will ignore "self" molecules and the "not self but safe" molecules, but the immune cells are terribly threatened by anything seen as "not self and dangerous," and they will vigorously attack these molecules in an attempt to damage or destroy the dangerous foreigner so it can't harm the body and endanger survival.

It's a good system—when it works. It helps to keep you healthy by attacking the legitimately dangerous viruses and bacteria that can invade your system. With autoimmunity, however, the wires get crossed and the immune cells mistake proteins that are genuinely "self" as foreign—more specifically as "not self and dangerous." The results can be devastating.

There are many ways this can happen:

• **Leaky gut:** The intestine, which should be tightly sealed to all but the smallest particles that are meant to leave the digestive tract, becomes permeable, allowing inadequately digested food proteins and bacterial fragments into the bloodstream, where they are not meant to be. When they show up in the bloodstream, the immune system becomes activated and, depending on your genetics, sensitivity to the food protein begins. The immune cells make antibodies that attack those food proteins and increase the production of inflammation molecules, leading to generalized inflammation and nonspecific feelings of fatigue, malaise, and poor mood. Leaky gut syndrome is the term used to describe this development of holes or leaks in the lining between the small bowel and the blood vessels. When these bowel contents show up in parts of the body they were never meant to be, this can be a trigger for the beginning of autoimmune disease, as the immune system rushes to attack these "invaders." Note that while leaky gut syndrome used to be something many doctors questioned as a legitimate process, more scientists and clinicians, including autoimmune specialists, now recognize that leaky gut is real . . . and a factor in developing autoimmunity. Many are now studying the connection between leaky gut, microbiome alterations, inflammation, oxidative stress, and cytokine levels, especially in autoimmune diseases.

This intestinal permeability can happen for many reasons, including microbiome imbalance (dysbiosis), food sensitivities and allergies, prescription and/or over-the-counter medications (especially antibiotics and acid-lowering medications), or inflammation for any reason (such as from an infection, allergic reaction, toxin exposure, or prolonged stress). There is even some evidence that food additives can increase intestinal permeability. There are many theories on why some people develop this condition—often called leaky gut syndrome—but it is often the first step in the development of autoimmunity. When the immune system detects these inadequately digested food proteins or bacterial particles in the bloodstream, it typically reacts by increasing inflammation and making antibodies to attack and then digest those protein fragments. One way this happens is by increasing the production of NF-kappaB and related proteins, which further worsen inflammation all over the body.

- **Dysbiosis:** Many things can disrupt the balance in the human microbiome—that collection of bacteria, fungi, viruses, and archaea (single-cell bacteria-like organisms living in our bowels that are even more ancient than bacteria) we all carry around within our gastrointestinal system. A poor diet, stress, and many of the same things that cause inflammation (listed above) can also disrupt that balance, causing an overgrowth of sugar-loving yeasts and bacteria and reducing the numbers of beneficial microbes. Having the wrong microbes living in and on our bodies can trigger abnormally aggressive immune cells that are hypervigilant. In addition, having the wrong microbes in our guts will change the production of neurotransmitters, leading to problems with mood and thinking. Dysbiosis has been linked to many chronic health issues, especially but not exclusively those related to the digestive system, such as Crohn's disease, ulcerative colitis, and celiac disease. It has also been linked to all other autoimmune diseases, including rheumatoid arthritis, systemic lupus erythematosus, psoriasis, and multiple sclerosis. Having an overgrowth of sugar-loving yeasts and bacteria contributes to an increasingly leaky gut, illustrating how many of these dysfunctional processes are interlinked.

- **Warped proteins:** Human proteins in tissues can change shape because of the addition of a side chain, so they no longer look like they belong in the body, making them appear foreign to the immune system and increasing the attack by the immune cells and the production of autoantibodies. These side chains can come from sugar, heavy metals, cigarette smoke, pollution, solvents, and other toxins. They can cause the immune system to turn on the body's own tissues and attack. This is why cigarette smoking and air pollution are associated with an increased rate of and more severe cases of rheumatoid arthritis, MS, and other autoimmune conditions.

- **Molecular mimicry:** Bacteria, fungi, viruses, or archaea (a small bacteria-like organism) that enter the body may have a similar amino acid sequence to human tissue. This can cause molecular mimicry. In an attempt to attack the bacteria and other microbes, the body also accidentally attacks the similar-looking human tissue. Antibodies made against food proteins and bacterial particles (depending on the person's genetics) may also cross-react with human tissue, leading to the autoimmune disease process.

- **Premature cell death:** Cells can die prematurely, spilling their contents into the spaces between cells. This spillage can include DNA, mitochondria, ATP (a vehicle for cellular energy), or other intracellular fragments, which can confuse the immune system, triggering the development of autoantibodies that will lead to an autoimmune disease process if left unchecked—and the eventual development of one or more full-blown autoimmune diseases.

- **Epigenetics:** Genetics play a role. Two people may have similar exposures, and one person will develop an autoimmune disease while the other will not. Some people are more prone to autoimmunity or to heart disease, cancer, diabetes, or obesity, as well as a practically infinite list of other health issues. But genetics isn't destiny. Those prone to health issues may develop them via triggering exposures (any of the other items on this list). Or (and this is an exciting developing area of research), reducing or eliminating the triggers could keep those disease-prone genes inactive for life.

There are likely multiple other avenues for triggering autoimmunity in the human body that we have yet to discover and describe, but the result is the same in all cases. The immune system, which is meant to protect the body, attacks the body. Which structures it attacks influences the nature of the autoimmune condition. For example, when the body attacks the myelin—the fatty sheath around nerve cells—resulting in nervous system damage, then we say that person has multiple sclerosis. If the immune cells attack the skin, resulting in rashes, blisters, and other visible skin conditions, we may name the condition psoriasis, eczema, or a blistering condition such as bullous pemphigoid. If the body attacks lung tissue, resulting in wheezing and constricted airways, then we call it asthma. If it attacks the thyroid, resulting in a wide range of symptoms related to thyroid function, then we may call it autoimmune thyroid disease. If it attacks the joints, resulting in pain and stiffness, then the person may be diagnosed with rheumatoid arthritis or systemic lupus. Although all these diseases present differently, the root cause for the more than 140 different types of autoimmune conditions is the loss of tolerance of "self" in the body, and the attack by the immune cells on "self," causing the symptoms of the disease.

Actually, autoimmune disease may be a factor in more diseases than previously thought. Research is revealing that there may be an autoimmune component to a host of other chronic conditions, such as heart disease and high blood pressure, migraines, and mood disorders. Research is ongoing in this area, and I believe we've only scratched the surface in understanding the effects of autoimmunity on our bodies.

Once it's happening, what do we do about it? There is a conventional view of autoimmune disease, and then there is a functional medicine view. Let's consider both.

The Conventional View of Autoimmune Disease

The conventional medicine view of autoimmune disease says that the body has lost the ability to recognize its own internal protein components as native components of itself, but that we don't know why. Scientists are aware that all chronic disease states begin as the result of broken biochemistry and confused signaling between cells. But the why is frustrating for scientists. Why is this dysfunction happening? Because medicine is a practice of action, rather than exploration per se, conventional medicine focuses on slowing the progression of disability, usually through drug therapy. If we can't know the why, we might as well focus on intervening in the middle of the process. This is the only proven way, according to published research, to make any consistent favorable impact on the progression of an autoimmune disease, so that is what doctors do: They try to help. They assess the patient, pull out their prescription pads (or laptop computers, as is increasingly the case today), and send their patients off to the pharmacy.

The drugs conventional doctors prescribe for an autoimmune disease make the immune cells weaker so that they cannot attack the body as vigorously. All of the disease-modifying drugs for MS and the other autoimmune conditions focus on blocking some part of the body's immune response, using various mechanisms. Some disease-modifying drugs for autoimmune disorders act as a poison to rapidly dividing cells (the immune cells are some of the most rapidly dividing cells in the body) so that they cannot work as effectively at attacking (or protecting) the body. Some disease-modifying drugs are designed to block a specific pathway in the immune process. Science continues to develop more and more specific drugs to work on specific areas of action, interacting with every step of the immune response, and these will likely get increasingly complex, going after specific receptors and molecules in our cells. As our understanding of our immune responses become more detailed and complete, our drugs become more powerful at blocking specific avenues of dysfunction. But none of them can attack the autoimmune response at every point in this complex process.

If these drugs simply arrested the progression of the autoimmune response, that might be just fine—we might figure out how to turn off the immune system entirely or to target certain problem pathways more efficiently. However, these drugs are not benign. The more we understand about molecular pathways, the more we can see how shutting off immune function can create serious problems in a complicated human body. For example, immune cells are critical to repair the wear and tear that occurs each day of our lives, so if you turn them off, you also turn off or markedly limit the maintenance and repair that our immune cells normally do for us each day. This leads to accelerated aging as well as a decreased ability to protect oneself from external threats like infections and internal threats like cancer. The more potent the drugs are, the more effective they are at stopping immune damage, but they also block the necessary maintenance, repair, and protection that our immune systems should provide.

The side effects aren't pretty, either. Because our immunity has evolved to play a protective role through multiple channels, all drugs that target our immune cells will have an extensive list of side effects, many of them having major negative impacts on quality of life. Remember, we are blocking a major natural function in the body, and even though this function isn't working properly, there are other functions that *are* working properly that will be taken offline. Some of the side effects of these drugs include fatigue, joint pain, achiness, depression, and mouth sores. There is a slightly higher risk of infection (because the immune system is being suppressed), as well as a feeling of general malaise, because making the immune cells less effective often results in making *all* cells somewhat less effective.

Essentially, autoimmune drugs blunt the body's activity in both a negative and a positive way. Symptoms of the autoimmune disease may improve, but people on immunosuppressive drugs may feel acutely worse in other ways while taking drug treatment, and some of those symptoms may involve lasting damage. Many stay on the treatment no matter how bad they feel because of the looming possibility of becoming progressively more disabled by the disease progression if the disease is unchecked, but it certainly doesn't feel like a way to thrive.

This is the treatment conventional medicine offers the autoimmune patient: a slowing of the progression of disability at the cost of feeling somewhat or even a lot worse right now, and perhaps for the rest of life.

The Functional Medicine Perspective on Autoimmunity

There is another view of autoimmune disease, and this is the view on which I've based the Wahls Protocol. The problem with the conventional focus on drugs is that study after study has shown that diet, toxin exposure, and activity level account for 70 to 95 percent of the risk for autoimmune disease, mental health issues, cancer, and in fact most chronic diseases. Drugs do not improve the quality of your diet. They do not reduce your toxin exposure; in fact they often increase it. And they certainly don't increase your activity level. Rarely will they help lower the chronic stress you feel in your life. To those of us practicing functional medicine, the solution to autoimmunity has been staring us in the face all along.

Functional medicine is more interested in the root cause of why the body has lost its tolerance to its own proteins in the first place, and recognizes the complexity of the body and the impossibility of finding solutions by treating symptoms only. We know that the immune system is attacking the body, mistaking "self" for "not self and dangerous." But instead of throwing up our hands at the why, we dive headfirst into it. What biochemical reactions have gone wrong that led to the development of these misshapen proteins? What is the exact nature of the broken biochemistry, and what are the environmental factors that triggered or worsened the condition? Functional medicine looks around and says: "What in life is causing this?" "Is it coming from inside or outside, or from the effects of the outside on the inside?" It is inclusive rather than reductionist.

This is why treatment of an autoimmune disease[1] with functional medicine involves several primary avenues: A more detailed patient interview and history, physical and laboratory testing to investigate how well the chemistry of life is working, and optimizing the body's environment to minimize immune hyperreactivity, as opposed to using pharmaceutical intervention as the first and only intervention. It may be that I include pharmaceuticals as part of the treatment plan. If I do, it is always as a part of a comprehensive plan that includes a therapeutic diet and lifestyle at its base.

This last avenue is the focus of the Wahls Protocol because lifestyle intervention is the best way to optimize the body's environment. We counsel our patients to provide the body with things it needs and remove things that cause harm: We institute a nutrient-dense diet of whole food relatively free of allergens and sugar, toxin elimination, appropriate physical activity, a rebalancing of stress hormones, and the resolution of chronic infections are the first lines of defense against autoimmune disease.

These environmental alterations help to restore tolerance in the body by slowly coaxing the body into an increasingly healthy state so it can solve its own problems. The lack of a precise environmental cause for autoimmune

WAHLS WARRIORS SPEAK

After the birth of my first son in 2006, I ended up in the hospital with a bad staph infection. After it was finally "gone," I started having weird symptoms: tingling in my back, breathing difficulties, and cold feet. I was told initially that I had anxiety or that I drank too much coffee. Finally, after my entire right side went numb in 2009, they did an MRI and immediately sent me to a neurologist, who just threw my chart on the table and said, "The good news is you don't have a tumor, and the bad news is you have multiple sclerosis. Would you like Copaxone daily injections or Avonex?" He told me I would be fine for about ten years, then slowly progress. Nice bedside manner. I was 27 years old.

I started the Wahls Diet in May 2012 and my progression has definitely slowed. My mood is 100 percent better, which is awesome, and I am able to exercise again, which I had not been able to do because of the fatigue. I now treat my food as my medicine, and if it is not going to heal me, I don't eat it. My family is so grateful for Dr. Wahls's work because they have their mom and wife back!

—Karen K., Elk Grove, California

diseases (and other chronic health problems) may be the reason few conventional physicians use therapeutic lifestyle changes—that is, diet, exercise, and meditative practices—to treat their patients. If research has not fully isolated a single intervention as effective against a single problem (which is currently the gold standard for proving efficacy), it is not generally recommended in conventional medicine. But there isn't as much money in testing for less profitable lifestyle changes like food, exercise, and stress reduction. Those interventions are about normalizing the body's environment so the body can work better to correct its imbalances. A functional medicine doctor may still recommend pharmaceutical intervention, but he or she does not limit the approach to this. We believe we can do more, and the results, like those from my clinical trials, prove it's true. In any case, no matter whether you elect to use conventional drug therapies for your autoimmune or other chronic disease(s), I strongly urge you to include a therapeutic diet and lifestyle intervention as part of your wellness and treatment plan.

In medical school, we are told to always use therapeutic diet and lifestyle first before using drug therapy, but alas, we have received very little training on how to actually do that in clinical practice. Prior to the 1940s and the development of antibiotics and the modern pharmaceutical and medical device industries, medicine used to be focused primarily on nutrition. Now we rush to giving people drugs, devices, and surgeries to fix their health challenges— this is where our training has been focused. Functional medicine, in contrast, focuses on therapeutic diet and lifestyle interventions. That is the crux of a functional medicine doctor's training, so if that is what you seek, that may be the medical approach you need from your primary care doctor. (For more about how to find a functional medicine practitioner, see page 415.)

WHEN I SAY "FUNCTIONAL MEDICINE DOCTOR" OR "FUNCTIONAL MEDICINE PRACTITIONER" . . .

Doctors are not the only health professionals who can practice functional medicine. Advanced practice nurse practitioners, chiropractors, physician assistants, and other experienced health professionals may also be useful and valuable additions to your health care team. Throughout this book, whenever I say "functional medicine doctor" or "functional medicine practitioner," please know that I mean any professional trained in functional medicine practices.

Do You Still Need Your Disease-Modifying Medications?

Many of the patients I see in my clinical practice have been able to steadily reduce their prescription medications the longer they are on the Wahls Protocol. I see the same thing in our clinical trials. As you feed your cells what they need, your cells will rebuild you molecule by molecule. Blood pressure improves, fatigue lessens, blood sugar normalizes, excess weight drops off without your being hungry, sexual function improves, pain abates, and the need for immune suppression, including disease-modifying drugs, typically declines over the next three years. This is true whether the disease is a classical autoimmune problem like multiple sclerosis; a chronic disease like obesity or diabetes; or a mental health problem like depression, anxiety, or posttraumatic stress disorder.

Note, however, that *we do not stop medications before cellular healing has eliminated the need for the medication.* Once blood pressure drops, blood sugars improve, mood brightens, energy is good, pain is resolved, and fatigue is gone, then and only then do I begin the process of tapering medications. When people start the therapeutic diet and lifestyle, I tell patients we must watch them closely so they do not develop side effects from the high blood pressure, high blood sugar, or pain medications that are no longer needed. As they continue to improve, then I may begin a conversation about what other drugs (such as immune-suppressing drugs) could be gradually, carefully tapered and perhaps, if all goes well, eventually stopped. This is not something for you to do on your own. This is critical!

It's important to understand why, for some patients, medication remains important. Abruptly stopping disease-modifying drugs in the autoimmune patient increases the risk of a serious acute flare of the underlying autoimmune disease, disease reactivation, and decline—in fact, research has shown that this happens in a statistically significant proportion of patients.[2]

WAHLS WARRIORS SPEAK

In December 2011, at the age of 56, I received my third diagnosis of relapsing-remitting multiple sclerosis [RRMS] since experiencing my first "diagnosable" episode in August 2011. After months of testing and obtaining second and third opinions, I accepted my diagnosis from a neurologist at Mount Sinai. I was shown on my MRIs that my lesions were significant, and some looked "old." I may have been living with RRMS for the past 30 years. In early January 2012, I began a treatment of Copaxone and

> *started the Wahls Diet. Over time, I was able to decrease the daily injections to weekly, and stopped them altogether in June 2012. My neurologist told me that whatever I was doing to heal, it wasn't the Copaxone. Everyone who has seen me this past year concurs that I am doing something right and am on the road to recovery and beyond!*
>
> —Debra K., Accord, New York

No one wants to have irreversible damage to their brain and other critical organs. If you are already on potent immunosuppressive drugs, stay on them as you adopt the Wahls Protocol. Eventually, as the body is rebuilt, replacing incorrectly shaped molecules with correctly made and shaped molecules, the rate of worsening slows, then stops, and as the cells continue to function more effectively, often better and better health and vitality ensue. Each person is unique, and how quickly his or her health is stabilized and improves will be unique. It will depend on the burden of less effective enzymes (DNA), the burden of poor lifestyle factors (diet, exercise, toxins, hormone balance, etc.), the burden of prior and current infection(s), and how much work the person does to optimize all lifestyle factors. Your personal physician or a functional medicine doctor is the one who can help you determine when and if medication should be reduced or tapered. (In chapter 10, I will discuss more about what factors to consider before discontinuing disease-modifying drug therapy after giving lifestyle interventions time to work.)

About Multiple Sclerosis in Particular

In this revised edition, I want to broaden my focus to include not just multiple sclerosis, but all autoimmune conditions, all neurological conditions, and indeed, all chronic diseases that can be transformed through my therapeutic diet and lifestyle changes (and that includes most of them). However, my core community is made up of people who share the same disease I have, so I do want to spend some time addressing this frustrating and debilitating disease specifically.

MS was first described by French physician Jean-Martin Charcot back in

TALKING TO YOUR DOCTOR ABOUT LIFESTYLE INTERVENTION

If you have an autoimmune disease, you and your doctor are likely to agree on one thing: You need disease-modifying therapy. The question is, what kind of disease-modifying therapy? It is my assumption that you want to arrest the progress of your disease. You don't want to experience continued flares and the damage they cause. You don't want to progress or relapse into disability. But you also don't want to suppress the parts of your immune system that are beneficial to you. If you are given an initial diagnosis and are not yet on any medication, one option is to propose to your treating specialist that you would like to try lifestyle modification for three to six months before starting disease-modifying drugs. Bring this book with you, to show your doctor what you intend to do. Most important, focus on a nutrient-dense diet, stop eating sugary foods and junk foods, and incorporate a regular exercise program and stress reduction into your life. These are all the things we know should be part of every chronic disease management program (and in my opinion, everyone's life, whether they have health issues or not). Be open to close follow-up to confirm that your disease is calming down and that there is no ongoing silent damage. You may still need medication after three to six months, but you may need less—and you may also find that closely following the Wahls Protocol (especially the Wahls Elimination Diet) may be enough to arrest your progression and reduce or even eliminate your symptoms.

1868, and although we've known about this condition for more than a hundred years, there is still a lot we don't understand about how the disease gets started and how and why it progresses. Although the majority of people with multiple sclerosis are diagnosed initially with relapsing-remitting multiple sclerosis, in which periods of disability come and go, within fifteen years of diagnosis, 80 percent will transition to the more severe form of the disease, secondary progressive multiple sclerosis, in which disability becomes permanent and inevitable in spite of therapy. (This is what happened to me.)

There are several theories about why someone develops multiple sclerosis, but MS is generally thought to be related to some genetic vulnerability that interacts with many unknown environmental factors (this is the epigenetic effect I explained earlier in this chapter). Numerous studies have shown that it is the interaction of multiple genes and the environment that determine whether someone will develop MS. There have been nearly a hundred genes identified that slightly increase the odds for getting MS. Yet no study has definitively identified precisely which problem is the cause of MS,[3] or why the problem develops in the first place.

When the disease is triggered, immune cells begin attacking and damaging myelin and other parts of the brain, leading to a shrinking brain and problems with balance, vision, and/or muscle strength. Over the years, as symptoms accrue, doctors are finally able to diagnosis these symptoms as multiple sclerosis.

The highest rates of MS are found in Europe, Canada, the United States, and southern Australia. Epidemiological evidence suggests that people who develop this disease probably acquired an infection before the age of 15 that, because of a genetic vulnerability, was not completely cleared from the body. If the person who suffered from the infection is also exposed to particular environmental factors (whatever they might be) and is genetically vulnerable (in some way not clearly understood), the immune system will begin destroying the brain and spinal cord. In other words:

genetic vulnerabilities + environmental triggers = onset of MS

That appears to be the formula, and the more genes you have that put you at risk (there isn't just one), the smaller the dose of environmental insults you will require to develop the symptoms (the prodromal state) that could ultimately be diagnosed as multiple sclerosis (the disease state). The disease may not rear its ugly head or show on the surface for decades, but inside the body, the process of silent damage has already begun its inexorable march.

As the immune cells attack the myelin, which wraps around the wiring connecting cells in the brain and in the spinal cord, the transmission of information down the long arms of the nerve cells slows. As the damage to the myelin progresses, the nerve cells can become so damaged that they can no longer transmit information at all. When that happens, the loss becomes permanent.

Types of MS

There are four *main* types of MS:

1. Clinically isolated syndrome (technically a pre-MS state)
2. Relapsing-remitting MS (RRMS)
3. Secondary progressive MS (SPMS)
4. Primary progressive MS (PPMS)

About 85 percent of people begin with **clinically isolated syndrome**. That is the first attack of neurological symptoms. Forty-five percent will have some type of motor or sensory problems. Twenty percent will have optic neuritis (visual problems), 10 percent will have brain stem problems (nausea, vomiting, and balance problems are the most common), and the remaining will have problems in multiple areas. The current standard is to recommend treatment with disease-modifying drug therapy at initial presentation, to lower the risk of permanent damage to the brain and spinal cord.

The subsequent disease course is most often (85 percent of the time) episodically worse (relapse), followed by periods of improvement (remission). This is why it is called **relapsing-remitting MS.** Approximately 10 to 15 percent experience gradual decline without any improvement (this is progressive multiple sclerosis). This form of the disease involves acute episodes of worsening symptoms, called relapses, which are followed by gradual improvements as the brain and spinal cord add sodium channels to the nerve cells, allowing them to transmit information again, albeit more slowly than before. In addition to the relapses, which have obvious symptoms, the person with RRMS will often develop silent lesions (lesions that have no apparent symptoms), which can be seen on MRI scans of the brain.

The majority of people diagnosed with RRMS will convert to a different form, called **secondary progressive MS (SPMS),** within twenty years of initial diagnosis. When that happens, the person often stops having acute relapses and remissions. Instead, there is a gradual worsening of the MS-related symptoms and increasing disability. There is only decline.

Approximately 10 to 15 percent of MS patients are initially diagnosed with another form called **primary progressive MS (PPMS).** They never have acute worsening and remissions. They experience only a gradual decline from the beginning.

Conventional Treatment for MS

Because multiple sclerosis is an autoimmune disease, the mainstay of treatment is suppression of the immune cells with progressively more potent drugs. For MS, the disease-modifying drugs that were initially used were the "ABC-R" drugs, which are Avonex, Betaseron, and Copaxone, or the drug Rebif. Today there are many more options for immune-suppressing disease-modifying drugs.

As scientists continue to try to understand the exact nature of what the genetic vulnerabilities are and why they are not all the same in every person with MS, several theories have emerged that currently influence treatment. One theory is that multiple sclerosis is actually a vascular disease. Dr. Paolo Zamboni has described chronic cerebrospinal venous insufficiency (CCSVI) in the setting of multiple sclerosis and as the cause of MS.[4] CCSVI is the narrowing of the veins that drain the brain. The consequence is that the backing up of pressure in the veins leads to an excess deposit of iron in the tissues, increasing inflammation and oxidative stress, thereby contributing to the development of MS symptoms.

Although the typical conventional treatment for MS often involves immune-suppressing drugs, Zamboni reported that doing angioplasty to open the blockages was associated with an acute reduction of MS-related symptoms. He further reported success in treating fatigue with angioplasty—that is, using a balloon or stent to open up the narrowed blood vessel in an outpatient procedure.[5] However, some experienced a relatively short-lived improvement from this invasive procedure, necessitating multiple angioplasties to reopen the blood vessels.[6] Furthermore, there has been controversy about whether CCSVI is present at an increased rate in those with MS over those without MS.[7] Subsequent studies have shown that rates of CCSVI increase as we age, and that CCSVI has not been consistently shown to be increased in

---

THE LATEST MS DRUGS

The following is adapted from the National MS Society web page. There are more than a dozen drugs available, with more in development. These are the available drugs as of 2019 (visit nationalmssociety.org for the most current information on drug treatment options):

- **Self-injected:** *Avonex, Betaseron, Copaxone, Extavia, Glatopa 20 mg and 40 mg, glatiramer acetate 20 mg and 40 mg, Plegridy, and Rebif.*
- **By mouth:** *Aubagio, Gilenya, and Tecfidera.*
- **Infusions:** *Lemtrada, Novantrone, Ocrevus, and Tysabri.*
- **Novantrone** *is FDA-approved for people with worsening relapsing-remitting MS (worsening in between relapses) and those with secondary progressive MS (started with relapses but are now worsening with no or few relapses). This DMT is used infrequently due to serious side effects and risks.*
- **Ocrevus** *was approved for the treatment of relapsing-remitting MS and primary progressive MS (progression without relapses since symptom onset).*
- **Zinbryta** *was approved by the FDA in 2016, but withdrawn by the manufacturer due to risks in March of 2018.*

Because of safety concerns, the FDA recommends that Lemtrada generally be reserved for patients who have had an inadequate response to at least two other disease-modifying therapies.

The MS disease-modifying treatments have side effects and risks that are different for everyone. Starting a DMT or switching to a different DMT are decisions best made by the person with MS and his or her MS doctor, after a conversation about how the medication works, its side effects, and costs.

RRMS patients.[8] Zamboni no longer recommends angioplasty or stenting for RRMS patients.[9]

Conventional approaches that prescribe only disease-modifying pharmaceuticals to relieve MS symptoms do not address the initial cause of the dysfunction, so they cannot ever actually cure it. Conventional medicine stops short at symptom relief—and when it comes to MS, symptom relief is notoriously ineffective.

As with all autoimmune disease (and all chronic diseases), functional medicine sees MS and its treatment in a different way.

The Functional Medicine Approach to Treating MS

Conventional medicine has divided MS into four types, but even within the four types, the way MS presents is widely variable because the damage can occur anywhere in the brain and spinal cord. If the damage occurs to the nerves that carry information from the sensory organs, then abnormal sensations will result. The person may have poor vision, poor balance, or problems with pain, like the face pain I experienced. If the damage occurs to the nerves that are going between the brain and the muscles, then problems with weakness and/or poor coordination will result, which often impedes mobility. Because the damage is often spotty, people can develop a uniquely abnormal pattern of walking, standing, or using their hands.

These are all characteristics of what we call multiple sclerosis, but here is the interesting part: When we look at this problem at the cellular level, all autoimmune conditions including MS share seven common characteristics, regardless of the specific diagnosis:

1. Mitochondria are strained, producing energy inefficiently and producing too much waste (as I explained in the last chapter). This leads to too many free radicals in the body, which damage the cells.
2. The immune cells are too reactive, leading to excessive inflammation throughout the body.
3. The immune cells specifically attack "self," or cellular structures that belong to us and cause further damage as opposed to repair.
4. Toxins such as lead, mercury, and pesticides stored in the body and chronic low-grade infections, such as Lyme disease or even periodontal (gum) infection, worsen autoimmune-related symptoms.
5. Low vitamin D, excessive stress hormone levels, and imbalanced hormones in general are often present, all of which worsen inflammation.
6. Deficiencies or excesses of particular vitamins, minerals, essential fatty acids, and antioxidant phytonutrient molecules are common.

7. Deficiencies in health-promoting microbes and excesses in disease-promoting microbes living in and on our bodies are also common and are associated with increased inflammation.

Because of these commonalities, functional medicine looks at MS less as a specific disease and more as a system-wide malfunction not unlike a broad range of other chronic diseases. This turns treatment on its head, because defining the problem and therefore the solution is no longer about which drugs relieve specific symptoms. It is much more about correcting:

- Mitochondrial strain
- Immune cell dysfunction
- Toxin load in the body
- Stress hormone and other hormonal imbalances
- Microbiome balance, by increasing health-promoting microbes and reducing disease-promoting microbes
- Immune cells' control of viral and other chronic infections.

WAHLS WARRIORS SPEAK

I felt immensely better within three weeks of beginning the Wahls Diet! My cognitive functioning and energy levels felt like they had returned to what they had been pre-MS diagnosis. I realized that I had not been aware of how foggy my brain had become until I was out of the fog. I no longer needed naps in the middle of the afternoon after moderate outings, exercise, or company. My balance is improving. Urinary frequency, urgency, and incontinence are fading. My double vision when overheated has changed to reduced color saturation in one eye. The nighttime muscle tension in my legs has significantly reduced. I have fewer issues with insomnia.

When I tell people how well I feel, they sometimes ask if I am in remission. I say no, I believe that I am actually healing. The most recent MRI showed no new lesions and my doctor allowed me to go off Betaseron.

—Sally B., Lansing, Michigan

Accomplish all that, and you can make significant headway in resolving the issues and symptoms controlled by a host of autoimmune and chronic diseases including but not limited to MS, as well as other chronic diseases like mood disorders, obesity, high blood pressure, and heart disease. You do that by fixing the cells, which can then fix the body.

We have observed the Wahls Protocol to be helpful for those with blood vessel problems—cerebrovascular, cardiovascular, and peripheral vascular disease. We have observed how it improves blood pressure, exercise tolerance, and mental clarity. How does that happen? Let's look at blood vessels that develop clogging, whether it is of the veins or arteries. Clogging happens for a reason. It is part of the blood vessel's attempt to heal and repair the damage caused by environmental insults, narrowing the artery or vein. Scientists have identified thirty-eight discrete steps that occur as blood vessels transition from healthy to being significantly clogged.[10]

Some of the insults that can contribute to the development of clogging of the veins or arteries include:

1. Toxins such as heavy metals, pesticides, and solvents[11]
2. Chronic low-grade infections such as Lyme, chlamydia bacteria, and Epstein-Barr virus[12]
3. Insufficient vitamins, minerals, antioxidants, and essential fats (micronutrients)[13]
4. Food allergies and sensitivities[14]
5. Hormonal imbalance[15]
6. Sleep disruption[16]

These are all the same factors that lead to mitochondrial dysfunction and that can be altered through environmental changes: diet, toxin removal, exercise, elimination of allergens—all the factors the Wahls Protocol addresses without drugs and without surgery.

Functional medicine's prescription—and my preference as both a physician and a patient—is to use intensive lifestyle management to allow blood vessels to begin healing and reopen any blockages there may be throughout their vessels—whether or not this is a particular "cause" of multiple sclerosis. (I believe it is more likely just another symptom of immune cells attacking the body inappropriately—in this case, the blood vessels.) Lifestyle management attacks biochemical dysfunction from multiple angles with a cascade of beneficial effects. This is why the Wahls Protocol is helpful for most autoimmune and most other chronic diseases. We are getting to the root causes of these cellular dysfunctions that lead to autoimmune and other chronic disease states.

Life is a series of self-correcting chemical reactions. Therefore, once you have optimized your cell chemistry, the body will often begin to heal itself in remarkable ways, even when scientists don't understand the exact nature of what was wrong in the first place. As functional medicine seeks to find an underlying cause, this complexity is the reason we are less focused on naming and categorizing and more focused on balancing and replenishing. Naming and categorizing and looking at symptoms in isolation result only in a narrowed and incomplete view of what is really going on.

What This Means for You
(No Matter Your Health Dysfunction)

As science advances and scientists consider chronic diseases at the cellular and biochemical levels, they are increasingly noting the commonality between chronic diseases—in particular, the common threads across the entire autoimmune spectrum. At the cellular level, there is nearly always mitochondrial strain leading to excess free radicals that damage cells, organs, and bodies, worsening the dysfunction. And there is almost always inappropriate excessive inflammation that also damages cells, organs, and bodies.[17]

When I was in medical school, I was taught to diagnose based upon the patient's story, a physical examination, and laboratory findings. I learned to distinguish many diseases that scientists who study the cellular biology and biochemistry of our diseases now recognize as different manifestations of the same illness. For example:

- Excessive inflammation is a factor in many if not all psychiatric disorders.[18]
- Excessive inflammation is also a factor in heart disease, high blood pressure, stroke, and cancer.[19]

- Inadequate vitamin, mineral, and antioxidant content in the blood increases the likelihood that an individual will have one of the top ten causes of death and disability.[20]
- Relatively low vitamin levels increase the probability of cancer, accelerated aging, and multiple chronic disease states by interfering with hundreds of steps in our biology.[21]
- High blood pressure, the clogging of arteries, and heart disease all exhibit strained mitochondria, too much inflammation, and immune cells that are attacking the blood vessels—and many are now theorizing that these conditions have an autoimmune component.[22]

Strained mitochondria, excessive inflammation, immune cells that are attacking other cellular structures, and toxin overload have been observed in obesity, metabolic syndrome, polycystic ovary syndrome (an increasingly common cause of infertility in women), hirsutism (excess facial hair on women), erectile dysfunction, sleep apnea, and fatty liver disease.[23]

One might even suspect that there are no individual diseases at all! If all disease boils down to broken biochemistry and confused signaling between our cells, resulting in excessive chronic inflammation and strained mitochondria, largely as a result of our lifestyle choices, then this may indeed be true.

What I see when I look at this picture is a very simple message: Your health and vitality are in your hands. You don't have to be a doctor or be able to diagnose yourself to start making changes in your own body at the cellular level. You don't even have to name your problem. No matter what details we tease out of the picture as we try to diagnose and distinguish one disease from another, the truth is that dysfunction starts at the mitochondrial and cellular levels. If we arrest it there, we open the door for the body to heal, and we prevent much of the damage that will inevitably occur if we start with symptoms rather than cause. If we do a better job of ensuring cells have the building blocks they need, slowly those cells will begin practicing the biology of life more correctly. Because our cells are a complex web of chemical reactions that are self-correcting, if we eat and live the way our DNA expects, our cells will slowly put our bodies back together again. If we don't—if we starve our cells for the building blocks they need—problems will occur. Of course they will! You are alive because your cells are self-correcting chemical factories. Your job is to facilitate that self-correction, not impede it.

As you institute the Wahls Protocol, more and more of your mitochondrial and cellular processes and chemical reactions will move toward a healthier range. As that happens, the symptoms of whatever disease your doctors have told you that you have will likely diminish. Your sense of health and vitality will slowly improve as your cells replace the broken, faulty, incorrectly built molecules with healthy, correctly built, functional molecules. In our clinics, our patients typically report noticing favorable changes within just a hundred days! The key is that the better the environment we provide for our cells, the more likely we will be to stop the accelerated aging and instead begin to "youthen." My patients often laugh and tell me the Wahls Protocol is the fountain of youth. They and their families are looking and feeling younger with each passing month that they are on the protocol. I think that is the future that we all want—to be as healthy as possible for as long as possible.

Chapter 3

GETTING FOCUSED: WAHLS PROTOCOL PREP

Y OU MIGHT BE ready to jump right into what you're supposed to eat and take and do to follow the Wahls Protocol. Change is exciting, and I know you want to start optimizing your cells, organs, and body as soon as possible. But before we get into the specific instructions for following the Wahls Protocol, it's very important to get something in order: your priorities.

This chapter's message is extremely important. Consider it a prerequisite of the Wahls Protocol. You might be thinking you can deal with the psychological and emotional aspects later. You want to get right down to business. I've found throughout the years of working with people, however, that unless they get their head in the right place, they are much less likely to comply with the plan. To do this, I'd like you to think about a few things, including what's really important to you and whether the way you are living your life *today* truly reflects these priorities.

Your Hero's Journey

The hero's journey paradigm has been very helpful to my patients in the VA, my clinical practice, and in my tribe. You may find it helpful as well. In his book *The Hero with a Thousand Faces*, literature professor and author Joseph Campbell detailed the concept of the hero's journey as it has been depicted across time and space and documented by the great religions and cultures of the world. The hero's journey has a common arc: Society is facing a struggle and is losing badly. The hero separates from society, studies deeply on his or her own, and learns some important truths. Then the hero returns to society to engage in the struggle. Society, led by the hero, makes significant gains in its struggle, thanks to the hero. In Western myths, the hero always wins. In other cultures, the hero may or may not survive, but the society always makes important gains in the struggle, and the hero is always honored for his or her contribution.

When I invite my patients to consider their own hero's journey, I ask them to acknowledge their struggles, their suffering—what they had to learn and what they now have to teach others about their experience. This gives them new meaning and new insights into the meaning of their illness and how they could be giving back to others.

I invite you to consider your hero's journey. What have you learned? How can you engage in the struggle and help your tribe? Finding ways to be helpful to others adds meaning to our lives. Finding ways to be helpful to others who have struggled as we have can be especially meaningful. In our clinics, when our patients worked through their hero's journey, it was consistently a turning point for them. It gave them inspiration, hope, and purpose—they found the meaning in their struggles. It gave them the energy and resolve to take on the hard work of tackling diet and lifestyle changes.

Know Your Higher Purpose

It's also critical to understand your motivation. Why are you doing the Wahls Protocol? The easy answer is to get better. But look beyond that. Why do you want to get better? You probably have more reasons than you might think at first. Maybe you want to set an example and be there for your children. Maybe a spouse or parent depends on you. Maybe you have something you still need to accomplish in this life. You aren't done living! Whatever it is, large or small, think of the motivation that is the most important to you—that will

WAHLS WARRIORS SPEAK

My husband has MS. He was diagnosed four years ago, but as I look back, he has had vague symptoms for years. His mother also had MS. She died in a very debilitated state. She lived with us for the first four years of our marriage, and I never understood her anger and emotional stages until now. My husband felt a lot of shock, anger, and emotional volatility after his diagnosis. He was very weak from the drugs he was given and we were scared, knowing the decline that my mother-in-law experienced.

I started searching for every possible avenue of healing. My husband was very resistant at first to diet change, and I was skeptical despite being a registered dietitian with a master's in nutrition because at the time I was really into low-fat/high-carbohydrate grains. However, the Wahls Diet has taken our entire family to another level of healing. No more stomach trouble, with great improvement in concentration and mood. Most of our autoimmune issues have either resolved themselves or are gradually lessening.

—Anne G., Deer Park, Illinois

drive you through this process, and that you can come back to time and time again when you are struggling and need inspiration.

In this chapter, I want to help you define what that thing is for you and help you to get your head in a positive space for maximum success. Let's call it your higher purpose.

I know your situation has profound challenges that are not fair. There are no doubt many difficulties for you and your family beyond your having a serious health condition. This is an opportunity to nail down that higher purpose for your existence. A study on the impact of this process demonstrated that those with a clear higher purpose in life had fewer strokes, suffered fewer heart attacks, and survived longer than those without a strong sense of purpose.[1] Furthermore, having a higher sense of purpose improves a person's resilience and personal and spiritual growth, despite declining health and increasing disability.[2]

> ## WAHLS WARRIORS SPEAK
>
> *Having a long-term perspective on life and future goals is really important. I remember thinking that this world is so much bigger than me and what I'm experiencing now. There was an initial shock at diagnosis where I was pretty depressed and kind of numb, and I wondered why this was happening to me. Dealing with cancer was a battle on four fronts: mental, emotional, spiritual, and physical. The mental side of it means making plans for the future and for a long life, thinking about the things I want to do and why I want to live. The emotional battle is dealing with anger, fear, jealousy, resentment, bitterness, and a lack of forgiveness. Negative emotions cripple your immune system, so they definitely had to go.*
>
> —Chris W., Memphis, Tennessee

Clearly articulating your own higher purpose can give you all these benefits and more. Don't worry that what you come up with is the one you will have to stick to forever. Your higher purpose will likely evolve over time, but what is it right now? Start thinking about this today.

Begin Your Wahls Diary

The next thing I want you to consider—and this is something that will be a great help as your higher purpose comes into focus—is to begin your own Wahls Diary. This is an important part of the process; I ask those in my clinic to do it. In fact, it is required for those in my clinical trials. Now I'm asking you to do it, too. Throughout this program, you'll keep track of a lot of things, including what you eat, your stress levels, your supplements, your pain and energy levels, and how you are handling each day and the various challenges in your life. When you have a medical issue or a health problem, monitoring your symptoms, medication, diet, and exercise and tracking your progress is crucial, not only for your own information but for your health care team. Your Wahls Diary can provide this service, but I hope it will play an even bigger role in your life. In it, you'll also monitor how you feel, how you deal with stress, what you do, what your relationships are like—all of it. This will become a record of your life, a snapshot into you as you are right now, and—even more important—an invaluable log that tracks your steady improvement as you embark upon the Wahls Protocol. This is too much to just keep track of mentally (and anybody with autoimmune-induced brain fog knows how difficult that would be!). Instead, I want you to keep a written record.

I also encourage you to take a picture of yourself and attach it to your Wahls Diary. My patients and study subjects enjoy being able to look back and see how much they "youthen" as time goes by on the Wahls Protocol. Do it right now if you can. Just snap a picture of yourself. A selfie with your phone will do. Print it out, if you can. Put it "in the cloud" so you can go back to it and share it with the right people. A few months—not to mention a few years—from now, that picture will be enlightening.

FROM MY WAHLS DIARY

Following my diagnosis in 2000, I realized my rules had changed. I had to redefine who I was and reinvent myself. I was still "Terry Wahls, doctor" and "Terry Wahls, mother" and "Terry Wahls, partner to Jackie," but the dynamics of all these relationships had changed, and I had to deal with that. The most dramatic of these was in the way I was able to parent.

I have always been a strong believer in the importance of teaching my children determination, resilience, and perseverance. I always planned to do this through athletic activities like camping and challenges like mountain climbing. As I became more and more disabled, however, I began to realize that my plans were going to have to change. Many of the things I'd planned to do, I soon realized would never happen. We weren't going to go mountaineering. We weren't going to compete together in martial arts. They wouldn't be cheering me on to any athletic victories. No family Birkebeiner races. No Nepali treks. All those dreams I'd had seemed lost. How could I be a role model for them? How could I teach them something I couldn't even do myself? But then I realized that MS could be a tool I could use to teach my kids about resilience in a completely different way.

One morning I saw my daughter, Zebby, who was only eight at the time, sitting and watching my every move. When I thought about it, I realized both my children, Zebby and Zach, often watched me to see how I would handle things. They were young and confused about their active, athletic mother losing her ability to do the most basic things. They wanted to know what I was going to do. They wanted to know how I would handle this new tribulation in my life. This was a wake-up call for me. I began to smile. I began to get out of bed with energy. I got into my Endless Pool, dialed up the current, and began doing the crawl stroke with the singular thought: *They are watching me.* I began to tell myself they were *always* watching me, because this changed my whole attitude and the whole way I went about doing things.

This was my motivation to keep pushing myself. I told myself that if I wanted them to learn to cope with difficult times, then I needed to show them how I was handling adversity. I realized that I could still be a role model with MS, and in some ways a more powerful role model with MS than without it. Climbing a mountain is tough, but getting up every day and going to work and staying engaged in life with multiple sclerosis is actually a hell of a lot tougher. This became my purpose and motivation to prevail over my condition rather than to lose myself to it. What can you do to give yourself purpose and motivation?

Your Wahls Diary will become an important, even essential part of your healing. Studies have demonstrated that people who journal have improved stress hormone levels, reduced disease activity, and higher life satisfaction scores. It's time to start writing!

What to Write

There are two aspects to your Wahls Diary: objective recording and subjective reflections and feelings. You don't have to start formally. Just tell some stories about yourself until you get used to writing. When you feel ready to get organized, here are some things you can include in your Wahls Diary:

1. What you eat each day, especially to make sure you meet all the daily food targets for the level of the Wahls Protocol you will choose to follow (you'll learn all about this in the next section of this book). For example, keep track of all your vegetable servings!

2. Any health measure and test results you get from your doctor.

3. A numerical rating for your daily mood, energy level, or pain level, and any other significant symptoms you want to monitor. This can be helpful to track as you begin to feel better, so you can look back and have a clearer picture of your progress.

4. Exercise. What did you do today to move your body? Even if it's just a slow walk down the street or some exercises in your home, write it down.

5. Write about your feelings today. Are you motivated? Nervous? Skeptical? Hopeful? What do you hope is going to happen on the Wahls Protocol?

6. Your hero's journey. It is your personal history. It doesn't have to be chronological, just describe important events in your past.

7. Look back at the way you've overcome past challenges and the positive aspects of those challenges. What did you learn? What do you need to learn next?

8. Make lists of what you are grateful for. This can help you find the gifts in your current circumstances including the people and things for which you are grateful, and that can add to your resiliency.[3]

9. Make a list of all the people you love.

10. Write down all the things you hope to do in your life.

11. Be honest: Write down all the things you miss from your old life.

12. Write down your short-term and long-term goals. Check them off as you meet them.

Don't let this list limit you, either. Much of the power of the Wahls Diary is in its psychological impact, and only you know what you need and want to record or write about. You are not just getting organized—you are getting things off your chest. This is your diary and your space to be yourself, but I would like you to use some of that space to tell the story of you. Not your entire life story—I'm not going to ask you to pen your memoir right now while you're dealing with everything else (unless you want to!). Instead, start small.

What challenges in your life come to mind first? Spend some time daydreaming about your past, and pick a story—any story. Then write it down.

Rather than trying to forget your former self, writing will help you embrace that self. Everything that has ever happened to you has become part of your story and has made you who you are today. And your story continues— every decision you make today influences who you will become tomorrow. Your Wahls Diary can lengthen and extend that space in a way that can help you to continue your personal growth, even as your chronic disease may make you feel like your growth has been stunted or arrested. Writing is your way out of mental traps that make you feel like you aren't moving forward.

You don't have to be good at writing to do this. You don't even have to use correct grammar and spelling. If a pen is too difficult, use your computer. Using a laptop computer in bed is a fine way to keep a journal. The medium doesn't matter. What matters is that you begin to write. Don't edit your words. Just write. Let them tumble out just as they are. No critique. No editing. I'd like you to get in the habit of journaling every day, even if you write just a few lines, a paragraph or two. What did you do? How are your stats? How do you feel? Sometimes you'll want to write more, sometimes less. It's the regularity of the writing that becomes so healing.

Throughout this book, I'll have a Wahls Diary Alert whenever it will be helpful to answer a question or record something in the Wahls Diary. Use these as starting points, as inspiration, or as a way to remember what you know you'll want to remember later. These will look something like this:

WAHLS DIARY ALERT

Answer some or all of the following questions in your Wahls Diary:

1. How do you feel today? Be specific.
2. What did you do just for yourself today?
3. What did you eat today? How did it make you feel?
4. Did you exercise today? What did you do? How did it feel?
5. For whom or what are you grateful? What matters most in your life?

6. What is your higher purpose or driving force in your life? This will change, but think about what it is today. Describe what it is in the form of a mission statement: My mission in this life is . . .
7. How long have you been treated with conventional medicine? How is that working?
8. Do you remember the first time you ever had a symptom of your condition? Tell the story.
9. What symptoms are most troublesome to you today?
10. Do you blame yourself for things? Like what? Is blame useful or hurtful?
11. How would you describe your stress level today? Did you take steps to lower it?
12. What could you do tomorrow to make it a better day than today?

Your diary will evolve, as will you. It will serve many purposes for you as you go through this book and begin creating health. Writing is the beginning of taking control, of finding purpose and meaning in your life as you know it now and in guiding you to your future.

Tracking Your Symptoms

I'd also like you to use your Wahls Diary for more quantitative information. Every day, keep track of what you eat, how much you sleep, and what you do for exercise. (I'll give you a template at the end of this chapter.) Also, right at the beginning, I'd like you to do a symptom assessment.

Keeping track of your symptoms is extremely important as you embark upon the Wahls Protocol. You will still have some bad days, and when you do, you might feel like you haven't progressed at all. This checklist, called the Medical Symptoms Questionnaire (otherwise known as the MSQ), will remind you how far you've come. Put it in your Wahls Diary and answer the questions every few months. Always include the date so you can look back on your very first questionnaire and all the others you filled out, can see improvements you might not feel or notice happening. This will give you strength and courage to keep going. You can point to an objective list and say to yourself, "I'm improving!"

This medical symptoms questionnaire comes from the Institute for Functional Medicine, and I've reprinted it with their permission. This is what I use with my patients in my clinics and the people enrolled in my clinical trials, and I have them fill it out periodically to monitor their progress, just as I would like you to do. Remember, your first questionnaire will be your baseline. You might want to do it twice, first to keep track of how you've been feeling for the past thirty days, and then to track how you've been feeling for the past forty-eight hours. Check the appropriate box for each one:

MEDICAL SYMPTOMS QUESTIONNAIRE (MSQ)

Name _____ Date _____

Rate each of the following symptoms based upon your typical health profile for:
☐ *Past 30 days*   ☐ *Past 48 hours*

Point Scale

0   *Never* or *almost never* have the symptom

1   *Occasionally* have it, effect is *not severe*

2   *Occasionally* have it, effect is *severe*

3   *Frequently* have it, effect is *not severe*

4   *Frequently* have it, effect is *severe*

Head

_____   Headaches

_____   Faintness

_____   Dizziness

_____   Insomnia

_____   *Total*

Eyes

_____   Watery or itchy eyes

_____   Swollen, reddened, or sticky eyelids

_____   Bags or dark circles under eyes

Blurred or tunnel vision (does not include near- or

_____ far-sightedness)
_____ *Total*

Ears
_____ Itchy ears
_____ Earaches, ear infections
_____ Drainage from ear
_____ Ringing in ears, hearing loss
_____ *Total*

Nose
_____ Stuffy nose
_____ Sinus problems
_____ Hay fever
_____ Sneezing attacks
_____ Excessive mucus formation
_____ *Total*

Mouth/Throat
_____ Chronic coughing
_____ Gagging, frequent need to clear throat
_____ Sore throat, hoarseness, loss of voice
_____ Swollen or discolored tongue, gums, lips
_____ Canker sores
_____ *Total*

Skin
_____ Acne
_____ Hives, rashes, dry skin
_____ Hair loss
_____ Flushing, hot flashes
_____ Excessive sweating
_____ *Total*

Heart
_____ Irregular or skipped heartbeat
_____ Rapid or pounding heartbeat

_____ Chest pain

_____ *Total*

Lungs

_____ Chest congestion

_____ Asthma, bronchitis

_____ Shortness of breath

_____ Difficulty breathing

_____ *Total*

Digestive Tract

_____ Nausea, vomiting

_____ Diarrhea

_____ Constipation

_____ Bloated feeling

_____ Belching, passing gas

_____ Heartburn

_____ Intestinal/stomach pain

_____ *Total*

Joints/Muscles

_____ Pain or aches in joints

_____ Arthritis

_____ Stiffness or limitation of movement

_____ Pain or aches in muscles

_____ Feeling of weakness or tiredness

_____ *Total*

Weight

_____ Binge eating/drinking

_____ Craving certain foods

_____ Excessive weight

_____ Compulsive eating

_____ Water retention

_____ Underweight

_____ *Total*

Energy/Activity

_____ Fatigue, sluggishness

_____ Apathy, lethargy

_____ Hyperactivity

_____ Restlessness

_____ *Total*

Mind

_____ Poor memory

_____ Confusion, poor comprehension

_____ Poor concentration

_____ Poor physical coordination

_____ Difficulty in making decisions

_____ Stuttering or stammering

_____ Slurred speech

_____ Learning disabilities

_____ *Total*

Emotions

_____ Mood swings

_____ Anxiety, fear, nervousness

_____ Anger, irritability, aggressiveness

_____ Depression

_____ *Total*

Other

_____ Frequent illness

_____ Frequent or urgent urination

_____ Genital itch or discharge

_____ *Total*

_____ **Grand Total**

Note that less than 10 = optimal
More than 50 suggests the presence of significant inflammation and/or toxic load problems.
Reprinted with permission from the Toolbox, Institute for Functional Medicine

Total up your score and use this as an objective measure of how you are feeling. As the weeks progress, I expect this score to go down. On some days it may go up a bit, but it should be a relatively steady downward slope as you follow the Wahls Protocol, if you were to track your numbers on a graph. What you fill out today represents today. How will you feel next week? Next month? Next year? The MSQ will help you answer those questions and step back to see the big picture.

But don't limit yourself to the MSQ when gauging your progress. Write about it, too: how you feel each day, as specifically or generally as you like. Or if you prefer, make your own questionnaire tailored more specifically to your issues. Either way, later you will be able to look back and recall how you used to feel and compare it to how you feel as you advance.

CALL TO ACTION

Go to terrywahls.com/bonus to download a copy of the Medical Symptoms Questionnaire that you can use again and again.

Structuring Your Diary

Some of my patients buy a nice bound book to handwrite their Wahls Diary. Others use something simple: a spiral notebook or even a legal pad. Many prefer to keep their diaries on their computers. They can then print out relevant parts to bring in to the clinic.

You may already have an idea of how your diary could look, but here is a suggestion. Each day I would like you to record any or all of the following details about your life. After that, you can add more, about whatever subject inspires you on that day, but having these details on record will be an immense help to you as you look back to see how far you've come. Your doctor may also appreciate this kind of specificity about your health.

Consider a format like this:

WAHLS DIARY ALERT

I use a number of tools in my clinics to help people assess their progress as they embark upon the Wahls Protocol. These are all publicly available, so you might want to do them all before you begin, record the results in your Wahls Diary, and then take them periodically to further gauge your progress:

- **Telomere length.** There are some commercial products that will measure your telomere length. Telomeres are caps on the ends of the chromosomes. With each cell division, the telomeres shorten; hence measuring the telomere length has become a more scientific method to measure the biological youth of your cells. Diet and lifestyle choices can lead to accelerated shortening of telomeres (more rapid aging) or lengthening of telomeres (what I call biologic "youthening"). I checked my telomere length using TeloYears (teloyears.com) and found that my telomeres indicate that I am biologically 10 years younger than my calendar years. This is remarkable, since one would expect anyone with progressive MS to have accelerated aging and a telomere age older than calendar age. This is an interesting test, but I do recommend following the Wahls Protocol guidance as a telomere therapy rather than the advice on the website, as it is not designed for people with autoimmune or other chronic diseases, like the Wahls Protocol is.

- **Biologic age calculator.** There are several online. They are not all compliant with the Wahls Protocol in their questions and recommendations, but their results can be illuminating nevertheless (although I do recommend you stick with the Wahls Protocol for guidance after you get your results, as it is specifically formulated to address chronic health issues, and most of these calculators are not). A few I like include sharecare.com/static/realage and biological-age.com.

- **Brain grade scale and cognitive training online.** There are multiple apps and programs that will train your brain. Some good ones currently available (some for free, some for a modest fee) include Lumosity

(Lumosity.com), Sudoku (websudoku.com), HAPPYneuron (happy -neuron.com), daily crossword puzzles (games.aarp.org/games/daily -crossword or look for the New York Times Crossword app in any app store), MyBrainTrainer (mybraintrainer.com), and Braingle (braingle .com). Training your brain will increase the brain growth hormones your brain needs to repair damage, build new connections, and grow more brain cells.

- **Nintendo DS Brain Age 2.** I also recommend Nintendo DS games in my clinics. You can use them to calculate your brain age and track your progress. When I first did the Brain Age game with my kids, my score said I was 85 years old. My kids howled with laughter, but I knew that my processing or thinking time was slow. Today my brain age is 40! Who's laughing now?

WAHLS DIARY DAILY TEMPLATE

Date: _____

Hours of sleep: _____

How did I feel when I woke up today? _____

Weight (at least once per week): _____

What I ate for breakfast: _____

Physical activity for the day (list all): _____

Supplements I took today, with times:

Time	Supplement

Medications I took today, with times:

Time	Medication

List all snacks:

What I ate for lunch: _____

What I ate for dinner: _____

For what or for whom am I grateful today? _____

What did I do today? _____

What helpful or happy social interactions did I have today?

_____

How would I rate my stress today on a scale of 1 to 10?   _____
(10 = lots of stress)

How would I rate my pain today on a scale of 1 to 10?   _____
(10 = lots of pain)

How would I rate my energy today on a scale of 1 to 10?   _____
(10 = lots of energy)

How did I feel today, overall? _____

What else do I want to write about today? _____

List one good thing that happened today: _____

I hope you're now inspired to start tracking your life, your health, your mood, your habits, your food, your supplements, your medication, and how your day went. Write about your challenges. Write about your passions. Write about the things that bother you, that upset you, that made you cry. Find your motivation and write about that, even if it changes over time. Remember why you want to live. Remember who needs you.

Remember what you still need to do. And always end with one good thing—a positive note to send you off at the end of the day will reduce your stress and make you feel better. That, of course, is the end goal, and having a higher purpose is the first step to getting there. You are on a sacred journey—your hero's journey. You can make your struggles count for something.

Part Two

EATING FOR YOUR CELLULAR HEALTH

Chapter 4

THE WAHLS PROTOCOL 101

D IET IS WHERE it all begins. It is the one most influential element about your environment that you can control, and it is therefore your most powerful tool in healing your MS or other autoimmune or chronic disease. I didn't come to this realization right away; in fact, developing the Wahls Diet plan as it exists today has been a multi-step process. Now it is refined to a great extent, and customizable, because you can choose which stage or level is right for you:

1. **Wahls Diet.** The most basic level kick-starts your system by infusing it with intense nutrition and removing dietary elements that could be contributing to your decline.
2. **Wahls Paleo.** The next level, and the level where many people choose to stay, provides more structure to further eliminate dietary elements that can compromise gut health.
3. **Wahls Paleo Plus.** This most challenging level is also the most therapeutic for those with autoimmune conditions and is particularly beneficial for anyone with neurological or psychological issues, whatever the underlying disease state, as well as for those with a history of cancer.

4. **Wahls Elimination Diet.** This is a new low-lectin diet that you can incorporate into any of the three levels of the Wahls Protocol. The purpose of the Wahls Elimination Diet is to intervene aggressively against inflammation by reducing foods that tend to promote inflammation, and to help pinpoint specific, individual food intolerances or sensitivities, for those who are still having problems or want to be even more personalized in their approach. This is a temporary diet meant to last a minimum of 12 weeks and ideally 6 months (or more), after which eliminated foods are gradually reintroduced one at a time while monitoring for symptom recurrence.

One Hundred Percent for One Hundred Days: Why It's Critical Not to Cheat!

I challenge my patients to do whatever level of the Wahls Protocol they have chosen 100 percent for 100 days. By 100 percent, I mean absolutely *no cheating.*

What's wrong with a little cheat? A cheat day here and there? Taking it "easy"? Every time someone with an autoimmune disease experiences a flare of symptoms (this could happen due to environmental exposure, toxins, over-training, stress, physical trauma, or eating a food to which the person is intolerant), inflammation levels increase. Much of the work we do with the Wahls Protocol is about decreasing excessive inflammation because *inflammation causes damage.* With every inflammatory flare, you increase the damage to your cells, which leads to the release of substances that further disorder your immune cell responses. Then your innate and adaptive immune systems trigger ever-increasing levels of inflammation, more autoantibodies, and worsening destruction with each successive exposure. This can trigger the development of damage that is so severe it becomes irreversible. You may even pick up a new autoantibody that attacks different cellular structures. As a result, you can acquire additional autoimmune disease(s) in the process. For this reason, you may not be able to regain the previous level you were at before your dietary indiscretions.

This is called epitope spreading, and it worsens the autoimmune disease state. This effect is one of the reasons why people often receive additional autoimmune diagnoses when they are not addressing the root causes for their cellular dysfunction and the development of autoantibodies in response to excessive and inappropriate inflammation. There is no guarantee that you will be able to get back to baseline or repair what has been destroyed. *Every flare worsens potentially irreversible damage.* It's hard not to cheat. When someone you love makes something for you (like a cake or a dinner containing gluten or some other food you know you shouldn't eat), it's hard to say no. You don't want to hurt their feelings . . . and the food looks so good! But remember what eating those foods will do to you. If you stopped taking your disease-modifying drugs and experienced a flare, any doctor would tell you, "You shouldn't have stopped taking the drugs!" It's the same thing when you cheat on your disease-modifying dietary intervention. This *is* your disease-modifying therapy—or a critical part of it. Don't go off your "medicine" by cheating on your therapeutic diet.

Those who are in my clinical trials are able to tell people that they are in a rigorous and strict scientific study and cannot disrupt the process with a cheat, but they love and appreciate the person's effort. You can do this, too. Consider yourself in a "clinical trial for life." You are the scientist, running interventions on yourself to determine what works best for you. My patients like the empowerment and exploratory nature of this point of view. Commit to being 100 percent compliant for 100 days, and see what happens. It's an experiment with big potential for positive change in your life.

While each dietary plan has very specific components, there are some underlying principles that are relevant to any and all dietary aspects of the Wahls Protocol. First and foremost, it is designed to maximize the vitamins, minerals, antioxidants, and essential fats that your brain and mitochondria need to thrive, based on what I've learned from functional medicine, my own review of the medical research, and an approximation of the natural diet that humans ate as hunter-gatherers. I believe it is important for you to understand why this is not only a healthful way of eating, but much closer to the diet your DNA expects, so let's look at some of the principles on which the Wahls Protocol dietary plans are based.

Principle 1: Paleolithic Nutrition

One of the basic ideas of the Wahls Diet is that it mimics some of the primary known aspects of the diets of the Paleolithic or hunter-gatherer people. Paleo-style diets seek to replicate the original human diet as closely as possible, taking into account the changes in the environment and food supply since Paleolithic times. The primary aspects of this diet are the elimination of most if not all grains, dairy products, and legumes, and of course all processed foods that are the product of modern technology. Instead, the emphasis is on green leafy vegetables, fruits, root vegetables, nuts and seeds, meat, and seafood—in other words, the foods our ancestors could have hunted or gathered tens of thousands of years ago.

Humans first began eating grain as a significant part of their diet approximately 10,000 years ago with the advent of organized agriculture, and they began eating dairy and legumes even more recently—approximately 8,000 years ago. These additions are very recent in human history compared to the 2.5 million years that the *Homo* genus (family) spent eating green leaves, fruits, roots, and meat. In our particular species, our direct *Homo sapiens* ancestors ate these foods for 250,000 years before the introduction of grains, dairy, and legumes. That's a pretty good test run for any diet. The modern version of a Paleolithic type of diet is a good, sound diet, in general. There are critics of this kind of diet, and also some misconceptions about it, but these are mostly by people who don't seem to know exactly what the modern version of a Paleolithic diet really is. Before I ask you to accept the concept, let's take a look at the arguments.

One argument is that there is no single Paleolithic diet. This is true. The original hunter-gatherers typically ate an estimated two hundred different plants and animals over a year's time. The foodstuffs our ancestors consumed were highly adapted to the specific regions they lived in, and each local society learned over hundreds of generations which plants and animals were associated with providing vitality for or bringing sickness to the clan.

Also, studies have shown that traditional diets are radically different between societies. For example, hunter-gatherers in the Arctic ate a pure animal-food diet ten months out of the year. Amazonian rain forest dwellers and African hunter-gatherers ate more insects, amphibians, and lizards, and hundreds of different plants. The Native Americans ate a mix of fish, meat, and hundreds of different plants and animals unique to their environment over the course of the year. All these diets were extremely local and seasonal. Because many different cultures have existed as hunter-gatherers, there are likely thousands of diets created by humans that maximize their vitamin, mineral, essential fat, and antioxidant intake per calorie based on the food available in any given locale and the biological needs of the people living in those particular environments.

However, all these diets have some commonalities. They are all packed with many more vitamins, minerals, and essential fatty acids than typical

HUNTER-GATHERER CHALLENGE: DIVERSIFY YOUR DIET

I try to eat a minimum of 200 different plant species over the course of a year. This can be a fun challenge to kick off each new year: Start a list and keep track of every plant species you eat. Challenge yourself to get to 200 . . . or beyond! Get your family involved and everyone can contribute their ideas and discoveries. Try new teas, herbs and spices (those count toward your 200—they are all unique plant foods), experiment with new vegetables and fruits you've never tried, and embrace a sense of adventure. It's also a good idea to vary your animal products as much as possible—try game meats, different kinds of seafood, even organ meats! The more variety in your diet, the more micronutrients you will get, providing your cells with nutrition from as many avenues as possible.

Also, be sure to take full advantage of locally grown or raised plants and animals. Delve into your local food scene—talk to gardeners, organic farmers, heirloom seed collectors, even restaurant owners with a local-food focus—to see what is native to your area that you could try. For example, if you live on the coast, explore the diversity of seafood and sea vegetables. If you live in the middle of the country, explore the diversity of wild game and heirloom varieties of vegetables and fruits, different kinds of mushrooms, and the bounty and diversity you can get from learning the art of foraging.

Westernized diets, which are filled with processed foods and refined ingredients such as white flour, high-fructose corn syrup, and other refined sugars. Remember, the healthier the diet, the more likely the reproductive success.

In addition to heavy processing, our modern diets also typically contain minimal vegetables and fruits and have far fewer vitamins and minerals.[1]

Many critics of Paleo-style diets miss this point. Emulating more closely the foodstuffs of our Paleolithic ancestors is a great improvement over what most people are doing now.

Another argument against the Paleo diet is that our world has changed and no food we currently eat resembles foods our Paleolithic ancestors ate. It's true that many of the foods we eat today have been altered through intensive plant breeding into foods that are much sweeter and richer in carbohydrates than they once were. Also, even natural, organic foods cannot escape containing some level of toxins because the world is now so polluted and pesticides from industrial farming can drift through the air and be carried through the water. Soil is also depleted, reducing the nutrient content of the food grown in it. Then there is selective breeding and genetic modification aimed at producing animals with more meat and fat and greater volumes of milk (often at the expense of quality of life for those animals) and a higher number of bushels per acre. The emphasis is not on improving vitamin or mineral content per bushel—it is about maximizing the yield of the crop, which leads to more profit, and this has impacted our food quality in ways we may not even understand yet.

And we are no longer acting as stewards of the soil. Franklin D. Roosevelt once said, "A nation that destroys its soil destroys itself. Forests are the lungs of our lands, purifying the air and giving fresh strength to our people." To look at the spirit of this quote from a more technical standpoint, the soil in which we grow all our crops has a microbiome of its own, just like we do. The soil microbiome consists of an extensive network of bacterial and fungal microbes that are essential for the health of anything growing in the soil—for instance, soil microbes help plants take in minerals and nitrogen. The use of glyphosate (Roundup) and other pesticides and chemical fertilizers (to replace older methods like crop rotation) has diminished the diversity of the soil microbiome, and in so doing, the health of the soil.

Plants depend on the soil microbiome to facilitate absorption of minerals and nutrients. Microbiome-depleted soils result in a decline in the nutritional quality of plants, which leads to less nutritious grains, vegetables, and meat produced on our farms.[2]

We do know that all of these factors have resulted in animals with fewer omega-3 fatty acids in their meat and more fat-soluble toxins inside them (grass-fed animals and wild-caught fish have better fat profiles and fewer toxins), as well as plants that are both chemically treated and less nutrient-dense than they once were. We can never go back to a planet as pure as it was in the Paleolithic era, but that doesn't mean we can't or shouldn't eat the best, cleanest, most nutrient-dense foods available to us. It means simply that we may need to eat even more vegetables and fruits to compensate for diminished nutrient levels.

Another criticism is that eliminating grains and dairy eliminates important sources of nutrition, and without them, deficiencies will result. This is simply untrue. You can get all the nutrients you need without eating grains, dairy, or legumes. A hunter-gatherer-style diet packed with a wide variety of natural plant foods and natural meats (from grass-fed animals, game meat, and/or wild-caught fish) contains all the nutrients you need. (To support this claim for the Wahls Protocol, we have included a dietary assessment in our current clinical trial[3] and we have investigated the nutrient density of each level of the diet.)

Finally, a common criticism is that people didn't live very long in the Paleolithic era. This is true: Our ancient ancestors had a mean age of death in their 30s, but this is because there was a 38 to 45 percent mortality rate for those under the age of 15. Those who survived childhood actually did quite well. Michael Gurven and Hilliard Kaplan studied this question extensively and published their findings in 2007. The results might surprise you. Hunter-gatherers historically often lived past 60 years of age, and the same is true in the current hunter-gatherer societies that have not yet adopted Western lifestyles.[4] These people are physically and mentally fit without medication, and many are thriving into their 70s and even 80s. The transition from hunter-gatherer societies was associated with loss of height, increased risk for degenerative arthritis of the spine, and tuberculosis, although fertility increased, which led to an increase in population, albeit a less healthy one.[5]

WAHLS DIARY ALERT

Answer any of these questions in your Wahls Diary:

- Are you feeling ready to begin your new dietary regimen? Are you excited? Nervous? How do you feel?
- After you finish this chapter, write about which level of the diet you think will suit you best, at least for now.
- What are your expectations when you change your diet? What do you hope to feel, specifically?
- Once you get started, remember to record how you react to the changes you make.

Those populations that converted to Western diets continued to do worse as "progress" marched on. The next major transition came with the Industrial Revolution in 1850, resulting in the wide availability of sugar, white flour, and a steady decline in breastfeeding. This was associated with another decline in health and an increase in chronic diseases, including heart disease, diabetes, and obesity.[6] Now, as societies move from developing economies to developed economies, the early mortality due to infectious disease is replaced by chronic diseases related to lifestyle—that is, diabetes, obesity, cancer, heart disease, and autoimmunity.[7]

These impact a population later, but the price is high. Consider obesity alone: According to the Centers for Disease Control and Prevention, in 2010, 69 percent of Americans were overweight or obese.[8]

Put more simply, the extension in the average age of life from the Paleolithic era to the current era has occurred because of the decrease in infectious causes of death, lower childhood mortality, and increased use of medical technology—not because we as a society are enjoying more vitality and vigor.

All these criticisms overlook a simple fact: The modern Paleolithic diet concept is not meant to exactly replicate what our ancestors ate. Instead, it is meant to take the general concepts and apply them to our modern food supply as well as we can in an effort to restore human health and reverse the epidemic of chronic diseases that have plagued humans since the agricultural revolution.

Why Paleo-Type Diets Are Superior Diets for Humans

Any logical person knows that just because humans did or didn't do something in early history doesn't automatically mean that this is the wisest course to follow. However, a hunter-gatherer type of diet isn't just good in theory. Research supports the positive effects of a hunter-gatherer-style diet:

- **Better health markers.** When healthy volunteers adopted a hunter-gatherer diet rich in animal protein, nonstarchy vegetables, and berries, they experienced a significant improvement in multiple biological markers of health status, including improvements in blood pressure, blood cholesterol values, and improved sensitivity to insulin.[9] In another randomized crossover trial, subjects were given a standard diabetic diet or a hunter-gatherer diet for three months and then switched to the other diet. Again, scientists found that the hunter-gatherer diet was associated with better blood sugar control, better blood pressure, better cholesterol values, and more weight loss than the standard diabetic diet.[10]
- **A better microbiome configuration.** Most people have more than 100 trillion individual bacteria and yeasts living in their bowels that help digest the food we eat, and whose by-products of the digestion of the food we eat have significant health effects on us, including on our digestive, immune, and even mental health. This internal ecosystem is called the microbiome, and we are only beginning to discover its significance for human health.

  A diet rich in natural animal and plant products is high in many of the compounds (from omega-3 fatty acids in fish to a wide variety of polyphenols in plant foods) that feed the beneficial microbes within us. Microbiomes are unique to individuals, and people who live in different parts of the world have different microbiome configurations, but natural whole-food diets (without sugar- and flour-based products) usually result in more diverse and robust microbiomes with an abundance of beneficial microbes that positively contribute to human health.

But like any ecosystem, we can be thrown out of balance. Stress, pollution, toxins, injuries, medications, and of course diet can all have a negative impact on microbiome balance, reducing both the diversity and the numbers of beneficial microorganisms, which gives more pathogenic species a foothold. We rely on more than a thousand different bacterial and yeast species to help ensure that we have all of the necessary building blocks for the optimal function of our cells, but when the wrong ones take over, the biochemistry of the body can begin to malfunction.

Grains, dairy, legumes, and sweeteners—all high in starches and/or sugars—feed the more pathogenic, typically more sugar-loving bacteria and yeasts. This not only reduces our microbiome's diversity (as with diet, diversity of species in our microbiomes is linked to better health), but specifically reduces many of the more than a thousand different beneficial microbial species that humans had living in their bowels for the first 2.5 million years that our ancestors existed—the ones suited to the original human diet that are part of the proper metabolism and chemistry that occur in our cells.

If our collective health as a society eating the standard Westernized diet with this new ecosystem was still excellent, this might not be much of an argument. Society, however, has been progressively less well. Our new ecosystem is off. Sugar-loving bacteria, like *Pseudomonas*, and yeasts, like *Candida albicans*, cause all sorts of problems for human bodies.

- **Better integrity of the intestinal lining.** Natural whole food promotes healthy digestion and a gastrointestinal tract suited to the digestion of this kind of diet—it keeps food sealed inside throughout the process of digestion, until that food is digested or broken down fully, at which point nutrients can be released so the body can use them. But a diet high in sugar and simple starches compromises this process by shifting the microbiome to favor sugar-loving bacteria and yeasts that can produce toxins capable of compromising the tightly sealed lining of the gastrointestinal tract. Lifestyle and enviromental factors like antibiotic use, the development of sensitivities to specific food proteins (like gluten in grain and casein in dairy products), and exposure to chemicals and toxins like tobacco smoke or food additives and emulsifiers can also impact the integrity of the gut lining. Eating foods that are conventionally grown using weed killers such as glyphosate disrupts the microbiome, increasing the probability of leaky gut and the development of food sensitivities. These toxins and toxic processes can interfere with the system that regulates the cement that holds the cells lining the small bowel together (called intracellular cement).[11] Zonulin is a protein that regulates how that intracellular cement functions. When the zonulin is activated improperly (due to these types of exposures), the cement that holds the cells tightly together begins to open little doors, allowing the bowel contents to leak into the bloodstream. The result of exposure to these things is a "leaky gut."

- **Better blood vessels, brains, and skin.** When your cells get everything they need, they build a body that works. But a poor diet doesn't provide all those requirements, and since the cement that seals the intestinal lining is the same stuff that lines all the blood vessels, if it begins to break down, you can bet that the lining of the blood vessels—including the ones that lead to the brain—are likely breaking down as well. You could have leaky gut, leaky blood vessels, and a leaky brain! You can also develop leaky skin. With leaky blood vessels, the immune cells will be more likely to burrow into the walls, deposit cholesterol and inflammation molecules into the blood vessels, and clog and narrow veins and arteries. In the brain, the blood-brain barrier that provides an extra layer of protection for the brain against infecting bacteria will become less effective. The brain is more likely to allow overactivated immune cells in, increasing the probability of inappropriate inflammation and worsening problems with mood disorders and neurological disorders like multiple sclerosis. In the skin, you are more likely to develop all sorts of annoying rashes and skin problems that come and go. This is why leaky gut is not just about gastrointestinal issues—it's about your entire system and your health overall. This is not a situation you want happening in your body! Yet it happens in many people, largely because of how far we have strayed from the diets natural to our human bodies and biochemistry.

WAHLS WARRIOR SPEAKS

I was diagnosed with RRMS when I was 19 years old, but except for an episode of optic neuritis, I didn't see another symptom until I was 30. I'm 33 now, and things got really bad for me in February 2012. I discovered Dr. Wahls's work in July 2012 when my sister sent me a link to the video "Minding Your Mitochondria." By the time I started the Wahls Diet in August 2012 and Copaxone in September 2012, I'd lost the ability to walk on my own after having been on multiple sports teams only three years before. In the time since starting the diet, I have noticed massive improvements in mental clarity, and I have times when I can walk around without my cane, feeling like a normal person again. Those times make it so worth it. I can give up cheeseburgers if it means I can walk again! I felt so good a few weeks ago that I reintroduced bread into my diet. I won't be doing that again. I felt sluggish and the spasticity in my legs came back. To find that a doctor out there who also has MS basically experimented on herself to find an optimal diet—it was so very inspiring. Thank you, Dr. Wahls.

—Natalie S., Halifax, Nova Scotia, Canada

The Wahls Diet: Beyond Paleo

You may be wondering whether you even need the Wahls Diet at this point. Can't you just do one of the other Paleo-type diets? There are a lot of versions of the original human diet currently available in books right now: the Paleo Diet, the Primal Diet, the Caveman Power Diet, etc. They all have some similarities and some differences, but Dr. Loren Cordain began the movement with his original book, *The Paleo Diet*, based upon medical anthropologic studies of people who lived more than 10,000 years ago and people who are still living as subsistence hunter-gatherers. The movement was largely popularized by Robb Wolf, the author of *The Paleo Solution: The Original Human Diet*, as well as by Mark Sisson, the author of *The Primal Blueprint: Reprogram Your Genes for Effortless Weight Loss, Vibrant Health, and Boundless Energy*.

I am a big fan of the Paleolithic-style diet, but I also want you to understand that the Wahls Diet is not "just another Paleo diet." It provides more structure and guidance to help you maximize your nutrition, which is critical for those with any chronic disease. Also, the Wahls Diet (Level One in particular) shares much in common with the Mediterranean diet, with its emphasis on a broad range of greens, sulfur-rich vegetables, and brightly colored vegetables and fruits. The Wahls Diet and the Mediterranean diet also share high polyphenol intake due to the large amount of fresh vegetables and fruits. They both also emphasize low meat intake and a lot of olive oil, which all result in favorable health outcomes. One study has even looked at how a Mediterranean diet affects multiple sclerosis risk, and found that this diet may indeed reduce risk.[12] But unlike both standard Paleo and Mediterranean diets, which can be excellent for healthy people, the Wahls Protocol is a more precisely organized and aggressive plan to restore your health. This was the crux of my research as I developed the Wahls Diet. Although I was on the Paleo diet for a long time (as originally detailed by Dr. Cordain), it was not enough to heal me. I needed more. You also may need to do more than just stop eating foods that may harm you. You also need to know how to maximize your nutrition for your cells and mitochondria.

Dr. Jayson Calton and Mira Calton did a micronutrient analysis of several current diets, including Diane Sanfilippo's Paleo diet as described in her book *Practical Paleo*[13] and Mark Sisson's Primal Diet for their book *Naked Calories: The Caltons' Simple 3-Step Plan to Micronutrient Sufficiency* (revised edition), and discovered that those diets were much more nutrient-dense than the standard American diet and in fact were among the most nutrient-dense diets that they analyzed. Great news! Both the Paleo and Primal diets, however, were still meeting only the recommended daily allowance (this is also known as the RDA) for fifteen of twenty-seven micronutrients and would have required more than 14,000 calories to meet all the RDAs. (The standard American diet would have required more than 27,000 calories!)[14] These Paleo-style diets are obviously far superior to the standard American diet, but without specific guidance to maximize the micronutrient content, anyone following these diets is still at risk for missing key brain and mitochondrial vitamins, minerals, essential fatty acids, and antioxidants. If you have an autoimmune or neurodegenerative disease (or any other major chronic disease, for that matter), this is a risk you simply can't afford.

What each level of the Wahls Diet plans seeks to replicate, in an attempt to avoid or repair these detrimental processes, is to fill your plate in a very structured way with foods that will ensure you get the maximum nutrition possible using agriculturally available products. Few of us are able to actually hunt and gather our food from the wild, nor do we have the exact knowledge our ancestors had about how to get the most nutrition from the foods growing in our locale. However, if you eat a diet heavy in leafy greens, nonstarchy vegetables, and fruits like berries—as well as animal protein (without including any of those more recent troublesome dietary additions, like gluten grains, dairy products, and at more advanced levels, legumes, all grains, and sweeter fruits)—you have the best possible chance at optimizing your health.

The main differences between the Wahls Diet plans and other Paleo-type plans are:

- **Nutrient density.** All levels of the Wahls Diet plans are rigorously and meticulously nutrient-dense. You will get a specific structure to follow to ensure maximum but not toxic vitamin, mineral, and antioxidant levels. I don't leave anything to chance, assuming you will eat enough fruits and vegetables or enough protein and/or healthy fat. You need a very specific nutrient load. Your body has been missing it. It is medicine for you.
- **A high level of fat.** The Paleo diet recommends lean meats, but the Wahls Paleo Diet, and especially the Wahls Paleo Plus Diet, ramps up healthy fat intake in a brain-beneficial way (in the form of specific kinds of fats, like those in oily wild fish, coconut oil, olive oil, and avocados). The brain is 60 to 70 percent fat. We need healthy fats to make the myelin insulation for the wiring in your brain, so you won't be skimping on the healthy fats.
- **Emphasis on seasonal and local.** I recommend expanding your palate and the food on your plate to include as many native/local/seasonal foods as possible. To me, this is the essence of eating Paleo—getting as close to how your Paleolithic forebears ate, living right where you live now, in each of your environment's seasons. Locally grown and seasonal foods tend to be more nutritious because you are likely to consume them shortly after harvest, at their most perfect ripeness. The longer food is stored, the more vitamin and antioxidant levels break down. Food out of season, shipped from across the globe, has far fewer nutrients. Also, native wild foods grow

in the soil and under the conditions most natural for them, so they are likely to be healthier plants. Healthier wild soils lead to healthier plants that are more nutritious to eat. They have built-in protections against native insects and have a much higher level of protective antioxidants and vitamins. I encourage my veteran patients to hunt, learn to forage for wild

WAHLS WARRIOR Q&A

Q: Why can't I eat eggs on the Wahls Diet? They are encouraged on the Paleo diet, and as long as they are organic and from free-ranging chickens, they seem like they would be a healthy addition.

A: The simple answer is that the Wahls Protocol does not include eggs because I have a severe egg allergy, and for our clinical trial I was specifically required to exactly replicate what I did to effect my own recovery. One of the things I did was to remove all allergenic foods from my diet, and this included eggs.

You may not be allergic to eggs, but many people are and don't realize it. For example, 60 percent of patients with inflammatory bowel diseases like Crohn's disease and ulcerative colitis have an abnormal aggressive immune response (IgG Ab) to eggs; 13 percent of people with seasonal allergies have a dysfunctional immune response to eggs; and the most common trigger for eosinophilic esophagitis (a chronic allergen-triggered inflammatory disease affecting the esophagus) is an allergic reaction from wheat, milk, or eggs.

The best way to know whether you can tolerate eggs is to remove them completely from your diet for a 100 days, then have a test meal. For example, have three or four eggs a day for two days, then see how you do. If you have an increase in any symptoms, you may be surprised to learn that you do react to the protein in eggs and you are better off leaving them out of your diet. If you have no increase in any negative symptoms over the next two weeks, then eggs may not be a problem for you, but I would strongly recommend choosing eggs from pastured chickens that eat grass and insects and forage for their own food outdoors, because these eggs will contain many good fats, vitamins, and protein.

foods, and add gardens and edible plants to their yards. The food obtained and the time spent being out in nature are both quite healing.

- **A willingness to work with you where you are.** No matter what your diet is like today, you can step into the Wahls Protocol at a level you can handle and progress from there, as you are ready. I am not going to give you a timeline. Your level of commitment and the speed at which you progress is completely up to you.
- **Important shifts beyond food.** The Wahls Protocol includes dietary guidance, but it also contains much more, including exercise recommendations, information about e-stim for muscle stimulation, discussions about physical, metabolic, and mental resilience, an emphasis on the critical element of stress reduction, and a host of other therapies to choose from (especially in Chapter 10).
- **No gluten, no dairy, no eggs, few if any legumes.** Some Paleo-style diet plans allow dairy (preferably raw organic), encourage egg consumption, and even permit some legumes. (Note that legumes and gluten-free grains are necessary if you are vegetarian.) I do not recommend these food items on the Wahls Diet. Gluten is completely out, but so are dairy and eggs. While legumes do contain some antinutrients, I'll show you how to reduce those antinutrients in the Wahls Paleo chapter if you need to eat legumes.

Now let's take a quick look at what differentiates each level of the diet.

Level One: The Wahls Diet

This is the most basic diet required in the Wahls Protocol. It involves just three primary elements:

1. Nine Cups of Fruits and Vegetables Every Day, Broken Down as Follows:

- Three cups tightly packed raw or cooked leafy greens, like kale, collards, chard, Asian greens, and lettuces (the darker, the better)
- Three cups deeply colored vegetables and fruits, such as berries, tomatoes, beets, carrots, and winter squash

- Three cups sulfur-rich vegetables, including broccoli, cabbage, asparagus, Brussels sprouts, turnips, radishes, onions, and garlic.

I recognize that 9 cups sounds like a lot, and there are two reasons for this. One, in order to get enough concentrated nutrition, you need to eat a lot of vegetables. Two, sufficient vegetable and fruit intake will fill you up so that you won't feel as much of a need to eat grains, sugar, and dairy. I want you to fill up mostly on vegetables, and this means learning to eat a lot of them. I also understand that for some people—especially those who don't often eat a lot of fruits and vegetables or who suffer from a delicate digestive system—such a leap in fiber consumption can be uncomfortable. In the next chapter, I'll give you more specific information about how to transition to eating 9 cups comfortably. You don't have to do it all at once.

2. Gluten-Free/Dairy-Free

The 9 cups puts nutrients into your body that you were missing, but this next step is about taking out what may be causing reactivity in your body, and that requires removing gluten and dairy from your diet. Unlike the first step, where it's okay to ease in, I recommend you go cold turkey on this one. Stop eating gluten and dairy *today*. It could be the most important thing you ever do for yourself.

WAHLS WARRIORS SPEAK

I eat fresh food and I eat in moderation, I enjoy fresh juices, and I stay away from wheat and soy. I meditate every morning and evening, and now I am able to listen to my body. I know not to push it to extremes. I feel like a normal person again, and my coworkers, friends, and family see the changes as well. This is the first year I have not had a relapse, and the only thing I changed was my eating and drinking habits. I am able to work six days a week again, and my energy level and mental state are clear and positive. In reality, overall I feel better than I did before I was diagnosed with MS!

—Ethel C., Little Rock, Arkansas

People with autoimmune disease are more likely to have a leaky gut, and if you have a leaky gut, gluten and dairy are particularly damaging. When the intestine has holes in it, incompletely digested wheat (gluten) and/or milk (casein) proteins can get into the bloodstream. These undigested particles are too large to be in the bloodstream. If you are genetically vulnerable to having your immune cells be activated by gluten and/or casein, this will cause even more issues. Twenty to 30 percent of those with European ancestry have the DQ2 or DQ8 genes, which put them at risk for developing gluten sensitivity.[15] (Five percent of those with abnormal immune responses to gluten do not have these genes, so other mechanisms do exist.) In these people, gluten and casein proteins in the bloodstream can trigger an inappropriate immune response. Both gluten and casein are metabolized into morphine-like compounds with an effect on immune, gut, and brain cells. For example, dairy products contain butyrophilin, a compound that is structurally similar to a compound in the myelin that surrounds nerve cells. Due to molecular mimicry, immune cells attempting to attack casein molecules that have leaked from the gut can also turn on myelin—a hallmark of multiple sclerosis. This can lead to a hyperreactive immune system that can then become supersensitive to other foods that weren't bothersome before, such as tree nuts, citrus, strawberries, or other vegetables and fruits.

How your body will react to a leaky gut is individual. You may not have the genetic predisposition to get into trouble or your responses may still be relatively mild. Others may have more dramatic reactions, including severe allergy or gastrointestinal symptoms that can eventually lead to more severe problems. If you have MS or another autoimmune disease, however, the likelihood that you will respond drastically to leaky gut is high.

WAHLS WARRIOR Q&A

Q: Is it okay to just reduce gluten and dairy, or to give up dairy but not gluten, or to give up gluten but not dairy? Or does it have to be complete?
A: It is very hard to give up the foods you love, especially comfort foods like gluten and dairy, but you need to do it 100 percent because even a

tiny amount of gluten or dairy could rev up the inappropriate immune response in your body if you have an unrecognized gluten or casein sensitivity. Do not assume you don't have a sensitivity. Gluten can be associated with an abnormal immune reaction in people with the DQ2 and DQ8 genes (although 5 percent of those with an abnormal immune response to gluten do not have these genes). Also, gluten and casein are both metabolized into morphine-like compounds with effects on immune cells as well as gut and brain cells.[16] Even if you don't notice any particular symptoms after eating gluten or dairy, your body may still be suffering from the effects of an intolerance, limping along under the daily assault of gluten and casein. Because of an amino acid sequence that is similar in both gluten and casein, most people who are sensitive to gluten are also sensitive to dairy, so I recommend giving them both up. You don't need gluten- and casein-containing foods in your diet in order to be healthy, and you have no idea how good you could be feeling without these foods.

For at least one month, take them out completely. You can tell yourself that if you turn out not to have a sensitivity, you can add them back in. Then have a test meal, testing one thing at a time. Try a test meal eating some dairy products, preferably fermented milk products like yogurt or goat's milk—these are the most likely to be tolerated. About 80 percent of people with gluten sensitivity will cross-react with dairy, but you might be in that 20 percent. If you have any negative response, cut out dairy for good. If you don't, you may be able to work it back into your diet. If, however, you can do only one thing right now, cut out gluten first. Because gluten products are the most likely to be associated with adverse reactions and so many people experience improvement when they eliminate gluten completely from their diets, I strongly urge going off gluten immediately and staying off it forever.

I ask you to give up these two things with the full awareness that this is extremely difficult. The reason gluten and dairy foods are considered "comfort foods" (think macaroni and cheese, cupcakes, and cheeseburgers) is because they actually have an opiate-like addictive effect in the body. (I'll talk more about this in chapters 6 and 8.) Giving them up can actually feel a bit like withdrawal. Once you get over the initial shock of removing gluten and dairy, however, you will start to feel better rapidly.

GLUTEN DETECTION

Because so many people are now recognizing that gluten causes adverse symptoms for them, several companies have come out with kits and devices that can detect gluten in food. This can make life easier, as you can test a food without having to rely on someone's assurance that something doesn't contain gluten. You can also check if you have gluten in your urine or stool. This can help you identify if you are still being exposed to gluten, which may explain why you may not have made as much progress as you have hoped. See the Resources section for links to some products that offer this service.

---

3. Organic, Grass-Fed, Wild-Caught

High-quality protein is the third crucial element on the Wahls Diet. While you can be a vegetarian or even a vegan at this first level—and I'll explain how in the next chapter—I don't recommend it. The next chapter also includes my detailed explanation of this controversial position. The highest quality protein sources for humans are organic, grass-fed meat, wild-caught meat (like game meat), and fish, and I strongly recommend that you eat them. Choose organic whenever you can, but don't go without high-quality protein.

Level Two: Wahls Paleo

Wahls Paleo is similar to the Wahls Diet, but it is slightly more restrictive and also more therapeutic. If you have severe autoimmune, neurological, psychological, or other chronic medical problems, I recommend moving quickly to Wahls Paleo quickly after adjusting to the Wahls Diet (highly motivated people may be able to start with Wahls Elimination or Wahls Paleo).

Wahls Paleo includes everything the Wahls Diet includes, with these added components:

1. Reduce all gluten-free grains (presumably you are completely gluten-free by now), legumes, and potatoes to just two servings per week.

It's preferable to eliminate grains and legumes entirely, but allowing two servings a week gives you more flexibility to be social with friends and family. That is what we have done in the second wave of our study. These servings are *not required* but they are allowed, should you feel the need. Even gluten-free whole grains, legumes like black beans and lentils, and potatoes contribute to increased carbohydrate load. You also get more lectins and phytates, which are antinutrients, in these foods. I encourage you to have more nonstarchy vegetables than gluten-free grains and to eat more vegetables than fruit. In addition, you can eat more meat as you further reduce the carbohydrates.

WAHLS WARRIOR Q&A

Q: The Wahls Protocol sounds great, but I'm not sure what my family will think of the food. Is it okay for them to go on the diet with me? What if they don't want to do this? Will I have to prepare separate meals for myself and the rest of the family?

A: It is extremely important to have family support when you embark upon the Wahls Protocol. I know from my observations that this must be a family decision. We tell our study subjects that we expect the family to eat only study-compliant food in the presence of the subject and to purge the house of foods that don't fit with the diet. Subjects whose families buy in and eat the same way as the study subjects are nearly always successful. Those whose families are not supportive and still eat the standard American diet are nearly always doomed to fail. For this reason, it's important to have a family conversation about food. What is everyone willing to do? What can everyone live with? This might take some negotiation, but fixing two different meals is not usually sustainable. We've had families go gluten-free while the study subject is on Wahls Paleo, but they may get gluten-containing foods when away from the study subject. That can work, but being surrounded by people eating the standard American diet while you are doing the Wahls, Wahls Paleo, or Wahls Paleo Plus Diets almost certainly will not. Fortunately, not only is the Wahls Diet healthful for any healthy adult, but it might even be preventive, staving off a future of chronic disease. It is also an excellent and beneficial diet for children, who tend (in our culture) to eat far too many processed carbohydrate and sugar-laden foods. Knowing that better health, more energy, and the loss of excess weight will likely accompany this dietary switch could help convince other family members to jump on board with you. And if you are the one doing the food shopping and cooking? You control what you buy. You can always decide not to subsidize health-compromising behavior by refusing to keep forbidden foods in your home. If family members want to eat those things outside the home, you may have less control over that, but if you can control your immediate environment, I suggest you do so. You decide what to pay for if you are eating at a restaurant. Don't fight with your kids about what they will order. If you have adolescent children, tell them that you will pay for foods that are compliant with the program. If they want to eat excluded foods, they will need to order and pay for them separately. (This is what I did, and my children, now adults, still agree that this is a reasonable approach for adolescent children.)

2. Add seaweed or algae and organ meats to your diet.

A lot of people balk at the notion of eating seaweed and organ meats. My patients who are suspicious of vegetables in the first place have a particularly hard time with seaweed and algae, and former vegetarians often have a really hard time with the concept of eating organ meats. Adding these two foods to your diet, however, is a potent healing step. Seaweed adds critical minerals, and organ meats add coenzyme Q10, both of which supply valuable nutrients for your mitochondria that can be difficult to get from more common foods. In chapter 6, I'll show you some palatable ways to try these foods.

3. Add fermented foods, soaked seeds and nuts, and more raw foods.

Enzyme-rich foods are an essential part of traditional diets, but much of our modern food is bereft of enzymes because of processing and cooking.[17] The best sources for enzymes are:

- Raw fruits and vegetables.
- Fermented foods like lacto-fermented sauerkraut, pickles, kimchi, and kombucha tea.
- Soaked and sprouted nuts and seeds. (Soak nuts and seeds in water for six to twenty-four hours before consuming; I'll tell you more about how to do this in chapter 6.)
- Raw animal protein such as sushi, steak tartare, and ceviche.

WAHLS WORDS

A ketogenic diet is extremely low in carbohydrate content (as low as 25 grams or even lower) and higher in fat to facilitate having the body burn fats instead of glucose. Functional medicine health care practitioners are using ketogenic diets to treat other progressive neurological conditions like Parkinson's disease and early memory loss.

Level Three: Wahls Paleo Plus

This is the most extreme and most intense level and the one I follow seasonally. I recommend it for my patients who aren't seeing enough progress with the Elimination version of Wahls Paleo level. This is an extremely low-carb, high-fat diet, similar to ketogenic diets already being used in a medical setting to treat epilepsy. It adds the following elements to the rules of the Wahls Diet and Wahls Paleo:

1. Eliminate all grains, legumes, and potatoes.

That includes nongluten grains like rice and quinoa. This may seem difficult, but once you get in the habit of not even considering grains on the menu, it won't seem so hard.

2. Consume at least 6 cups of vegetables, divided evenly between greens, color, and sulfur vegetables.

You won't be as hungry on Wahls Paleo Plus, so you won't be able to eat as much, so you are cutting back on your vegetable consumption somewhat but still eating enough to get dense nutrients. You still need those crucial micronutrients!

3. Eliminate cooked starchy vegetables and fruit other than berries.

Instead of cooked starchy vegetables, eat starchy vegetables raw, which makes those carbohydrates less digestible by you and more digestible for the beneficial bacteria in your microbiome. If they are deeply colored (such as yams, beets, and carrots), you can count them in your servings of color for the day. Also eliminate all fruit other than a maximum of one serving per day of berries. The amount of berries you can have depends on you—for some people, even a single serving of berries can be too much. How many carbohydrates you eat in order to achieve and stay in ketosis depends on your genetics and your microbiome. If you find you are not in ketosis, reduce or even eliminate berries as well.

4. Add coconut oil and full-fat coconut milk or olive oil depending on your lipids.

Wahls Paleo Plus is a high-fat diet, which, contrary to what you may have read about good health, is not automatically harmful to your heart. In fact, a high-fat diet coupled with a relatively lower carbohydrate intake will actually provide the most intensive nutritional support for your brain and your heart. This diet is even closer to how our ancestors ran their metabolisms for 2.5 million years. The fat in the diet is converted to ketones, which are excellent sources of energy for our mitochondria, brain cells, and muscle cells. This is why our species could survive and even thrive during the winters, which are typically a time of very limited carbohydrate intake, and during famine and war. You will however need to check your fasting lipids to confirm whether you will be stressing coconut fat or olive oil. If your lipids (cholesterol and trigylcerides) are too high, it is better to rely on olive oil and time-restricted feeding to achieve ketosis.

5. Eat just twice (or even once) per day and fast 14 or more hours every night.

You will not be as hungry on Wahls Paleo Plus, because eating protein and fat with relatively fewer carbohydrates will tend to suppress your appetite. During the long periods between breakfast and dinner, and between dinner and breakfast, your body can focus on processing and eliminating toxins, making hormones, and healing. If you find it uncomfortable to eat just twice a day, go ahead and keep having three meals when you really need them, but always be sure to wait 14 hours between dinner and breakfast. This significantly increases the vigor and the number of mitochondria in your cells. Your brain will love it!

Level Four: Wahls Elimination Diet

This variation of the diet can be incorporated into any of the other three levels. It is greatly reduced in lectins, which are compounds in plants that can cause inflammation and food reactivity for people who are sensitive to them. For these people, lectins can lead to damage to the gastrointestinal lining, causing leaky gut and increasing the risk of autoimmunity.

This diet is intended to be followed for 100 days minimum, but ideally for 6 months. It can take 6 months to eliminate the memory your immune cells have to react to lectins. This is a big ask, I know—this level is quite restrictive. However, if you are not seeing results on Wahls Paleo or Wahls Paleo Plus, lectins may be the reason. It's definitely worth giving the Wahls Elimination Diet a try. The Wahls Elimination Diet can also help you to pinpoint other specific foods that are causing a problem for you.

After the 100 days to 6 months, you will begin reintroducing food ingredients, one per week, starting with the things you miss the most. Take note of any symptom recurrence—it is a sign that you are sensitive to the food you introduced, and it should probably not be a part of your diet. It is very important not to have even one bite of any of the eliminated foods during the elimination period, as this can compromise the results of your reintroduction testing.

The Wahls Elimination Diet can teach you a lot about yourself and the foods that work for you. You will probably not need to stay on it permanently. Most people are able to successfully reintroduce most of the foods (other than gluten and dairy) after their inflammation has been significantly reduced. The people most likely to continue to be sensitive to nightshades and find that they do better continuing to exclude them (or always cooking them in a pressure cooker on high) are those with an autoimmune problem involving the joints (such as rheumatoid arthritis, systemic lupus erythematosus, or psoriatic arthritis) and those with inflammatory bowel disease.

Since this diet can work with any of the other diets, all the information about how to do it is here (it does not have its own chapter).

I specifically recommend the Wahls Elimination Diet for people who are most prone to problems with lectins, including people who:

- Have rheumatoid arthritis, or any autoimmune disease with the involvement of the joints. These people will especially benefit from the elimination of nightshade vegetables.
- Have inflammatory bowel disease (IBD). These people should also avoid all raw foods until their bowel movements are consistently formed (some may <u>never</u> tolerate many or any raw salads, vegetables, or fruits).
- Are still symptomatic even after being on Wahls Paleo (level 2) for a few weeks.
- Have severe symptoms, since this is the most aggressive way to reduce inflammation.

Note that I do not typically start most people out with the Wahls Elimination Diet, because 80 percent will experience marked improvement with the Wahls Diet or Wahls Paleo and will never need the Wahls Elimination Diet. Going from the standard American diet to the Wahls Diet (level 1) is challenge enough for many families, and the Wahls Elimination Diet is the most challenging to implement. However, I do offer it because it is the version with the highest response rate.

How to Do the Wahls Elimination Diet

You can do the Wahls Elimination Diet at any level of the Wahls Protocol. Keep the same rules as for the Wahls Diet, Wahls Paleo, or Wahls Paleo Plus, according to which one you have been doing, with the following additional restrictions:

Eliminate all nightshade vegetables: tomatoes, peppers, eggplant, and potatoes (sweet potatoes are okay) and spices made from nightshades (all pepper-based spices).

These vegetables are particularly high in lectins, and lectins are most concentrated in the seeds and skins of these vegetables.

Eliminate all nuts, seeds, and seed spices (any spice that is a seed, or a ground seed, such as cumin, caraway, coriander, mustard, black pepper, etc.).

Note that seed spices do have a very low dose of lectins, so you may choose to keep some of these in your diet—it really depends on how rigorous you want to be and how severe your symptoms are.

Eliminate any food you suspect you may be sensitive to, in addition to the above foods.

For example, you may have a sensitivity to oxalates, histamines, sulfites, or FODMAPs (see the following box), or you might just suspect a certain food bothers you, such as citrus fruits, lamb, or pistachios. The Wahls Elimination Diet is customizable to your sensitivities, no matter what they are. Then after the elimination period, you can reintroduce them according to the reintroduction instructions below, as you would the other foods listed above.

After 3 to 6 months on this diet, you may begin reintroducing foods you would like to have back in your life. Introduce one food ingredient per week, starting with the things you miss the most. This is the procedure:

1. Take your pulse for 60 seconds and write it down.
2. Take a mouthful of the food. Chew it thoroughly, then swallow it.
3. Immediately take your pulse again for 60 seconds. If it has increased by 10 points or more, that is an adverse reaction. Remove it for another 6 months before trying it again.
4. If your pulse did not jump 10 points or more, have up to ¼ cup more of the test food. Chew thoroughly, swallow, and check your pulse again. If it has increased by 10 points or more, that is an adverse reaction. Don't try that food for six more months.
5. If your pulse did not jump, you may have 1 cup of the food item. Repeat the process, taking your pulse after eating 1 cup of the item.
6. If your pulse did not jump, you can have this food two or three more times that day.

7. For the rest of the week, observe your symptoms. Do you have any recurrence? Do you have any symptoms involving your skin, gut, breathing, any other physical symptoms, or any mental health symptoms like anxiety, depression, or brain fog? Asks the people who live with you and know you best if they notice anything different that you might not have noticed. Any changes indicate an adverse reaction. Don't try that food again for six more months.

8. If all goes well, you can begin reintroducing the food. For example, you may test tomato sauce, and if it goes well, try organic heirloom tomato slices, to see if you can tolerate tomato skins and seeds in small amounts. If you pass that test, you know you can eat the food once a week and do well. If that goes well, you can gradually reintroduce the food two or three times a week, but always stay attuned for any symptom recurrence, which means you have overdone it and should back off again.

A few tips:

- If you want the best possible chance of tolerating a nightshade vegetable, remove the skin and seeds (for example, as in tomato paste or sauce) and cook them in a pressure cooker.
- If you want the best possible chance of tolerating legumes and gluten-free grains, soak them for 6 to 24 hours, rinse them, and cook them in a pressure cooker.
- You do not need to go into ketosis unless you are doing this Elimination Diet at the Wahls Paleo Plus level (see chapter 7). The Wahls Elimination Diet can be done at all three levels of the Wahls Protocol.
- If you are a vegetarian, you can still do the Wahls Elimination Diet and incorporate some gluten-free grains, legumes, nuts, and seeds, *only if* you do one of the two following things:
  - Soak them for at least 24 hours first, then rinse them well before using or drying them in a dehydrator or an oven set at a low heat (see page 211 for instructions).
  - Cook them in a pressure cooker (such as an Instant Pot type of device) using high pressure, which denatures all lectins except gluten and

casein. (I highly recommend all vegetarians use pressure cooking to cook their gluten-free grains and legumes.)

- If you are doing the Wahls Paleo Plus level of the Wahls Protocol, you may find that you don't need to go into ketosis while on this Wahls Elimination Diet because it is the most anti-inflammatory level of the diet. However, there are circumstances where ketosis may be helpful, if you are doing the Wahls Elimination Diet at the Paleo Plus level, such as having a seizure disorder in addition to an autoimmune condition, or having inflammatory bowel disease, rheumatoid arthritis, or lupus with significant neuropsychiatric symptoms.

OTHER ELIMINATION OPTIONS: OXALATES, HISTAMINES, SULFITES, AND FODMAPS

Lectins aren't the only compound that can be inflammatory for some people based on genetics and their microbiomes. Some people are allergic to citrus fruits, spinach, or carrots—there is research that suggest this is due to cross-reactivity between the proteins in these foods and certain mammalian proteins. If you have systemic lupus erythematosus and are still symptomatic while following the Wahls Elimination Diet, I suggest removing spinach and carrots as well for 100 days and assess your response.

Other food categories that can trigger reactions and inflammation in sensitive people include oxalates, histamines, sulfites, and FODMAPs. Your medical team may have already instructed you to avoid these foods, or you may suspect on your own that you are sensitive. Let's look at each of these:

Oxalates

Oxalates are naturally occurring compounds in foods that can bind to calcium so they can't be used by the body. This calcium oxalate can form crystals and accumulate in the kidneys. If you have a history of oxalate kidney stones, you may have been instructed to avoid oxalates. People with autism spectrum disorder may have high oxolate levels and may also do better on a low oxalate diet. If you have an overgrowth of *Candida albicans* yeast in the bowels, you are more likely to have a problem tolerating high oxalate foods. For a detailed list of foods that are high in oxalates such as spinach, beets, and rhubarb, see this list: pkdiet.com/pdf/LowOxalateDiet .pdf (page 154 has some more tips for better tolerating oxalates).

Histamines

There is increased awareness that for some people, eating foods that are high in histamines increases their symptoms of headache, fatigue, malaise, bloating, itching, and congestion. People with seasonal allergies, skin that flushes easily, an itchy throat or runny nose while eating, or a diagnosis of mast cell activation syndrome (MCAS) are particulary sensitive to high-histamine foods such as fermented foods, cured meat, soured foods, aged cheese, certain nuts, eggplant, and smoked fish, as well as foods that trigger the release of histamines, such as bananas and shellfish, and foods that block diamine oxidase (DAO), which helps to control histamines— examples include alcohol and green tea. We all have histamines to fight allergens, but in these people, the body overreacts, producing too many histamines. This is especially likely during allergy season, when histamine levels may already be higher than normal. If you suspect a histamine intolerance, try adding high-histamine foods, histamine-releasing foods, and DAO-blocking foods. Note that if you perceive that the fermented foods are giving you a problem, fiber may be your only strategy for supporting your microbiome until the histamine sensitivity quiets. Often after addressing all of the other lifestyle factors and following their Wahls Protocol diet for several months, people find that their histamine tolerance gradually improves and they can begin to add small amounts (a forkful) of fermented foods. If you believe that histamine has become a problem for you, look for a nutrition professional who can assist you with reducing your histamine intake and work with your primary care provider. An antihistamine may be beneficial in reducing symptoms after consuming a foodstuff that is high in histamine.

For a complete list of foods you could add to your elimination diet, see amymyersmd.com/2017/10/histamine-intolerance.

Sulfites

Sulfites are chemical preservatives that are found in certain foods such as wine, beer, dried fruit, potatoes, and shrimp. They are also in many medications. They can cause asthma-like symptoms. If you want to add sulfite-containing foods to your elimination list, look for anything that contains sulfur dioxide, potassium bisulfite, potassium metabisulfite, sodium bisulfite, sodium metabisulfite, or sodium sulfite. See myclevelandclinic.org/health/articles/11323-sulfite-sensitivity for more information.

FODMAPs

FODMAPs are fermentable oligo-, di-, and monosaccharides and polyols. These are all types of fermentable sugars in many plant foods, from wheat and rye to legumes and onions. They also occur in dairy products. Many people are sensitive to some of these FODMAPs but not all. Digestive distress is the main symptom. You can test different categories in your elimination diet to find out if you are sensitive. For a list of foods with the different types of FODMAPs, see thepaleoway.com/wp-content/uploads/2015/11/TPW_FODMAP-FoodsList.pdf

Although your conventional physician may not believe food sensitivity testing is helpful,[18] it may help you pinpoint troublesome foods. Although there is limited published research documenting the validity of the tests, a handful of studies showing diet modification based on food sensitivity testing using food-related IgG antibodies is helpful in reducing symptoms and improving quality of life for those with asthma, allergies, irritable bowel syndrome (IBS), depression, and obesity.[19] Many have also found them helpful in determining which foods to remove from the diet when adopting an elimination diet (for more information on food sensitivity testing, see the Resources at the back of this book).

Microbiome testing is another option—this can help you get more precise recommendations for the amount of dietary fat you should be eating, whether you are likely to be sensitive to gluten, or to provide other specific dietary recommendations. I predict that in the future, we will be able to assess and monitor our own DNA, microbes, microbial DNA, and metabolites, to identify if we can tolerate grains, dairy, saturated fat, and other foods. This will make us better equipped to create personalized eating plans best suited for optimal health. For more information about these tests, see page 349, as well as the Resources.

WHY TAKE YOUR PULSE?

The Pulse Test is an interesting strategy for understanding sensitivity/allergy to foods and inhaled proteins.[20] The Pulse Test was created by the allergist Dr. Arthur F. Coca and it is a way to determine whether the pulse and/or heart rate increase after exposure to a food item or anything else, such as a personal care product or something in the environment. While I use this in the Wahls Elimination Diet, it can also be used more comprehensively. This involves monitoring the pulse every two hours for three days to see what the low and high pulse rates are and recording everything that you eat or that comes into contact with your skin at the same time. Using the Pulse Test can be a bit tedious, but if you are willing to do the work of recording and to look for the patterns, it can be a very helpful tool.

Your Transition

If you are in my clinical trial, the rules are strict: You have to implement the study diets from day one. There is no easing into it. We do a two-week test to see whether participants can adopt the diet successfully. Those who are successful continue in the study for the next three years. It is a huge change in eating habits for most people, but they are highly motivated and are usually quite successful.

In my clinical practice, I am not so rigid. My practice style is to educate patients about the connection between diet and health and the four diets. I advocate for the diet that I think is most appropriate for them. I take into consideration their clinical issues and their desire to eat meat or not (the Wahls Diet, Wahls Paleo, Wahls Paleo Plus, and the Wahls Elimination

WAHLS WARRIORS SPEAK

I do not have MS, but my son does, so I follow the Wahls Protocol, too. In the beginning, I did so as a show of support for my son. I soon found, however, that my overall health was in much better shape. My body tells me very quickly if I stray back to my old eating habits. Now, at age 68, I am 116 pounds and I have a nice flat tummy, energy to burn, and blood tests and blood pressure readings that are all normal. I've never looked or felt better! This diet is good for everyone to follow as a way of life. Stop eating processed crap! You do not want to outlive your health!

—Liz B., Halifax, Nova Scotia, Canada

Diet); then I give them options and subsequently ask them what they have learned and what their goals are. I do find that most of my patients are able to make the drastic change all at once because they are highly motivated and their families are fully supportive. Most of us, myself included, come to the diet that is most therapeutic for us gradually, step by step. Some choose to simply ramp up the vegetables, some choose to also go gluten- and dairy-free, and others choose to go all the way to Wahls Paleo Plus or Wahls Elimination to get control of their bodies and the disease process as quickly as possible. Don't be too hard on yourself and your family if it takes a few months to fully implement the Wahls Diet, Wahls Paleo, Wahls Paleo Plus, or Wahls Elimination. But do begin. Then if you still aren't achieving the health outcomes that you are looking for, advance to the next level, or try the Wahls Elimination Diet for at least 100 days at 100 percent compliance, to get to the bottom of why you are not improving.

Anyone can benefit from the Wahls Diet, Wahls Paleo, Wahls Paleo Plus, or the Wahls Elimination Diet, but if you have MS or another autoimmune disease, the benefits will likely be dramatic. You will lose excess weight and gain energy and vitality. Take the steps one at a time, but if you have an autoimmune disease or any type of brain disease or chronic medical problem, the most important thing you can do is to adopt at least the Wahls Diet immediately: Eat the 9 cups (or proportionately what you can)

WEIGHT LOSS AND
THE WAHLS PROTOCOL

I did not design the Wahls Protocol for weight loss, but weight loss has been a side effect for a vast number of those I have monitored who were carrying excess weight and did the diet at any of the four levels. There is already a lot of research showing that a diet lower in refined carbohydrates and sugar and higher in fat is conducive to weight loss, but I believe that the Wahls Protocol is also effective for weight loss because it provides the body with all the nutrition it may have been missing. A properly working, fully functioning body will typically calibrate itself back to a healthful weight. If your primary goal in following the Wahls Protocol is to lose weight, I predict you will be successful and improve your health, too. Who knows— you may even ward off a chronic disease you might have developed in the future because you are taking better care of yourself in the present.

---

and go gluten- and dairy-free *today*. Progress from there according to the steps laid out in the next five chapters. Your journey has officially begun.

Which Way Is Right for You?

You may be convinced that the Wahls Way is your way, but what level should you try? For my clinical trials, participants must follow specific parameters, strictly adhering to the study diet; but in my clinics, patients have a choice. Do they want to try the Wahls Diet, or jump right into Wahls Paleo? Or go to Wahls Elimination? Or do I think they could benefit from trying Wahls Paleo Plus?

I educate my patients about exactly what we know and what we don't know about these various levels of diet, and whether I think the Wahls Elimination Diet may be the most optimal. I tell them why I am recommending the specific diet I suggest for them. We also talk about financial concerns. Remember, I took care of patients in the VA system, and many of them had limited financial means. We routinely talked about how to make things work with their financial resources. That meant some people were using pressure cookers and eating more gluten-free and legume-based proteins, to make it more affordable. Then I let them decide which diet plan will work for them. I make recommendations, but in the end it is their choice, just as it is yours.

In general, however, I do tailor my recommendation to people's specific health issues and what they and their families are open to doing. The more ill people are, the more strongly I encourage them to start with Wahls Paleo or Wahls Elinination, and as they adopt the diet and adjust to the changes, I encourage self-reflection. Are they satisfied with their health, or could they improve more? We talk about what dietary changes they'd like to tackle next. Once they have been successful in fully adopting Wahls Paleo, if they still are not as well as they want to be, then I may discuss Wahls Elimination. If people are still having symptoms on Wahls Elimination, then we talk about the Wahls Paleo Plus version of Wahls Elimination. Some of these symptoms might include:

1. Persistent brain fog
2. Neurobehavioral symptoms that persist following a traumatic brain injury
3. Neurological problems and neurodegenerative diseases (such as chronic headaches, seizures, movement disorders, Parkinson's, cognitive impairment, and Alzheimer's)
5. Psychiatric diseases that have not shown satisfactory improvement on Wahls Paleo or Wahls Elimination
6. A strong family history (or personal history) of cancer
7. Fatigue that persists
8. Autoimmune brain-related problems that are not showing improvement
9. Obesity, particularly if not losing weight on Wahls Paleo

Wherever you decide to start, you can always shift your plan if you aren't getting results. If the change to this way of eating will be a big one, you might start with the Wahls Diet. If you want results fast, you might start with Wahls Paleo. If you aren't getting results from Wahls Paleo, you may want to try the Wahls Elimination Diet or Wahls Paleo Plus. Start where it feels right to you, and do what you think you can achieve. Ask for support. And don't fear change! You are reclaiming your health.

Chapter 5

MASTERING THE WAHLS DIET

I F YOU ARE ready to change your life, improve your health, feed your cells, strengthen your mitochondria, and begin the process of reversing chronic disease in your body, begin here. The Wahls Diet is a beginning. Once you've mastered it, you may decide to move on to the next level, Wahls Paleo, or the final level, Wahls Paleo Plus, or you may want to try Wahls Elimination, but first you need to understand how to fully implement the components of this most basic dietary adjustment.

The Wahls Diet involves two primary components, and a third optional but strongly recommended component:

1. Adding certain foods to your diet
2. Taking certain foods out of your diet
3. Improving the quality of the food you eat

You will be amazed at the difference in how you feel by doing these three simple things. If you have an autoimmune disease, I recommend you begin the Wahls Diet *today*, to minimize any further damage, but even if you don't have an autoimmune disease, you can start to feel better almost immediately by instituting these changes.

WAHLS DIET

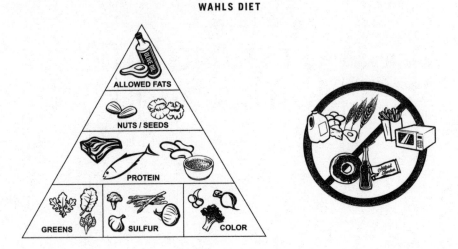

Before we get into the specifics of the Wahls Diet, let me assure you that I do not recommend these changes lightly. There are very good reasons for what I will be asking you to do. One of the most critical, in terms of intervening into your health issues, is that you will be significantly increasing the nutrients in your diet.

To show you what a difference you will be making by changing your diet according to the guidelines in the Wahls Diet, I have added charts at the beginning of each diet program chapter. These charts will show you how the three levels of the Wahls Diet stack up against the standard American diet in terms of nutrient density (based on a 1,759-calorie diet, which is the average caloric intake for my personal age and gender). The recommended daily allowance (RDA) is the amount of a specific nutrient that should meet the needs of 97 percent of the population. These values are set for every major nutrient by the Food and Nutrition Board of the National Academies of Sciences, Engineering, and Medicine and reviewed every few years. We compared the mean intake of the nutrients identified by medical literature as being key to optimal brain health to the reported average recorded intake of a woman my age.

Because there are established nutrient guidelines, dietitians and nutrition experts are often reluctant to cut out major food groups like gluten-containing grains, dairy products, and eggs, since these foods are sources of many vitamins and minerals. For example, the average woman gets most of her

B vitamins through the consumption of flours that have had synthetic B vitamins such as folate, riboflavin, thiamine, niacin, and iron added to them.

But I maintain that food, rather than synthetic supplements sprayed onto processed food, should and can provide all the essential nutrients you need for optimal health. The Wahls Diet goes beyond "adequate" levels of nutrients. It provides 1.5 to 8 times more vitamins, antioxidants, and minerals than the standard American diet does, even without enriched flour. The Wahls Diet is packed with what your cells need to thrive, without relying on synthetic added vitamins.

Wahls Diet		
Nutrient*†	*U.S. Diet (%)*	*Wahls Diet (%)*
Vitamin D	31	75
Vitamin E	55	143
Calcium	74	126
Magnesium	88	174
Vitamin A	100	340
Pyridoxine	121	626
Folate	122	207
Zinc	123	178
Thiamine	128	741
Vitamin C	133	514
Niacin	154	452
Iron	164	235
Riboflavin	175	827
Vitamin B$_{12}$	201	704

* *Compared to dietary reference intakes. Recommended dietary allowances (RDA) for females 51–70 years; Wahls Diet adjusted for 1,759 calories (National Academies of Science, Engineering, and Medicine, Institute of Medicine; Food and Nutrition Board)*

† *Average nutrient intake from food for females 50–59 years (What We Eat in America, NHANES 2009–2010, ars.usda.gov/SP2UserFiles/Place/12355000/pdf/0910/Table_1_NIN_GEN_09.pdf, accessed May 25, 2013)*

CALL TO ACTION

Many of my followers put a one-page summary of the diet on their refrigerator. You can pick up a colorful version of the Wahls Diet chart at terrywahls.com/bonus.

Part One: The 9 Cups

Let's begin with what you will be adding to your diet. The cornerstone of the Wahls Diet is the addition of 9 cups of vegetables and colorful fruits every day. Nine cups! It sounds like a lot, and for some people it's a daunting amount. If you are up for it, I would suggest adding in the 9 cups right away. It's the first thing you can do to start infusing your body with intense nutrition, and it will make a profound difference in how you feel. But not everyone is up to such a drastic change all at once. Although people in my study have to start in one fell swoop, people in my clinics more often work up to this amount over a seven-day period.

Use whichever approach seems most reasonable for you and your family. If you aren't eating much fresh produce at all right now, you could start with 3 cups per day, then gradually but persistently work your way up to 9. There is no need to stuff yourself, however. If you are too full to eat 9 cups, just remove

WAHLS DIARY ALERT

As you begin the Wahls Diet, it is important for you to begin writing down what you are eating and how you are feeling. You will begin the journey of learning what your body is telling you about your environment by tracking this information every day. The food you eat, the water you drink, the air you breathe, and what you are putting on your skin can all affect how you feel and how healthy your cells are. You will begin to notice how you respond to that environment. If you have symptoms, you will be able to look at your Wahls Diary to see what you have eaten that you might be reacting to. You will also begin to take responsibility for learning how to eat and live for maximal health and vitality. (Remember that the majority of people who are sensitive to a food will have some problem within seventy-two hours, although in a few cases it can take as long as two weeks for symptoms to show. Always look back at the last three days when you have a problem to see what the potential triggers may have been.)

the sugar, gluten, dairy, and eggs, and eat the vegetables proportionately in the three groups I describe next. This can help set you on the right track and keep you from quitting the diet because you think you can't do it or it's too much. Small steps are better than quitting because small steps will lead to better health, and quitting will do nothing to help you.

I don't want you to eat 9 cups of apples and iceberg lettuce, however. The

WAHLS WARRIOR Q&A

Q: I'm not crazy about vegetables. Can't I just take supplements to get all those vitamins and minerals?

A: People often ask me if they can just take supplements instead of eating all these vegetables. The answer, in a word, is no! By eating 9 cups of vegetables and fruits every day, you will be effectively dosing yourself with vitamins, minerals, and phytochemicals (plant-based micronutrients) that your body has likely been missing, in the most natural way your body can receive these compounds. The vitamins and antioxidants that naturally occur in food are more effective at supporting your cells when the whole family of related compounds is present. Vegetables and colorful fruits each have hundreds of related compounds in them, acting synergistically in the body to support the cell functions, and the vitamins and antioxidants are a far more effective support for your cells when they are taken with the hundreds of other antioxidants and phytonutrients in the whole plant. No supplement could ever fully imitate what's in that natural package.

Also, the vitamins, amino acids, and antioxidant supplements you take in pill form are typically synthetic. The synthetic forms of vitamins and other compounds do not have the same shape as the naturally occurring compounds, and they are not accompanied by all of the related compounds existing in whole food that contribute to the body's ability to use them. As a result, synthetic vitamins do not have the same properties and are not as effective at supporting our cells. For much more information about supplements, see chapter 10.

9 cups are organized in a specific way, for maximum nutrition per calorie (which the registered dieticians and nutritionists call nutrient density). You must divide your vegetables into three equal parts:

1. Three cups of leafy greens
2. Three cups of deeply colored vegetables and fruits
3. Three cups of sulfur-rich vegetables

The 9 cups are incredibly important for success on the Wahls Diet. In fact, it may just be the most important piece of the protocol overall.

ANCIENT NUTRITION

Our ancestors have been consuming phytonutrient-rich plants for millions of years. Although science is only beginning to discover what various phytonutrients can do for us, there are thousands of articles that support the health benefits of phytonutrients for everything from antibiotic and antioxidant properties to properties that do things like keep the blood vessels more elastic, facilitate toxin removal in the body, regulate various aspects of immune system function, and improve brain function.

This is the primary way to provide your cells with everything they need to work at maximum efficiency, for the benefit of your health.

Let's look more closely at how to divide up the 9 cups, and what you are getting when you let yourself indulge in this cornucopia of produce.

1. Three Cups of Leafy Greens

Leafy greens are nutritionally dense phytochemical factories. They are an excellent source of vitamins in the B group, especially folate (also called vitamin B_9), as well as vitamins A, C, and K. Think Green-BACK for vitamins B, A, C, and K. These four nutrient groups are incredibly important for anyone suffering from MS, as well as any other autoimmune or other chronic diseases:

- **B vitamins.** Your body needs many of the B vitamins for healthy nervous system functioning. For example, you need folate (vitamin B$_9$) to make myelin, the fatty insulation around your nerves that is attacked and degraded when you have multiple sclerosis. Anything to shore up your myelin production is a good thing!

- **A vitamin precursors (carotenoids).** Greens are also rich in alpha- and beta-carotene, precursors for vitamin A, which you need for (among other things) healthy retinas, the sensory membranes lining the inner surface of the back of the eyeball, which are stimulated by light. Many people with MS suffer from macular degeneration and other diseases involving the retina. Having more greens in the diet will improve the health of the retina and the optic nerves, lowering the risk of visual impairment. Vitamin A is also important for immune cell function. (Don't be confused about autoimmunity: Your immune system may be overactive, but vitamin A won't increase harmful immune activity. Instead, it will help your body to recalibrate its immunity back to a normal, healthy state.) Vitamin A also helps improve the strength of your bones and the flexibility and elasticity of your skin, helping you "youthen" as you adopt the Wahls Diet.

- **Vitamin C.** Vitamin C is crucial for healthy immune cell function as well as healthy skin and gum tissue. Vitamin C is also a potent antioxidant that helps lower the risk of developing cancer. Although cancer may be the last worry on your list of health concerns right now, know that antioxidants work in your body to keep cell function normal, and that's important for anyone with any type of chronic disease.

- **Vitamin K.** The vitamin K in greens is converted by health-promoting bacteria in the intestine to other, more potent forms of vitamin K that can work to reduce your risk of high blood pressure and calcification (hardening) of the blood vessels and heart valves. Even more exciting, vitamin K has been linked to the prevention of the onset of MS in experimental autoimmune encephalomyelitis in mice, an animal model of MS.[1] Scientists are increasingly aware that vitamin K is very important in mineralization of teeth and bones as well as for brain health, including in the production of myelin.[2] Vitamin K should be high on your list of important nutrients if you have MS or any other autoimmune condition or brain-related problem.

- **Magnesium and calcium.** Because the Wahls Diet plans eliminate dairy, it may not contain enough of these minerals. Eating more greens ensures a good supply of magnesium and a moderate supply of calcium. The magnesium in particular can help reduce muscle spasms and excess excitation in the brain.

But green leaves are also so much more than "green-BACK." When you eat a big plate of kale salad, you get thousands of compounds that wouldn't be present in supplements for folate, vitamin A, vitamin C, and vitamin K. Scientists can't even name them all yet. All these substances work together in the body to give your cells what they need, but for those with MS, the potential benefits for preventing MS and/or replenishing myelin cannot be ignored. Eat your greens: 3 cups cooked per day. (Or go by the rule that 2 cups raw equals 1 cup cooked, and measure them according to what they would be cooked—you could potentially eat 6 cups of raw leafy greens every day.)

Some great choices (the * indicates high in calcium):

- Arugula*
- Beet greens
- Bok choy* and other Asian greens
- Chard, all colors
- Collard greens*
- Dandelion greens*
- Kale, all types (curly; lacinato or dinosaur; red; etc.)*
- Lettuce, all types of deep green, bright green, or red leaf lettuce (no iceberg)
- Mustard greens*
- Parsley
- Spinach*

Note: Food lists in this chapter are not necessarily complete. They are here to give you examples of types of vegetables and fruits. Find a more comprehensive food list at the back of this book if you have questions about any foods that aren't listed in this chapter.

GOOD GREENS

Greens are rich sources of powerhouse phytochemicals. Known benefits of these nutrients include:

- Anti-cancer properties
- Anti-inflammatory properties
- Better brain health
- Cell protection
- Stronger, more elastic skin
- More balanced hormones
- Heart health
- Improved liver function

Adapted with permission from Phytonutrient Spectrum Comprehensive Guide, Institute of Functional Medicine, 2015.

2. Three Cups of Colors

The next 3 cups in your 9 cups should consist of brightly colored vegetables and fruits. Choose those that are colored all the way through, like carrots and beets, rather than brightly colored only on the skin, like red apples. In fact, fruits that are white on the inside, like apples, pears, and bananas, do not count toward your 9 cups. You can still eat them on the Wahls Diet, but not until you've had your 9 cups of approved vegetables and fruits. Save that apple or banana for a treat!

The big benefit of deeply colored produce is that the color is a sign of antioxidants. When the vegetable or fruit is colored all the way through, the concentration of the health-promoting antioxidants is the highest. Free radicals cause internal damage, but antioxidants nullify those free radicals before they can cause too much trouble.

So eat your colors! Fortunately, deeply colored vegetables and fruits are some of the best-tasting of all. Aim for eating at least three different colors daily. Some great choices include:

ANTIOXIDANT POWER

Antioxidants will help protect you against more than autoimmune disease. There are hundreds of studies showing that diets rich in the antioxidants found in brightly colored vegetables and fruits are protective against cardiovascular disease, cancer, and dementia.[3] For example, studies of the consumption of beetroot juice demonstrated an association with more nitric oxide production and healthier endothelial cells (the cells that line blood vessels, directly impacting blood vessel function). You want the linings of your blood vessels to be elastic, resilient, and impenetrable to troublemakers like artery-hardening debris. Antioxidants do this job, and they do it well, especially if you eat a lot of them in the form of natural food. In the beetroot juice study, participants had lower blood pressure and less sticky blood cells, which naturally improves blood pressure and reduces the risk of clogging of both arteries and veins.[4]

Green

(Although they are white inside, cucumbers and zucchini are permitted here if you eat the skins because they are low-starch vegetables and the skins are packed with antioxidants.)

- Artichokes
- Avocados
- Bean sprouts
- Beans, green
- Bok choy
- Broccoli
- Brussels sprouts
- Cabbage, green
- Celery
- Cucumbers with skin
- Grapes, green
- Green peas
- Kiwi, green
- Leafy greens
- Lettuce
- Limes
- Melons, honeydew
- Okra
- Olives, green
- Peppers, green
- Snow peas
- Watercress
- Zucchini with skin

Red

- Beets
- Blood oranges
- Cabbage, red
- Cherries
- Cranberries (fresh or frozen without sugar)
- Grapefruit, pink or red
- Grapes, red
- Onions, red
- Peppers, red
- Plums, red
- Pomegranates
- Radicchio
- Radishes
- Raspberries, red
- Rhubarb
- Rooibos tea
- Strawberries
- Tomatoes
- Watermelons

Blue/Purple/Black

- Aronia berries (grown throughout North America and Europe)
- Black currants
- Black mulberries
- Blackberries
- Blueberries
- Boysenberries
- Dates
- Eggplants
- Elderberries
- Figs, purple
- Grapes, black or purple
- Huckleberries
- Kale, purple
- Marionberries
- Olives, black
- Plums, black
- Prunes
- Purple heirloom carrots
- Purple yams or potatoes (remember these are starchy—and these must be pigmented all the way through in order to count in this category)
- Raisins
- Raspberries, black

Yellow/Orange

- Apricots
- Cantaloupe
- Carrots
- Ginger root
- Grapefruit, yellow
- Kiwi, golden
- Lemon
- Mangoes
- Muskmelons
- Nectarines
- Oranges
- Papayas

- Peaches
- Peppers, orange and yellow
- Persimmons
- Pineapples
- Pumpkins

- Squash, summer and winter
- Starfruit
- Sweet potatoes and yams
- Tangerines
- Turmeric root

INCREDIBLE COLOR

Different colors of vegetables and fruits indicate different properties and different combinations of phytochemicals. Here's a breakdown of just some of the benefits you're getting when you eat brightly colored vegetables:

- Anti-inflammatory properties
- Anticancer properties
- Stronger, more elastic blood vessels
- Better cognition
- Healthier brain cells
- Healthier cells
- Improved prostate health
- DNA protection
- Antibacterial properties
- Immune system health
- Skin health
- Reproductive health
- Eye health

Adapted with permission from Phytonutrient Spectrum Comprehensive Guide, Institute for Functional Medicine, 2015.

3. Three Cups of Sulfur-Rich Vegetables

Finally, I want you to eat 3 cups of sulfur-rich vegetables, which, in addition to antioxidants, also have health-promoting sulfur compounds in them. Sulfur may not get the media attention that antioxidants do, but it is an incredibly important compound for health. Sulfur-rich foods nourish cells and mitochondria, and specifically help the body to be more efficient in eliminating toxins. Sulfur is also important for synthesizing protein and for producing collagen, which makes up all your connective tissues. If you have joint issues, you need sulfur! It also helps give you strong, beautiful skin, hair, and nails. Diets containing sulfur have been associated with improvement in skin disorders and arthritis. Many arthritis sufferers take a supplement called MSM (methylsulfonylmethane) to help with joint pain, but I like to get my sulfur on my dinner plate, so it comes in its natural and complete package.

There are literally thousands of studies showing the health benefits of the compounds in the sulfur-rich family. One of the most relevant pathways for research in sulfur-rich vegetables involves their contribution to blood vessel

WAHLS WARRIORS SPEAK

I have highly active remitting multiple sclerosis with mobility impairment. Other than mild depression, I have no other symptoms. I was initially admitted to hospital with a suspected stroke with only four-fifths power in my right leg, but after three months of further tests, lesions were found in my brain and I was diagnosed with multiple sclerosis. I've been trying to follow the Wahls Diet to the letter for ten weeks. Before going on the diet, I had begun to deteriorate rapidly and my friends were noticing the decline. Almost within days, I began to feel better and now my thinking is clearer, I have less spasticity, my sleeping is better, and I feel much more positive about life and its possibilities. My friends remark how they can see a marked improvement in my well-being. I am enjoying food so much more because I can now taste the real flavors and I am better overall: I have lost weight, my hair feels healthier, I do not have dry scalp anymore, I have better libido, and I wake up refreshed every morning. I am grateful for many things in my life, and now I add Dr. Wahls to my list because she had the courage not to give up when faced with multiple sclerosis. Because of her, I now feel better equipped to deal with my own adversity.

—*Richard J., London, England*

health. This should matter a great deal to anyone with multiple sclerosis as well as those with other autoimmune problems. In addition, people with systemic lupus and rheumatoid arthritis have a higher rate of atherosclerosis than the general population, leading to narrowing of the blood vessels.[5] Sulfur-rich vegetables are crucial for them as well. Eat to keep the endothelial cells that line the blood vessels in a state of optimal health to reduce the risk of atherosclerosis.

Good sources of sulfur include the cabbage family, the onion family, and the mushroom family. All three have a long history as important medicinal foods in the Asian cultures. Let's look at these valuable vegetables more closely.

The Cabbage Family

The cruciferous, or brassica, family is also called the cabbage family and includes kale, collards, broccoli, cauliflower, Brussels sprouts, turnips, rutabaga, and radishes. The brassica family of vegetables are rich in many organic sulfur

VARIETY IS THE SPICE OF HEALTH

It is very important to rotate the vegetables you eat for more variety. All vegetables and most fruits have some toxins in them as part of their protection against the animals that would eat them (that includes you and me). In fact, these very chemicals stimulate our cellular machinery to operate at increasing efficiency. If you eat the same plants every day, the toxins can build up and have a negative health impact; but if you rotate your foods, you get all the benefits without the risk. For example, I eat greens in rotation: kale one day, lettuce the next, then spinach, and then beet greens or chard. The wider, more diverse the foodstuffs you eat, the more health-promoting benefits and the fewer negative benefits you will experience. Our ancestors would have eaten two hundred or more different plant and animal species each year. Think about it. How many different species are you eating? Kale, as much as I love it, should not be eaten day after day. Mix it up and you will be healthier.

compounds, including diindolylmethane (DIM), indole-3-carbinol (I3C), and sulforaphane that, in many animal studies, has been shown to be beneficial in supporting detoxification processes, reducing oxidative stress, and protecting brain cells by inducing the production of glutathione, a potent intracellular antixodant.[6] Cabbage family veggies are greatly valued across many cultures and are some of the most potently nutritious of all the vegetables. They are an important key to detoxification, which is critical for people with chronic disease. (I will talk more about these vegetables in the detoxification chapter.) These compounds are also potent antioxidants, which are linked to a reduction in the risk of heart disease and cancer.[7]

The Onion Family

This family includes all types of onions as well as garlic, chives, leeks, and shallots. Members of the garlic and onion family are rich in allicin sulfides (when the garlic or onion is crushed, these compounds transform into diallyl sulfides), which also have a long history of medicinal use across many cultures because of their antibacterial properties and blood- and blood-vessel-health-promoting properties. Regular consumption of these vegetables is also associated with a reduced risk for heart disease, cancer, and dementia.[8]

There are many studies showing that using aged garlic extract is associated with healthier blood vessels, less atherosclerosis, less clogging of the vessels, and greater fluidity of the blood.[9] While one could take aged garlic extract or L-arginine (the active compound in the extract), I prefer to see people rely on whole foods over extracts as a more comprehensive therapy. The extracts require processing and purification and likely lose useful elements during that process. The best and safest approach, in my view, is to eat more garlic, onions, and sulfur-rich vegetables.

The Mushroom Family

The last category of sulfur-rich vegetables consists of mushrooms, which are not only rich in sulfur but also in B vitamins. Mushrooms in particular have been used medicinally in Asia for thousands of years. We know they contain beta-d-glucan and fucogalactans, components of the cell walls of mushrooms,

STOP THE WASTE!

Buying fresh fruits and vegetables can be expensive, especially if you throw away nutritious parts or don't eat them before they spoil. Stop wasting your money and medicinal food with these strategies:

- When vegetables begin to look a bit stale, chop them and put them in a slow cooker with water or broth. Cook on low all day to make vegetable soup.
- Don't throw away the leaves on radishes, beets, or turnips. These can be used in smoothies or cooked and enjoyed. They are highly nutritious and count toward your daily quota of greens. The leaves on cauliflower, broccoli, and kohlrabi are also edible. Use them in smoothies and soups, and eat them steamed.
- Two easy ways to use greens: (1) Put them in a blender with fruit (green grapes, oranges, or other fruits) or coconut or nut milk and ice and blend on high to make a green smoothie. (2) Sauté onions and mushrooms in coconut oil, add chopped greens, and stir until wilted (just a minute or two). If the greens seem bitter, add more fat or a source of acid such as citrus or apple cider or balsamic vinegar.

and that these compounds stimulate the natural killer cells that help balance the immune system and are protective against cancer[10] and autoimmune disease.[11] There are many types of mushrooms, from common white "button" mushrooms and portabellos to more exotic types like shiitake, maitake, oyster, wood ear, and more. Each have their own specific therapeutic properties. Mushrooms are an excellent and delicious addition to the diet, but with one caveat: Rarely, some individuals with autoimmune disorders are sensitive to mushrooms. I'll talk more about this in chapter 6 when I discuss fermented foods, but if you perceive that you have more headaches, fatigue, or worsening of any brain symptoms after consuming mushrooms, I suggest removing them from your diet, at least temporarily. You may be able to introduce mushrooms back into your diet after six months on the Wahls Diet to see if you tolerate occasional use, but don't have them more than once a week. Fortunately,

SUPERIOR SULFUR-RICH

Known health benefits of sulfur-rich foods include:

- Anticancer properties
- Antimicrobial action
- Blood vessel health
- Cell health
- Detoxification
- Gut health
- Heart health
- Hormone balance
- Immune cell action support
- Liver health

Adapted with permission from Phytonutrient Spectrum Comprehensive Guide, Institute of Functional Medicine, 2015.

you've got plenty of other sulfur-rich foods to choose from, so have 3 cups' worth each day.

Here are some choices of sulfur-rich vegetables. You will note some crossover with other lists: some foods—like kale, which is a sulfur vegetable and a leafy green—fall into multiple categories. Include these in one or the other group as you assemble your 9 cups—your choice:

- Asparagus
- Bok choy
- Broccoli
- Brussels sprouts
- Cabbage
- Cauliflower
- Chives
- Collard greens
- Daikon
- Garlic, all types
- Kale
- Leeks
- Mushrooms, all types
- Onions: red, yellow, and white
- Radishes
- Rutabagas
- Scallions
- Shallots
- Turnips and turnip greens

WAHLS WARRIOR Q&A

Q: I can't eat FODMAP foods without digestive trouble. Can I still do the Wahls Diet?

A: FODMAPs (fermentable oligosaccharides, disaccharides, monosaccharides, and polyols) are short-chain carbohydrates such as fructose and lactose. Examples of FODMAP foods are wheat, rye, legumes, onions, garlic, mushrooms, avocados, stone fruits, and apples. These compounds are not generally absorbed in the small bowel but instead are further digested by bacteria in the colon through fermentation and then absorbed. In many people this will cause irritable-bowel-like symptoms (such as bloating, diarrhea, constipation, and belching). In my clinical observation, the irritable bowel problems of my patients and followers are nearly always resolved by reducing carbohydrates, eliminating gluten, and reducing or eliminating even gluten-free grain products as well. For many, adopting the Wahls Paleo Diet (see chapter 6) resolves the trouble. If for some reason you still have trouble, I would advocate reducing carbohydrates further by adopting Wahls Paleo Plus (see chapter 7). The micronutrients from organ meats and natural high-quality fats at that level tend to be well tolerated by people with irritable bowel issues. You may also find that the low lectin version of the diet, Wahls Elimination, is very helpful at reducing symptoms.

Making the Most of Your 9 Cups

It's not easy to just start eating 9 cups of vegetables and fruit every day. Where and how often should you buy them? How do you store them to keep them fresh? How should you prepare them for meals and snacks? What if all those vegetables give you a stomachache? Let's talk about these questions.

Where and How Often to Buy

Because the vitamin and antioxidant content in fresh vegetables and fruits degrades over time, the first thing to think about is buying your food locally when possible (getting your vegetables locally minimizes the time between harvest and consumption and maximizes the vitamin and mineral content of your food), and always choosing the freshest options. Farmers markets and farm stands are excellent sources for your 9 cups when it's the right season for these things. Buy vegetables and fruits at least once a week. If you are able, several times a week or even daily when convenient is even better. There is nothing nicer than eating a big plate of vegetables that were picked that day, or the day before, and not transported across the country or globe.

Even better, you can grow many of your own vegetables in your backyard if you have the available space. Ideally, you could walk to your deck or out to your yard to pick your food for supper. There is no fresher way to eat, and I believe that growing more of your own food is an important strategy for re-claiming your (and your family's) health and vitality.

Of course, becoming a backyard gardener takes some work, but perhaps less than you think. Many of your 9 cups can easily be grown in container gardens hanging from or sitting on your deck. This includes greens like spin-ach, kale, collards, chard, and lettuce, as well as other vegetables like onions, garlic, chives, tomatoes, and strawberries. You can also begin to add vegeta-bles and fruits into your existing landscape in low-maintenance ways. Berry bushes, for example, require very little care after planting.

Some people worry about the physical strain of gardening, but raised beds can put your vegetables at waist level. You won't even have to bend over to weed them. Raised beds also allow you to improve your soil quality, because you can fill up the beds with higher-quality soil and enrich it with compost and natural fertilizer. Your family might also enjoy lending a hand. Gardening is extremely rewarding and a good stress reliever—another important part of the Wahls Protocol that I'll discuss later.

If you live in an apartment, you may be able to join a community garden. Or if you can't or don't want to grow your own food, consider joining in the community-supported agriculture (CSA) movement. In a CSA, you purchase a share from a farmer in that year's crop. You then get a weekly box of freshly picked vegetables and fruit from the farmer throughout the growing season. Some CSAs are only for the summer, but an increasing number now have spring, fall, and even winter shares. It's fun to see what you will get each week and to think of ways to cook and eat all the different vegetables. It's also a great way to add more variety and rotate your vegetables. I recommend finding a CSA that is organic. Look online for CSAs in your area. You can also grow less traditional foods, like sprouts and mushrooms. Kids often enjoy growing these foods. See the Resources section at the back of this book for good sources to buy supplies for growing sprouts and mushrooms. Another fun family activity is looking for edible wild foods that grow throughout North America, especially in empty lots in cities and towns and along roadways. Remember, however, that you do have to be careful to identify the plants correctly, as some plants and mushrooms are poisonous. (See the Resources section for information about where to learn about foraging.)

WAHLS WARRIOR Q&A

Q: Does juicing the 9 cups of vegetables and fruits have the same impact as consuming the whole food?

A: No. If you use a juicer that extracts and removes the fiber, the juice will have a very high glycemic index and will cause your body to manufacture more insulin in response. The juice will be rapidly absorbed along with the vitamins and enzymes. I'd rather you use a high-speed blender such as a Vitamix or HealthMaster to make a smoothie. Smoothies retain the entire fruit or vegetable including the fiber, which results in a slower rise in blood sugar. If you add a generous amount of water to liquefy the vegetables and fruits, a smoothie can seem just like juice, but it will have a much more beneficial effect in your body because you have not converted your produce into a high-glycemic form. We have had subjects in our trial who are very petite and could not eat 9 cups of vegetables. They ate 4 to 6 cups and made the rest into a smoothie using a Vitamix. This can be a good solution for those who have trouble eating the 9 cups. Remember, there is no need to stuff yourself. Remove all the excluded foods and you will have more room for vegetables. If you do have to reduce the amount, do so proportionately from the three groups.

The rank order of preference for best nutrition from your vegetables and fruits are:

- Picked from your garden and consumed the same day
- Purchased from a local farmer (or picked up from a CSA) and consumed on the same day or next day
- Purchased fresh from a store, from a regional farmer, picked that week (not always possible to determine this)
- Frozen or fermented (often preferable to fresh that is shipped from a distance)
- Purchased fresh from a store, from a farmer across the country (like from the coast if you live in the Midwest, or from one coast to another)
- Purchased fresh but from overseas
- Canned

Remember, the farther food travels and the more often it is heated, the more vitamins and antioxidants it will lose. Note: If food is dried at 105 degrees or less, it is as good as fresh as long as it is kept dry and below 85 degrees.

Produce Prep

When you bring home your vegetables, consider preparing them immediately. Fill the sink with water and wash everything. You can rinse with water alone or add a tablespoon of vinegar to two quarts of water. Dry with paper towels and put vegetables and fruits into Ziploc bags or clear plastic containers so everything stays clean and is easy to see. For an even easier time later, prepare your produce: Scrub and trim off ends of root vegetables, snap the ends of beans, and tear up lettuce so it is salad-ready. Break apart broccoli and cauliflower into florets. If you can open a neat crisper drawer and see all your vegetables nicely arranged and ready to eat, you will be much more likely to make a salad or stir-fry, or just snack on raw vegetables than if you know you have to start from scratch, scrubbing, trimming, peeling, coring, seeding, and chopping everything. Don't forget to reserve the outer leaves: Throw them in the slow cooker (or freezer) for vegetable soup stock. For your berries, it is better to wash and prep them just prior to eating. Also, berries have a shorter shelf life and are best consumed within one or two days of purchase.

If you buy or harvest too much produce to eat at once, preserve your produce for later. I recommend washing, deseeding and coring, and freezing it in heavy

Ziploc freezer bags so you can defrost and enjoy good local produce all year. Canning is another option, although it is a lot of work and not everyone will enjoy it. Another great option: Learn how to use lacto-fermentation to store your food and increase its nutritional quality. You'll find some fermented recipes in the recipe section at the end of the book. (Of course, you can also buy high-quality organic frozen or fermented fruits and vegetables in the off-season.)

When the 9 Cups Are Too Much or Upset Your Stomach

You don't think you can eat all those vegetables! I understand. I hear this all the time. First of all, you might find that this problem solves itself as you implement all parts of the Wahls Diet, including the elimination of gluten and dairy foods. (I'll talk about this later in this chapter.) Most people eat so much grain-based and dairy-based food that eliminating these food categories leaves a lot of room in your stomach. How better to fill it than with vegetables and fruits?

I also understand, however, that this is a major dietary change. For some people, gastrointestinal distress is a problem that comes with the sudden increase in vegetable matter. You may have gas, stomach cramps, diarrhea, or even constipation as your body adjusts. If you have MS or an autoimmune disease, you may have more serious GI issues as well, such as inflammatory bowel disease, making eating all those vegetables difficult. A GI work-up may be in order to evaluate for a gastrointestinal disorder like inflammatory bowel disease (IBD) or irritable bowel syndrome (IBS). Some people may also be sensitive to oxalates, a compound in many vegetables, including leafy greens. (See page 126 for more about oxalates and a low-oxalate diet.) Or, depending on your unique enzymes, it may be that you need a lower dose of sulfur or a lower dose of greens. For example, some people do not tolerate 6 cups of raw greens or sulfur-containing vegetables, but they may tolerate cooked greens or a smaller dose (such as one cup of cooked greens or sulfur vegetables to start).

If you need to reduce one category of vegetable (I outline the categories on page 138), I encourage you to increase the vegetables in the other categories so you still aim for 9 cups (or slightly more or less based on your size). Normally I advise keeping all three categories in proportion, but it's okay to vary these proportions due to intolerances, or as you are adjusting.

In most cases, cooking greens or sulfur-rich vegetables, eating them in smaller amounts, and then working up to 3 cups will work just fine. If you aren't sure, talk to your doctor about whether this amount of leafy greens or sulfur-containing vegetables is okay for you. Otherwise, you may just need to ease in, and this is absolutely acceptable. Better to go slowly than to start suddenly and then quit. If you are having a lot of GI issues, I have two suggestions:

1. First, begin by eating 1 to 3 cups of homemade bone broth (see the recipe section at the end of this book) and some coconut milk every day to help heal the lining of your gut.
2. Start eating your vegetables in the form of vegetable broth. First, add vegetables to water and simmer for twenty minutes. Strain out the vegetables and add the vegetable broth to your bone broth. Once this is going well and you've adjusted, begin pureeing the vegetables and adding them to your soup. Start with smaller amounts and work up. Your body will get used to the nutrition, but the fiber will be broken down and the vegetables will be easier to digest.
3. As you get accustomed to this, you should be able to start adding more cooked vegetables into your diet without pureeing them, but go as slow as you need to. Steamed vegetables are usually well tolerated. With more time you will likely do well with salads, smoothies, and raw vegetables. Up your vegetable and fruit intake gradually as your tolerance increases. However, some people may never do very well with raw vegetables. Others will find they feel just fine with this stair-step approach.

The reasons for the difference in tolerance to vegetables have to do with your digestive enzymes and which bacteria are living in your bowels. We all have unique DNA and a unique mix of microbes living in our bowels, and therefore a unique balance of digestive and toxin-processing enzymes. I have observed that some people can't do 3 cups of greens because of diarrhea but do fine if they cook their greens instead or eat just 1 to 2 cups of salad greens a day. For people with inflammatory bowel disease or any kind of abdominal issues like irritable bowel syndrome, having vegetables as soups and stews is the easiest way to get in all the vegetables. As you advance, steamed vegetables are usually well tolerated, and then eventually you will likely do well with salads, smoothies, and raw vegetables. Take your time and increase your vegetable and fruit intake as your tolerance improves. Your digestive enzymes and the bacteria living in your bowels will adjust as your health improves, although the adjustment can be slow. However, depending on your unique microbiome and enzymes, it may be that you will never tolerate raw vegetables. Pay attention to your response and work with your primary care team if you are experiencing difficulty.

WAHLS WARRIOR Q&A

Q: What is your advice for people on medications (like Coumadin) that make it problematic to eat a lot of dark leafy greens and other healthy foods?
A: Coumadin thins the blood through its interference with the vitamin K1 pathways in the liver. For this reason, it is very important to have a consistent intake of vitamin-K-rich foods like greens every day. However, you must eat the same amount of greens every day (such as the 3 cups specified on the Wahls Diet), so that the dose of Coumadin can be adjusted to match the daily intake. If you eat a plateful of greens once or twice a month and avoid greens all the other days, you could experience wild swings in the blood-thinning effect (also referred to as prothrombin time) of your Coumadin on the days you eat a lot of greens.

Unfortunately, many people believe that this means they have to avoid vitamin-K-rich foods entirely. This is a mistake. Avoiding greens will, over time, lead to multiple vitamin and mineral deficiencies. As the micronutrient deficiencies pile up, the prothrombin time often fluctuates widely, making the management of the Coumadin dose increasingly difficult. In fact, when this happens, it's a sign that multiple nutrient deficiencies are present, and this increases the risk of developing calcium deposits on heart valves and in blood vessels, leading to aortic stenosis (often severe enough to need heart surgery) or worsening high blood pressure that requires more and more medication.[12]

My recommendation to patients on Coumadin is to talk to your prescribing doctor and explain that you want to increase your vegetable intake and that you will need more frequent blood checks as you do this so your dose can be appropriately adjusted. Then eat the same amount of greens every day. This method should allow you to fully nourish your body with all the goodness greens provide while you continue to benefit safely from your medication. Another option for people taking Coumadin is to take a daily dose of menaquinone-7 (vitamin K2) so that you have a consistent intake of vitamin K, so the Coumadin dosing can be safely adjusted. This will lessen the risk of having your heart valves and bloods vessels hardened by excessive calcium depositions as a result of vitamin K depletion. I also recommend taking vitamin K2 if you are taking 5,000 IU vitamin D or more, to reduce the risk of ectopic calcification, but talk to your doctor before starting this supplement. You must always work with the physician who is managing your Coumadin dose so that she or he is aware that you're working to maximize your nutrient intake.

If you have a marked adverse reaction to a specific food, recognize and respect that by avoiding it for three months. Practice the other aspects of the Wahls Diet, and in three months you may have healed sufficiently to tolerate a small amount of the offending food once a week. If not, continue to avoid it. The Wahls Diet contains many choices, so you can always eliminate those with which you perceive you are having trouble. There are plenty of other vegetables and fruits from which to choose.

Part Two: Gluten-Free/Dairy-Free

Now that we've talked all about what you get to eat, let's talk about what's off the list, and the reasons for that. Giving up gluten, which is the protein in wheat, rye, and barley, as well as casein, which is the protein in dairy foods, seems like a pretty tall order. You love bread! You love cheese! How can you live without these comfort foods?

Although they might not seem to be related on the surface, gluten and casein molecules have a similar amino acid sequence, so to our immune cells, they often appear to be equivalent. When we eat these foods, our dopamine levels rise, making us feel good—even doped up and high. (Think about how you feel when you eat a gooey, cheesy pizza, an ice cream cone, or a chocolate chip cookie.) Our brains get addicted to that dopamine-induced high, so we seek more, and more . . . and often end up eating too many calories and not enough nutrients. Gluten and casein interact with the same receptors that are stimulated by narcotics: the opioid receptors.[13] (Refined sugars and processed foods are addictive, too. They have been specifically designed to stimulate our pleasure centers, making us feel good, so we want more and more.[14]) But addictions can be broken, and they must be if you want to stop suffering from the ill effects of unhealthful foods. It's time to go cold turkey. That means no foods containing wheat (including white and wheat flour, or multigrain flours containing wheat), barley, rye, spelt, or any of the other gluten-containing grains and nothing made with milk from animals, including cheese, yogurt, cream, and ice cream. The Wahls Diet is your path!

This is not as difficult as it sounds. Now that you are eating 9 cups of fruits and vegetables a day, markedly increasing the nutrient density of your diet, you will feel full and nourished. Most starchy foods—especially grains and potatoes—as well as dairy products have a lot of calories and are quickly converted to glucose as your body digests them. These foods have relatively few vitamins, minerals, and other micronutrients compared to greens, colors, and sulfur-rich produce. By replacing the grains and white potatoes with vegetables, deeply colored fruits, and berries, you will get a lot more antioxidants and other phytonutrients each day, and fewer empty calories.

GLUTEN-FREE/DAIRY-FREE: FAD OR LEGITIMATE HEALTH STRATEGY?

There is a lot of buzz in the media these days about going gluten-free and/or dairy-free. There are some recognized conditions, like celiac disease and lactose intolerance, which require taking gluten and/or dairy off the menu, but what about all the other people going gluten-free and dairy-free, claiming vague symptoms and self-diagnosed "intolerances"? It's become a fad, no doubt, and some physicians have become concerned that many perfectly healthy people are removing wheat and dairy from their diets needlessly. I would argue that many people can benefit from removing all sources of gluten and casein from their diets, whether or not they have a diagnosed allergy, reactivity, or sensitivity. The truth is that for people with chronic disease in particular, gluten and casein can be very problematic. Food allergies and sensitivities are difficult to diagnose and are much more common than is generally medically recognized, especially in people with chronic disease. You may not have any indication that you have a problem with gluten and casein, because 90 percent of the time there are no acute abdominal symptoms. Instead, the symptoms are insidious, coming on gradually and resulting in a wide variety of manifestations: unexplained fatigue, unexplained rashes that come and go, headaches, and mood problems. Unrecognized gluten and/or casein sensitivity has been associated with a wide variety of health problems,[15] including but not limited to:

- Allergies
- Asthma
- Autism and other brain disorders
- Chronic migraine
- Eczema and other skin disorders
- Infertility
- Inflammatory bowel disease (IBD)
- Irritable bowel syndrome (IBS)
- Psoriasis
- Psychiatric disorders
- Thyroid disease

In fact, for many with chronic unexplained symptoms and those with autoimmune problems, food sensitivities may be one of the root causes for many of their symptoms. In North America, no food sensitivities are more common than those to gluten and casein.[16]

Because you have been consuming grain and/or dairy most of your life, you don't know if you have sensitivity issues or not and you may not realize how many of your symptoms may be related to food sensitivity to gluten and/or dairy. Your body is in a steady state based on what you are eating now and has adapted to the damage that is being done. You are used to feeling the way you feel. Get ready to start feeling a lot better.

These are the items that contain gluten that you should avoid:

- Barley and anything containing it (including most beer, as well as barley malt and malt extract, such as in malt vinegar)
- Bulgur (the wheat grain in tabouli salad)
- Cereal containing wheat, barley, or rye (hot or cold)
- Couscous
- Matzo flour/meal/bread
- Panko (most breading contains gluten)
- Pasta made from semolina and/or durum (both of which are wheat)
- Rye and anything containing it
- Seitan (pure wheat gluten)
- Udon noodles
- Wheat and anything containing it, including wheat bran and wheat germ. That includes anything made with wheat flour, such as most bread, bagels, crackers, muffins, cookies, cake, and pastries.
- Wheat cousins: spelt, triticale, faro, Kamut (Khorasan wheat), einkorn, and freekeh.

Note that because there are no standards for gluten-free labeling, even foods that are labeled gluten-free may contain trace amounts of gluten. That is one reason why some people go grain-free and avoid all flour-based products—they realize they feel better than when they were consuming gluten-free products. You could also use gluten detection kits, which detect gluten in your urine or stool, as well as gluten tests that test food for the presence of gluten, so you can know if it is safe for you to eat. You can find information about these in the Resources section at the end of the book.

Another potential problem is that when people continue to consume four to five servings of gluten-free products per day, they are taking in too many processed, refined carbohydrates. You will have a much more nutrient-dense diet sticking primarily to vegetables, berries, and your protein sources (Wahls Paleo is designed more along these lines—see the next chapter). Gluten is also hidden in many things you might not think about, like deli meats, condiments, communion wafers, salad dressings, soups, soy sauce, and even medications, cosmetics, and envelope glue! If you aren't sure if something contains gluten, look on the label for a gluten-free statement, or call the company.

Now for the good news: There are still grains and starches you can eat, at least at this level of the diet! I will restrict grains and starches much more at the next level, Wahls Paleo, but for now, in limited amounts, you may eat these gluten-free grains and starches:

Wahls Diet–Approved Grains and Starches

- Amaranth
- Arrowroot
- Buckwheat
- Chickpea flour and other legume-based flours
- Coconut flour
- Corn
- Flax meal
- Millet
- Nut flours (like almond flour)
- Packaged foods labeled "gluten-free" (in moderation)
- Potato flour
- Quinoa
- Rice, all types
- Sago
- Sorghum
- Soy flour
- Tapioca
- Teff

WHY NO OATMEAL?

I no longer recommend oats, even those that are certified gluten-free. Up to 30 percent of those with gluten sensitivity have an adverse reaction to oats, even when they are gluten-free. If you don't think you are sensitive to gluten-free oats, at the very least, I recommend being vigilant about any symptoms that could be related to oat consumption. Caution is warranted!

These are the dairy foods you should eliminate from your diet:

- Cheese made from cow's, goat's, or sheep's milk
- Cream (heavy cream, whipping cream)
- Dairy ice cream
- Dairy yogurt
- Half-and-half
- Milk chocolate and many other forms of chocolate and candy (Read the label: Many dark chocolate varieties still contain milk.)
- Milk that comes from cows, goats, sheep, or mares (Once you have been weaned, I don't recommend consuming milk products again, with the exception of ghee, or clarified butter, which has the milk proteins removed.)
- Nondairy creamer (Although it is labeled nondairy, it does contain milk derivatives.)
- Nondairy "whipped topping"
- Packaged food with milk, casein, whey, caseinates, or hydrolysates in the ingredients list
- Vegetarian "cheeses" that contain some milk solids (read the label)
- Whey

WAHLS WARRIOR Q&A

Q: I know there are a lot of problems with dairy products, but what about raw milk? Many diets similar to yours recommend raw milk products.

A: When milk is pasteurized and homogenized, the shape and availability of the protein and fat molecules are slightly changed. That is why some people report that milk has many more health benefits when it is raw. I do agree that raw milk may be better nutritionally than pasteurized and/or homogenized milk, but it still has casein, which increases the risk of food allergy and sensitivity and has the potential to transmit infection if the milk is from an unhealthy cow. For this reason, milk, cheese, yogurt, ice cream, whey (as in whey protein powder), and all other dairy products (except for clarified butter/ghee) are not part of the Wahls Diet, Wahls Paleo, Wahls Paleo Plus, or Wahls Elimination Diet.

Wahls Diet–Approved Milk Substitutes

Fortunately, there are many dairy substitutes that are just fine on the Wahls Diet. Read the labels to see what has been added and to minimize exposure to high-fructose corn syrup, sugars, and other foodlike compounds that are added to the product (often to give it a better "feel" in the mouth). The emulsifiers in these milk substitutes have, in some studies, increased the leakiness of intestines, leading to leaky gut and more lipopolysaccharides (LPS) in the bloodstream, increasing the risk for autoimmunity, so I do recommend moderation or making your own nut milk at home. The commercial nut milks and coconut milks do give people a nondairy milk option, however, for those who miss dairy or need help transitioning.

The exception to my "no additives" advice is the addition of calcium citrate for the additional calcium content; this is fine. I suggest unsweetened varieties with short lists of basic ingredients you recognize, or you can make your own by combining nuts or seeds and water in a high-speed blender and straining the liquid.

Enjoy any of these:

- Almond milk
- Coconut milk—canned full-fat coconut milk is just fine. (You can also buy packets of powdered coconut milk. I travel with these, as they are very convenient.)
- Hazelnut milk
- Hemp milk
- Rice milk (organic preferred)
- Soy, almond, or coconut-based coffee creamer (marked "vegan")
- Soy, almond, or coconut yogurt
- Soy, almond, or coconut frozen desserts (ice cream substitutes) with unrefined sweeteners
- Soy milk (organic only)
- Soy, nut, or other nondairy cheeses that are labeled "vegan"

You may also enjoy dark chocolate if it doesn't contain any milk products. For the best nutritional benefit and an intense chocolate taste, choose 75 percent or higher cacao content.

WHEN ORGANIC MATTERS: SOY!

Any soy product you choose to consume should be organic to reduce exposure to the toxic herbicide glyphosate (Roundup). This is also one more reason to avoid grains and legumes since, along with soy, they are crops that are sprayed with this toxic herbicide.

VEGETARIAN ADVICE

You can be a vegetarian on the Wahls Diet, although you cannot progress to the next two levels if you remain a vegetarian. If you are at an ideal body weight and enjoy excellent health, then you can simply stay at the Wahls Diet and you will still reap immense benefits. I urge you, however, to read the Wahls Paleo chapter to learn about the benefits of seaweed and soaking grains, legumes, and nuts even if you do not plan to begin eating meat. If you experience a decline in health, however, I urge you to consider Wahls Paleo.

I do not recommend vegetarianism, and the next chapter will also offer my reasons. However, your diet is your choice, and that's why I give you three dietary levels for the Wahls Protocol. I understand that some people have strong beliefs that necessitate vegetarianism, and I respect that. If this is you, then in order to get sufficient protein and calories, you will need to eat more grains and legumes than I would regularly recommend. The amounts below are based on a 2,000 kcal diet and USDA dietary guidelines:

- Protein foods, 5.5 ounces per day (a one-ounce-equivalent portion would be 1 tablespoon of peanut butter, ½ ounce nuts and seeds, ¼ cup cooked dried beans or peas, ¼ cup tofu, or 1 ounce veggie meat). I recommended rotating your protein sources for more variety and less concentration on any one item.
- Grains (choose gluten-free varieties), 6 ounces per day.

- Calcium-fortified vegan "dairy" products, 3 cups per day (such as calcium-fortified soy, rice, or almond milk; calcium-fortified soy yogurt; or tofu made with calcium sulfate.

Because of this higher grain and legume consumption, I also strongly recommend that all vegetarians soak their grains and legumes before eating. There are some very important reasons for this, which I will talk about in the next chapter, but in brief: Germination decreases the activity of antinutrients like phytates, lectins, and trypsin inhibitors that occur naturally in grains and legumes. Soak your grains and legumes in water, in a bowl or jar, for twenty-four hours before preparing. Drain and rinse well. This causes the grains and legumes to produce phytase, which neutralizes some of the antinutrient action. An added perk: Soaking decreases cooking time.

Using a pressure cooker (such as the Instant Pot) is another excellent way to reduce lectins—and it's quick. Pressure-cooking grains and legumes denatures the lectins (although not gluten or casein), so I highly recommend that vegetarians in particular cook all their grains and legumes this way.

Part Three: Organic, Grass-Fed, and Wild-Caught

The last component of the Wahls Diet isn't about what you can and can't eat but about the quality of the foods you choose. I understand that it isn't always affordable or even available, but whenever possible I want you to choose organic vegetables and fruits, organic grass-fed meat, wild game, and wild-caught fish.

Some people believe that terms like *organic, grass-fed,* and *wild-caught* are pure marketing ploys that drive up cost without any real benefit. While it's true that fruits and vegetables as well as animals and fish raised without chemical intervention are more expensive, there is good reason for this. While all vegetables, fruits, meat, and fish may be healthy in essence, what conventionally raised food also contains is not so good for you.

Organic produce is easy. It's widely available in health food stores like Whole Foods and other local grocery stores and food co-ops, but these days, even regular grocery stores are stocking more options. Aldi has gone organic, and even Walmart carries options. You can grow organic produce in your yard or buy it at the farmers market. If you can't afford it all the time, go organic where it really matters. The Environmental Working Group (ewg.org) has several food guides to help identify which produce items have the most pesticides applied to them and which have the least, so that you can prioritize your shopping. (Look for their current list of the Dirty Dozen and the Clean Fifteen, updated yearly.)

Aside from the Dirty Dozen, there is one area where reducing chemicals matters most: meat and fish. This is because of something called bioconcentration. The chemicals in an animal's feed are concentrated in the meat of the animals you eat. This happens in nature, too, because of the pollution on our planet. A very small fish, for example, will eat plant matter and may absorb a tiny bit of mercury and other chemicals from a polluted environment. When a larger fish eats that fish, it not only gets mercury and chemicals from living in a polluted environment but takes in all the mercury and chemicals concentrated in the smaller fish it eats. As you work your way up the food chain, with successively bigger fish dining on other fish, the concentration grows. This is why the largest fish have the highest rates of mercury and other chemicals in their flesh.

And guess who is at the top of the food chain? Us, of course. If you eat conventionally grown meat and aquaculture ("farmed") fish, you will be exposing yourself and your family to the growth hormones, antibiotics, and pesticides used to grow that animal. The highest bioconcentration of toxins are in your fat, and remember that your brain is 60 to 70 percent fat.

WAHLS WARRIOR Q&A

Q: How do people who are allergic to fish get omega-3 fats in their diet?
A: If you do not tolerate even fish oil, then see if you can tolerate algae DHA oil. If you can't take that, either, then it is important to take 2 tablespoons of flax oil daily. It will also be even more important for you to have grass-fed meat. Another option is getting checked for an egg allergy and/or sensitivity. If you are not sensitive to eggs, you may be able to eat eggs that are DHA-enriched.

The meat our Paleolithic ancestors ate was very different from the meat we eat today. Animals did not contain much saturated fat until late summer and fall, in preparation for winter. Throughout the rest of the year, the animal was very lean and more of the fat contained unsaturated omega-3 fatty acids. The fall animals were valued for the increased fat. Coastal communities ate much more seafood from much cleaner waters. The result was a diet higher in both protein and omega-3 fatty acids in comparison to the modern Westernized diet, and one that contained far fewer toxins.

When I was growing up on the family farm, most of the farms in this country were run by families like ours. The average farm size was 170 acres. These farms were typically diversified into several crops. People had small herds of dairy cattle, beef cattle, and hogs. Crops included corn, soybeans, alfalfa, and oats. We had a huge garden and picked wild plums, grapes, and berries that grew around the yard, in the farm along the fencerows, along streams, and in the local woodlands. We also raised flocks of chickens, ducks, and a couple of turkeys each year. But we were also beginning to use chemical fertilizers, herbicides, and pesticides that were becoming popular because they increased production.

I remember that my dad had a sprayer that he used to spray atrazine over the corn and a broadleaf herbicide over the thistles in the pastures. He also used antibiotics for the livestock to combat infections, and he dewormed all of the animals annually. He fed corn to the hogs, to fatten them for sale to the slaughterhouse. My father sold beef calves in the fall to other people who then fattened them with corn on a confinement lot somewhere else. The dairy herd was milked twice a day. The cows ate from lush pastures in the spring and summer and had corn and hay during the winter. It was a farm experience on the cusp of modern technology—one foot in the old ways, the other foot in the new.

Today, farming is much different. There are far fewer small family farms, with the average size of the corporate farm steadily rising. Meat is produced efficiently and relatively inexpensively. Most of the meat you see in the supermarket comes from animals grown in large confinement systems. The animals are often kept indoors or in crowded outdoor pens, and fed rations to maximize growth in the shortest number of days. These rations contain antibiotics and growth-promoting hormones, *and* the grain (and often the hay) these animals consume has been doused with glyphosate (found in Roundup). When livestock eat grain grown with glyphosate, the glyphosate residue in the grain negatively impacts the diversity of the microbiome for that livestock, contributing to health problems in the livestock, and adds to our glyphosate exposure. When we eat grain and legumes grown with glyphosate, that also negatively impacts the diversity of our microbiome.

The result is that nonorganic, conventionally raised meats and farmed fish almost always contain chemical toxins that you will have to process and eliminate via your liver and kidneys, and that disrupt your microbiome. A healthy body may be able to tolerate the chemicals for a while, but eventually the harmful substances in conventionally raised animal and fish products are likely to begin wreaking havoc in your cells, leading to a variety of diseases. Which particular disease you get depends on your particular genetic vulnerability, which toxins are accumulating, and which hormonal imbalances are occurring in your body. If you suffer from an autoimmune condition like MS, your body is already clearly imbalanced, so you of all people should be particularly careful about what's in your meat.

This is why you want to eat the healthiest, most vigorous, least polluted animals. If you were a Paleolithic human, you would be getting your meat and fish from the unpolluted wild, but this is a lot more difficult today. However, you can definitely increase the purity and nutrient density of your animal protein if you select it from the right sources.

- **Do you hunt, fish, or know a hunter or someone who fishes?** These practices can make some people squeamish, but they are how our ancestors survived, and there is no fresher, more natural way for acquiring your animal protein.
- **Do you have access to products from a game farm that lets its animals forage?** Bison farms, deer farms, and elk farms all sell delicious meat with minimal toxic residue and a higher concentration of healthy nutrients like omega-3 fatty acids. Be sure to find out whether the animals ate grain. If the animal ate grass for a few weeks, then switched to grain for finishing (the final "fattening up" before slaughter), the fatty acid ratio in the meat will match that in grain-fed animals. Grass-finished animals are the best choice.

WHERE TO GET YOUR MEAT

Ideally, all of your animal protein will be organic, grass-fed, and/or wild-caught. Here are explanations of various sources for animal protein:

- **Conventional.** Conventionally raised animals are grain-fed, often with genetically modified corn, typically confined to small living spaces, and usually given hormones to make them grow faster, as well as antibiotics to fight infections caused by living in close quarters.
- **Farmed fish.** Farmed fish are raised in netted cages in coastal waters. They are sometimes fed grain products, which make their omega-6 levels higher, and they are more likely to contain contaminants like neurotoxic polychlorinated biphenyls (PCBs), hormone-disrupting polybrominated diphenyl ethers (PBDEs), antibiotics, and pesticides that are used to control infestations of sea lice.
- **Grass-fed/grass-finished.** Grass-fed, grass-finished animals are fed only grass and forage from weaning to harvest. Look for meat from animals that are both grass-fed and grass-finished. (Note: Some game and bison are grown on tallgrass prairie, which provides more nutrients than grass.)
- **Grass-fed/grain-finished.** These animals ate grass after weaning but were fed grain, typically corn, the last six weeks before slaughter. This is enough time to change the fatty acid composition of the animal to increase the amount of omega-6 fatty acids and decrease the amount of desirable omega-3 fatty acids, losing much of the benefit of grass feeding.
- **Organic.** Organic meat is raised without hormones and antibiotics, but these animals may still be fed grain and have too many omega-6s. Some small family farms that do not have USDA organic certification nevertheless choose to raise grass-fed, free-range animals without hormones and antibiotics. Talk to the farmer.
- **Wild.** Wild game and fish are not domesticated or contained by humans and they find their own food sources. Try to find a friend who hunts and you can often get all the venison or elk that your freezer can hold.

- **Do you have access to a farm that raises grass-fed, grass-finished, pastured free-ranging chickens and organic, pastured domesticated animals?** Organic animals cannot be fed any hormones or antibiotics, and their feed must also be organic. Grass-fed organic farms are more common and easier to find than ever before, especially since you can mail-order some of these products if they aren't available near you.
- **Can you find meat from grain-finished animals that is organic?** This is still superior to conventional meat.
- **Can you find wild-caught fish, shrimp, and other seafood?** Choose smaller fish to stay lower down on the food chain, ideally from family fisheries bringing in small catches from cold waters. These will be the least contaminated and most natural fish options.
- **Avoid conventionally raised meat from feedlots, confined poultry, and farm-raised fish (according to your financial means).** These are the most polluted sources of animal protein.

It can be difficult to find these foods, and if they are out of your budget, please know that getting your 9 cups and going gluten-free and dairy-free are the essential elements of the Wahls Diet. You can do this without going organic, or going organic according to what your budget will allow. Priority number one with the Wahls Diet is to get those nutrients into you *now* and to stop causing an attack response in your body with gluten and dairy. These two steps alone have effected dramatic changes in the many thousands of people following the Wahls Diet, and you can expect dramatic changes, too. Many of our patients at the VA adopted the dietary principles while living on food stamps. They were not buying organic foods, yet they were able to implement these concepts in rural Iowa, living on a budget, and experiencing remarkable health transformations. Do the best you can, given your financial circumstances. If they can do it, so can you!

Additional Prescriptions

Although adding the 9 cups and avoiding gluten and dairy are the keys, I would also like you to consider eliminating a few more things at the Wahls Diet level that will help reduce the chances of food sensitivity reactions:

- Eggs. As I've mentioned before, I recommend giving your body a break from eggs (100 days) to really know for sure whether you are sensitive to eggs. Many people have annoying symptoms such as headaches, fatigue, mood problems, rashes, and other symptoms that resolve once they remove eggs from their diets.
- Nonorganic soy (which can lead to excess inflammation)
- Nonorganic soy or rice milk
- High-fructose corn syrup
- Refined sugar (like white and brown sugar)
- Artificial sweeteners and monosodium glutamate (these can lead to excitotoxicity—overstimulation of brain cells—as well as an unfavorable gut bacteria balance, similar to what you would develop on a high-sugar and high-carbohydrate diet)
- All trans fats or partially hydrogenated oil
- Any refined vegetable oil, especially corn, soybean, canola, grape seed, and palm kernel (we'll discuss oils and fats more in chapter 7)
- Any soda, including diet soda

In addition, I prefer that you not eat food that has been irradiated or microwaved. My preference is to have food that is in as natural a state as possible. Treating food with either microwave energy or ionizing radiation reacts with the food at the molecular level to either heat it (microwave) or kill microbes (ionizing radiation). I'd rather eat food that is fresh, local, and handled and prepared in ways that food has been prepared (raw, cooked, roasted, steamed, boiled, fried in saturated fat, or fermented) for hundreds of generations. Personally, I also think microwaved food tastes strange.

Wahls Diet Meal Plan

Now you know the basics and the reasons behind them. Let's get to how you can put all this into practice in your life. Here is a sample seven-day meal plan to launch you successfully into the Wahls Diet.

Helpful hint: If you usually have things like pancakes or toast in the morning, your breakfast is probably going to change. You will be dropping the emphasis on grains (although some breakfasts do include nongluten whole

WAHLS DIET AT A GLANCE

Note: Eat to satiety. You may increase or decrease the amount of vegetables, fruit, and meat you eat according to your size, but make sure to do so in proportion.

- Consume 9 cups of vegetables and fruits daily, divided as follows (or proportionately to what you can consume without feeling gorged):
  - 3 cups green leaves
  - 3 cups sulfur-rich (cabbage family, onion family, and/or mushrooms)
  - 3 cups bright color (green, yellow-orange, red, or purple-blue-black)
- Eat grass-fed or wild-caught meats and fish (6 to 12 ounces per serving, depending on your size and gender). I recommend minimizing processed meats like sausage, ham, bacon, or salami, but if you like them, look for gluten- and nitrite-free and monosodium-glutamate-free products.
- If you are a vegetarian, consume adequate calories and eat a varied diet including vegetables, grains, legumes, nuts, seeds, beans, and soy. You should take 2 tablespoons of flax, hemp, or walnut oil daily. You may include soy in your diet, but it should be organic and non-GMO (i.e., not a genetically modified organism—the package should state that it is non-GMO). If you are a vegetarian and consuming soy frequently, I recommend you prioritize fermented soy, like tempeh, pickled tofu, natto, or miso. (You can read more in chapter 6 about why fermenting is important if you eat soy regularly.)
- You may eat gluten-free starch, like gluten-free grains or potatoes, but try not to overdo it. Ideally, don't have these starchy foods every day. Vegetarians, however, will need to eat more gluten-free grains to ensure complete protein.

What you can enjoy in moderation:

- Apples, bananas, and pears, although they do not count toward the 9 cups and should be eaten only after meeting the 9 cups goal.

- Nuts and seeds, preferably raw, preferably soaked and sprouted (see page 211). This includes raw almond butter, tahini, and sunflower seed butter. Have up to 4 ounces per day.
- Non-grain-based alcohol (like wine, preferably organic, or gluten-free beer), up to 1 serving per day (optional)
- Sweeteners, up to 1 teaspoon per day (optional—choose honey, molasses, real maple syrup, raw sugar, or natural evaporated cane juice)
- Omega-3 oils (flax, hemp, walnut), cold only (do not cook with these!), and no more than 2 tablespoons per day (unless directed otherwise by your physician). These are good to put on salads or into smoothies.
- Other oils (olive oil should be the default—it's okay to use sesame oil and avocado oil occasionally). Choose cold-pressed organic non-GMO brands.

Forbidden foods:

- All gluten-containing foods
- All dairy-containing foods
- Eggs
- Nonorganic soy or rice milk
- White sugar, high-fructose corn syrup, and artificial sweeteners, including soda and diet soda
- All trans fats, partially hydrogenated oil, and omega-6-rich vegetable oils (such as corn, soybean, canola, grape seed, and palm kernel)
- Preservatives and flavor enhancers, including monosodium glutamate
- Microwaved and irradiated foods

grains). Instead, you will be focusing on vegetables, fruit, and high-quality protein.

Note to vegetarians: Even if you are vegetarian and therefore do not plan to progress beyond the Wahls Diet level, please read the other diet plans in the next two chapters; there is still a great deal of information there that is highly relevant to you.

Wahls Diet Week

All foods that have corresponding recipes at the end of this book are marked with an asterisk (*). Also note that I sometimes recommend almond milk, soy milk, or coconut milk. This is for the sake of variety, but you may substitute any of these for any other at this stage of the diet. Just remember that it is always a good idea to rotate your food, rather than eat the same thing every day.

	Breakfast	*Lunch*	*Dinner*
Day 1	Smoothie: • 1 cup kale • 1 small orange • 1 cup pineapple • 1 cup unsweetened organic soy milk • 1 tablespoon nutritional yeast 1 serving Rosemary Chicken* (prepared the night before, or substitute organic chicken sausage)	Salad: • 2 cups kale • 1 cup bok choy • 1 small tomato • 2 teaspoons extra virgin olive oil • rice vinegar to taste 4 ounces sardines in tomato sauce 1 cup raw turnips 1 medium peach	1 serving Red Chili with Beans* 1 cup brown rice ¼ Hass avocado Salad: • 3 cups romaine lettuce • 1 medium stalk celery • ½ cup mushrooms • 1 clove garlic • dried basil to taste • 2 teaspoons extra virgin olive oil • rice vinegar to taste 6 ounces plain coconut milk yogurt ¾ cup blackberries Tension Tamer, chamomile, or other herbal tea

	Breakfast	Lunch	Dinner
Day 2	Smoothie: • 1 cup parsley • 1 cup green grapes • 1 kiwi • 1 tablespoon nutritional yeast • water/ice 1 cup brown rice hot cereal • 1 teaspoon blackstrap molasses • ⅓ cup raisins • 2 tablespoons chopped walnuts ½ cup unsweetened organic soy milk	1 serving Basic Skillet Recipe* (Ham and Collards) 1 cup chopped baked sweet potato • 1 teaspoon extra virgin olive oil • ⅓ teaspoon cinnamon 1 cup raspberries 1½ cups unsweetened organic soy milk	1 serving Basic Skillet Recipe* (Lamb Chops with Broccoli) Salad: • 4 cups spinach • ½ cup orange sections • ¼ cup sliced assorted mushrooms • ¼ cup chopped onions • 1 tablespoon extra virgin olive oil • vinegar to taste 1 medium apple with skin 1 serving Wahls Fudge* peppermint herbal tea
Day 3	Smoothie: • 1 cup spinach • 1 cup honeydew melon • 1 kiwi • 1 cup unsweetened almond milk • 1 tablespoon nutritional yeast 1 serving leftover Basic Skillet Recipe* (Lamb Chops with Broccoli) ½ cup sliced carrots 6 dates	1 serving Salmon Salad* 8 gluten-free rice crackers Salad: • 3½ cups spinach • ½ cup raspberries • ½ cup raw zucchini slices • 2 teaspoons extra virgin olive oil • balsamic vinegar to taste Fruit cup: • 1 cup watermelon • 1 cup honeydew melon 1 cup unsweetened almond milk	1 serving Basic Skillet Recipe* (Steak and Mustard Greens) 1 serving Quinoa and Red Peppers* 1 cup cubed winter squash 2 teaspoons clarified butter 1 serving Wahls Fudge* 1 medium pear 1 cup unsweetened organic soy milk Detox herbal tea

	Breakfast	Lunch	Dinner
Day 4	Smoothie: • 1 cup kale • 1 small orange (1 cup) • 1 cup unsweetened organic soy milk • 1 tablespoon nutritional yeast 1½ ounces raw almonds 6 dried apricot halves 4 dried prunes	1 serving Wahls Pizza* 1 medium raw carrot 1 cup black grapes 2 cups unsweetened organic almond milk	1 serving Seafood-Tomato Soup* ½ cup boiled potato with skin Salad: • 3½ cups romaine lettuce • ½ cup cilantro • 1 garlic clove • ¼ cup green peas • 2 teaspoons extra virgin olive oil • lime juice to taste 6 ounces almond milk yogurt 1 cup strawberries ½ cup banana Throat Coat herbal, licorice, or other herbal tea
Day 5	Smoothie: • ½ cup raw beets • ½ cup mango • ½ cup blueberries • 1 cup unsweetened organic soy milk • ½ teaspoon grated gingerroot • 1 tablespoon nutritional yeast 3–4 ounces sardines canned in oil 2 slices gluten-free bread ½ cup celery	Wahls Spaghetti: • 1 cup cooked spaghetti squash • ¾ cup marinara sauce • 3 ounces ground beef • ¼ cup mushrooms • 2 tablespoons Rawmesan* 1 cup green beans Salad: • 3 cups bok choy • ½ cup summer squash • 1 clove garlic • 2 teaspoons extra virgin olive oil • lime juice to taste 2 medium plums 1 cup unsweetened organic soy milk	1 serving Algerian Vegetarian* 1 serving Quinoa and Red Peppers* 1 cup cooked butternut squash Salad: • 3 cups bok choy • ½ cup tomato • ½ cup sliced or diced cucumber with peel • ½ cup grapes • 1 clove garlic • 3 teaspoons sunflower butter • lime juice to taste 8 ounces coconut milk yogurt 1 cup peaches 2 tablespoons almonds chamomile herbal tea

	Breakfast	Lunch	Dinner
Day 6	Smoothie: • 1 cup cilantro • 1 small orange • 1 cup pineapple • 1 tablespoon nutritional yeast • water/ice 1 cup whole grain grits ½ cup pink grapefruit sections 1 cup unsweetened organic soy milk	Salad: • 3 cups bok choy • 2 cups romaine lettuce • ¼ Hass avocado • ½ cup tomato • ½ cup sweet red peppers • ½ cup mushrooms • 2 tablespoons almonds • 2 teaspoons extra virgin olive oil • lime juice to taste 1 medium chicken breast without the skin Fruit cup: • 1 medium banana • ½ cup grapes	1 serving Basic Skillet Recipe* (Salmon and Mustard Greens) 1 serving Mashed Turnips* 1 teaspoon extra virgin olive oil 1 cup green peas Fruit cup: • 1 medium peach • ½ cup unsweetened cherries 1 cup unsweetened organic soy milk rooibos or other herbal tea
Day 7	Smoothie: • 1 cup collards • ½ cup watermelon • ½ cup cantaloupe (muskmelon) • 1 cup unsweetened organic soy milk • 1 tablespoon nutritional yeast 6 ounces almond milk yogurt • ½ cup unsweetened cherries • 4 tablespoons chopped walnuts	1 serving Vegetarian Kale Soup* 15 gluten-free rice crackers Salad: • 2 cups spinach • 2 cups kale • 4 florets cauliflower (½ cup) • 1 clove garlic • ½ cup raw mushrooms • 2 tablespoons chopped almonds • 2 teaspoons flax oil • Bragg apple cider vinegar to taste (lime juice would work as well) 1 cup pineapple	1 serving Basic Skillet Recipe* (Pork Chops and Red Cabbage) 1 small (2-inch diameter) baked potato with skin 1 teaspoon extra virgin olive oil 6 medium spears asparagus 1 cup blueberries herbal tea

SNACK IDEAS

- Dried raisins and nuts
- Fresh raw walnuts, almonds, or sunflower seeds
- Sliced apples (after your 9 cups are in!) dipped in organic almond butter
- Dried mango slices
- Dehydrated kale chips
- Pickled herring and gluten-free crackers
- Guacamole and sliced raw vegetables
- Eggplant dip (roasted eggplant and crushed garlic and olive oil blended in a food processor) with raw vegetable slices (turnip, rutabaga, kohlrabi, celery)
- Fresh fruit
- Nitrite-free deli meat rolled up with a lettuce leaf, pickle, and mustard
- Green tea sweetened with fruit juice
- Green tea with coconut or nut milk

Chapter 6

WAHLS PALEO

Now that you are on the Wahls Diet, you are likely already experiencing some benefits. Maybe you feel a change in your energy or your mental clarity, or maybe you are already noticing some mobility differences. If you are feeling good, you may decide it is time to take it to the next level. Or maybe you have decided to start here because you want to see faster results. Either way, welcome to Wahls Paleo, my most popular diet plan and favorite level of the Wahls Protocol!

I would estimate that most of my patients end up settling in at this level. They want a more powerful plan than the Wahls Diet, but they aren't quite ready for the extremes of Wahls Paleo Plus or Wahls Elimination (see chapter 7). If you stay here, at the level of Wahls Paleo, rest assured you will be getting powerful medicine in the form of food, and your body will finally break free of many of the toxins that have hindered your healing in the past.

Wahls Paleo is a potent dietary intervention into the disease process. Since the first edition of this book was published, there has been a lot of research published about the benefits of eating this way, although studies specifically examining the effect of a Paleo-style diet on autoimmune disease is still an area where there is much to be explored. There is some research out there, including research linking diet to improvements in inflammatory bowel disease[1] and psoriasis,[2] as well as my own research on multiple sclerosis (see the Introduction and the Preface to the Revised Edition), and the results are promising. I am continuing to research, and my research is now being cited by others, and we are always writing up the results from our previous studies (so keep an eye out for more), but there is already a lot of research looking at how Paleo-style diets improve many different measures of health in people with a broad range of chronic conditions. Paleo diets have been associated with relief of a broad range of symptoms, better lab results, reduced fatty liver,[3] improvements in metabolic syndrome,[4] and improved insulin sensitivity, glycemic control, and fat mass,[5] and improvements in body composition.[6]

There are many different ideas about what constitutes a "Paleo diet," and Wahls Paleo is more highly regulated than some, since its purpose is to intervene in chronic disease, rather than simply for general health improvement (for example, the 9 cups is unique to the Wahls Diet; it is not a part of the Paleo diet). Wahls Paleo contains all the elements of the Wahls Diet, but with the addition of a few more elements. You will still eat your 9 cups of fruits and vegetables a day, keep gluten and dairy out of your diet, and consume high-quality protein. You'll also be doing these four things:

WAHLS PALEO DIET

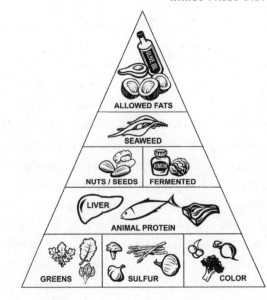

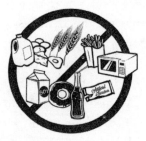

1. Reduce all remaining grains, legumes, and potatoes in your diet to just two servings *or fewer* per week.
2. Eat animal protein every day. You'll be eating more at this level than on the Wahls Diet. Shoot for between 9 and 21 ounces per day. (Adjust that according to your weight and gender. Small women may eat closer to 9 ounces, larger men may eat closer to 21 ounces, particularly if you are physically active.) Sixteen ounces per week of this allowance should be wild-caught cold-water fish or pastured, grass-fed and grass-finished meat.
3. Add seaweed and organ meat to your diet: ¼ teaspoon powdered kelp or 1 teaspoon dulse flakes per day, and 12 ounces of organ meat per week. (Organ meat is also included as part of your animal protein allowance.)
4. Add fermented foods, seeds and nuts (preferably soaked), and more raw foods to your diet. (I'll explain in this chapter how soaking can reduce the antinutrients in grains and legumes, for those who continue to avoid animal protein for spiritual reasons.)

Wahls Paleo		
Nutrient*†	U.S. Diet (%)	Wahls Paleo (%)
Vitamin D	31	52
Vitamin E	55	108
Calcium	74	70
Magnesium	88	138
Vitamin A	100	523
Pyridoxine	121	638
Folate	122	251
Zinc	123	351
Thiamine	128	703
Vitamin C	133	661
Niacin	154	531
Iron	164	303
Riboflavin	175	781
Vitamin B$_{12}$	201	850

* Compared to dietary reference intakes, recommended dietary allowances (RDA) for females 51–70 years; Wahls Diet adjusted for 1,759 calories. (National Academies of Sciences, Engineering, and Medicine; Institute of Medicine; Food and Nutrition Board)

† Average nutrient intake from food for females 50–59 years. (What We Eat in America, NHANES 2009–2010, ars.usda.gov/SP2UserFiles/Place/12355000/pdf/0910/Table_1_NIN_GEN_09.pdf, accessed 5/25/13)

WHY NOT 100 PERCENT OF THE RDA?

Technically, the Wahls Paleo diet does not reach 100 percent of the RDA for vitamin D or calcium. I've already talked about the best ways to get vitamin D naturally through light exposure, which can make up for this deficiency (pages 326 to 327) but in short, we manufacture vitamin D in our skin as a result of ultraviolet light exposure to bare skin. Thus it is not critical to get vitamin D from our food. (I do recommend everyone monitor their vitamin D exposure, however.)

Also, if you are getting enough vitamin D you will experience improved absorption of calcium in the gut, so you may not need as much actual calcium in your diet. In this way, getting your vitamin D through light exposure may also help correct any dietary calcium insufficiency. Also, retinol via liver or cod-liver oil along with weight-bearing exercise and/or regular use of a vibrating platform will naturally strengthen and protect bones, and a good dose of daily greens can also improve natural intake of calcium as well as magnesium. (This is one of many reasons I push more greens in my diet than other diets do.)

Taking calcium supplements is associated with higher ates of ectopic calcium in the heart valves and blood vessels, as well as kidney stones, which is why I do not recommend taking them. Instead, I recommend taking vitamin K2 (see the Resources section for good sources). Recommended daily intake for calcium has been steadily increased in the United States in an effort to reduce the risk of osteoporosis, but my interpretation of the root cause of osteoporosis has not been low intake of calcium, but rather, low intake of vitamin K. The vitamin K1 is converted to K2 by our gut bacteria, and the vitamin K2 helps the body absorb the ectopic calcium from the blood vessel walls and heart valves, supporting an influx of calcium into teeth and bones instead.

One last note: One of the main reasons I include (soaked/sprouted) nuts and seeds in the Wahls Protocol is to provide a boost of another important vitamin, Vitamin E.

Let's look at each one of these items in turn. As in the last chapter, I have compared the average American diet to the mean intake on Wahls Paleo, and once again, you can see that Wahls Paleo has markedly more nutrition for your cells!

Part One: Reducing Grains, Legumes, and Potatoes

At the Wahls Diet level, you eliminated gluten and dairy because of their potential for causing food sensitivities. Now it's time to cut the carbs down further. In our study, we allow people to have two servings of starchy nongluten grains like brown rice, starchy vegetables like potatoes, or legumes like lentils or chickpeas each week, but acknowledge that going entirely grain-, legume-, and potato-free is ideal. (I'll encourage you to do that at the Wahls Paleo Plus level, but it's never required. I understand how life can be in the real world!) Many of our subjects are mostly grain-, legume-, and potato-free but have these foods only very occasionally, usually when social situations make it difficult to say no. Feel free to be similarly strict if you are so inspired.

This limit sometimes surprises people because they believe that foods like brown rice, lentils, and potatoes are healthy foods. In some ways, they are. They contain vitamins, minerals, and protein, and they are gluten-free. Even gluten-free whole grains, legumes like black beans and lentils, and potatoes, however, contribute to increased insulin demand because they are

WAHLS DIARY ALERT

If you decide to transition from the Wahls Diet to Wahls Paleo, be sure to track exactly what you change in your diet and report how you feel. Do you notice any improvements in your symptoms? Any side effects? This can help you pinpoint which foods work best for you and also encourage you to stick with your new level of dietary commitment. Stay inspired!

also high in carbohydrates. Your pancreas still needs to manufacture and dump insulin into your bloodstream to keep your blood sugar stable as your body digests those carbohydrates, making you more likely to develop insulin resistance (more on this later in the book), which may increase your risk of early cognitive decline, depending on your genetics and other environmental risk factors. When you are battling chronic disease, especially one with brain symptoms, you don't need to do anything to diminish your brain's capacity for healthy functioning, and one of the primary goals of the Wahls Protocol is to maximize, not compromise, your brain function. Reducing your carbohydrate intake will also help reduce inflammation and improve your gastrointestinal health. Too many high-carbohydrate foods, even those that don't contain gluten, can also be detrimental to the balance of your microbiome (the bacteria in your gut) because the carbohydrates can act as fertilizer to sugar-loving bacteria and yeasts, and that can lead to many other health problems (particularly for those with a sensitivity to FODMAPs—see page 128).

Nonstarchy vegetables and colorful vegetables and fruits like winter squash, beets, and berries also have carbohydrates, but they have far fewer carbs than grains, legumes, or potatoes, and often have more vitamins and minerals per calorie, which gives them a higher nutrient density than grains, potatoes, or legumes. For this reason, you may keep enjoying these vegetables and fruits at the Wahls Paleo level—those 9 cups are still part of the plan! All vegetables and fruits can increase insulin demand, but at a much more moderate level. We're working the worst things out of your diet a little at a time.

Most of all, I encourage you to enjoy more nonstarchy vegetables (like green vegetables) than starchier choices like cooked beets and squash, and to enjoy those starchy vegetables raw or gently boiled or steamed, so that the food doesn't become completely soft and mushy. When starchy vegetables remain a bit crunchy, the starch in the vegetable is not so readily converted to sugar in the bloodstream. I also encourage you to begin eating a much greater percentage of vegetables than fruit at this level of the diet. To really ramp up the positive effects of Wahls Paleo, you are best off getting most of your nutrients from lower-carbohydrate, less-insulin-demanding sources.

Part Two: Eat Animal Protein Every Day

If you aren't a vegetarian, you might already be doing this, but now I want to be sure that you're not only getting animal protein but getting *enough* animal protein. Animal protein is an incredibly important component of Wahls Paleo. You should eat 9 to 21 ounces of meat each day, according to your size, gender, and physical activity level. Remember to choose organic, grass-fed, and wild-caught whenever possible, within your financial means.

Meat and fish are an essential part of the Wahls Paleo plan because of their unique nutrient profiles, yet I have found that even regular meat eaters tend to feel like they probably shouldn't be eating meat. They feel guilty. We have been indoctrinated to believe that a vegetarian diet is healthier, so I want to talk in a little more depth about meat as well as about vegetarianism.

For more than a decade I did not eat any meat, poultry, or fish, but I am now a firm believer in the importance of animal protein, especially for people suffering from chronic health issues. I recognize this is a controversial

WAHLS WARRIORS SPEAK

I am a family doctor in the Netherlands and I was diagnosed with secondary progressive MS in 2011. For about three years, I noticed a progressive deterioration in my walking ability. I began to limp with my right leg, but I was still able to walk without help. In September 2012, I learned about Terry Wahls, and my wife and I decided that something had to be done about my health. We started following the recommendations Dr. Wahls formulated and eating more of a Paleo-style diet. We eat lots of fruit and vegetables, fish and organic meat, and nuts. I completely abandoned eating grains, potatoes, pastas, and dairy products. Since then, I've noticed a marked improvement in my vitality, and my gait is really improving as well. For us, this is very encouraging! It is time for medicine to focus much more on nutrition and lifestyle. I thank Terry Wahls and her team for giving us much more insight and understanding of health and disease.
—Marco J., Maastricht, the Netherlands

position, so I want to give you my reasons. Let's start by looking at the great benefits you will receive from eating animal protein.

Animal Protein Benefit 1: Complete Protein

Our bodies need to manufacture proteins to conduct the business of life and manufacture our cellular structures, many of which require complicated protein molecules. Those proteins are all manufactured from amino acids, which are classified in three ways: essential, conditionally essential, and nonessential. We must get the essential ones in our diets because we lack the machinery or enzymes to manufacture them internally. *Conditionally essential* means that we can manufacture the amino acids ourselves under the right conditions. Our body can manufacture nonessential amino acids, so we needn't get them from food.

Because there are so many amino acids we need, our bodies will go to drastic measures to get them if we don't provide them. For example, if we don't have the correct amino acids to make the proteins we need, we will resort to autophagy ("eating of self"), meaning that we begin "eating" or digesting some of our own muscle and organ cells.

The body takes what it needs for its most essential tasks, even if it means sacrificing parts of itself that it deems less essential. This may be beneficial to us in, for example, a time of famine or starvation. This is an evolutionary adaptation for times when food was scarce, but it is obviously very harmful in the long term, compromising the body's ability to maintain its own muscle and organ integrity, leading to muscle wasting, weakness, and internal organ damage. High-quality proteins are essential for optimal health and function!

The great thing about meat is that it contains all of the essential amino acids. You get everything you need. Plants, however, do not contain all the amino acids necessary for your body. Grains are limited in their supply of lysine and/or threonine, and legumes are limited in the sulfur-containing amino acid methionine. That is why vegetarians need to eat a combination of grains and legumes to have all of the essential amino acids necessary to make complete proteins. You can do it, but it's trickier. If vegetarians eat only grains or only legumes, they are not consuming a complete protein and will need to digest some portion of their own bodies to get the missing amino acids

AFFORDING QUALITY ANIMAL PROTEIN

I prefer to spend my money in my community. Buying meat from a local farmer and paying a local butcher to process it keeps the money local and is often cheaper than buying meat in a supermarket because you can buy in bulk. In order to find farmers who are growing grass-fed, hormone-free meats in your area, contact your local county extension office. Many of the farmers who practice community-supported agriculture (CSA) for vegetable produce are also producing eggs and meat. If not, they will likely be aware of the farmers in the community who are and can give you recommendations about local farmers. You can even go out to the farm and see the operation itself to know that the farm animals are being raised humanely. I buy the majority of my meat directly from farmers I know. That way I know the animal was fed organic rations; lived outside, eating grasses and prairie plants; and most important, was healthy. I also make sure the animals have not been given antibiotics or hormones. In addition, organic organ meats are often much less expensive than the organic muscle meat.

(usually methionine, lysine, or threonine) to manufacture the proteins necessary for life.

Animal Protein Benefit 2: Essential Fatty Acids

Essential fatty acids are the fats that our cells need but cannot make themselves. We must consume them or we can become deficient, to the detriment of our own health. These include alpha-linolenic acid (ALA), an omega-3 fatty acid, and linoleic acid (LA), an omega-6 fatty acid. In addition, there are two conditionally essential fats: docosahexaenoic acid (DHA), an omega-3 fatty acid, and gamma-linolenic acid (GLA), an omega-6 fatty acid. The conditionally essential fatty acids, DHA and GLA, are more likely to be required if the person has developed a brain problem, autoimmune problem, or disease involving too much inflammation.

For the first 2.5 million years of the human genus, *Homo,* and the first

500,000 years of our species, *Homo sapiens*, humans ate these omega-6 and omega-3 fatty acids at roughly a 1:1 ratio. We ate things like plants and seeds that had omega-6, but we also ate a lot of wild animals that foraged for grasses, other greens, and wild fish, all of which contain omega-3 fatty acids. This provided us with that 1:1 balance[7] associated with a lower risk of both neurological and cardiovascular diseases.[8]

Today life, as well as the human diet, is much different. That ratio has been skewed in favor of omega-6 fatty acids, and the amount of omega-3 fatty acids has dramatically declined.[9] The introduction to the human diet of seed oils such as corn oil, soybean oil, and canola oil—which were originally considered waste products until World War II—as well as an increase in feeding animals grain rather than grass (reducing the omega-3 fatty acid content in their meat) led to the increase in omega-6 consumption. The current omega-6 to omega-3 ratio for some Americans is as high as 15:1 or even 45:1!

When the ratio shifts so far toward omega-6 fatty acids, many of our chemical pathways tilt toward inflammation and the development of chronic disease.[10] As a result, we are much more likely to develop excessive inflammation in our blood vessels, leading to higher rates of autoimmune problems, atherosclerosis, heart disease, and mental health problems.[11] This can easily be reversed, however, by ramping up the amount of grass-fed meat and wild-caught fish in your diet (while simultaneously eliminating or markedly decreasing the amount of vegetable oil). On a vegetarian diet, it is especially difficult to achieve a 1:1 balance. (I'll explain this in more detail momentarily.)

Fish Sources of Omega-3 Fatty Acids	
(Adapted from the "Toolbox for Clinicians" from the 2013 International Symposium for Functional Medicine, June 1, 2013, held by the Institute for Functional Medicine)	
Fish (4-ounce serving)	**Omega-3 fatty acids (grams)**
Chinook salmon	2.1
Herring, pickled	1.9
Scallops	1.1
Halibut	0.6
Shrimp	0.4
Snapper	0.4
Tuna, yellowfin	0.3
Cod	0.3

FATTY ACIDS VS. NF-KAPPAB

The human body has an innate immune response that recognizes the amino acid sequences in proteins to determine whether they are foreign and dangerous to health. This is a survival mechanism to protect us against threats. One of the key players in it is a protein complex called NF-kappaB, which responds to threats in the body. In the case of an infection, an injury, a disease process, or even chronic stress, NF-kappaB activates and triggers the release of inflammatory substances. However, NF-kappaB should not cause ongoing chronic inflammation. When that happens, it creates inflammasomes—cellular mechanisms that cause inflammation to persist instead of resolving and completing the repair process or healing. In the case of many autoimmune diseases, the autoinflammation process is made more severe and resistant to treatment by overly activated NF-kappaB and inflammasomes.

Many anti-inflammatory medicines and supplements target NF-kappaB, as it is considered one of the major causes of excessive inflammation. The goal is to activate resolvins, which are signals that help stop the inflammation cascade driven by NF-kappaB and inflammasomes. The primary resolvins are the omega-3 fatty acids EPA and DHA, which is why anyone with an autoimmune disease, as well as anyone with a chronic infection or other chronic disease, should be sure to get enough EPA and DHA. Eating high-quality fatty wild-caught seafood and grass-fed and grass-finished meats is an excellent way to accomplish this. In Chapter 10, you can find a list of many additional substances that can also contribute to resolving signaling and effective inhibition of NF-kappaB.

Animal Protein Benefit 3: Bone and Joint Strengthening

When traditional societies ate meat, they used the entire animal to maximize the health of the clan. Today we tend to focus on muscle meat only, but many other parts of an animal, such as chicken or pig feet and the gristly, sinewy parts contain beneficial nutrients that aren't contained in the muscle.

Bones, sinews, gristle, and cartilage were staples in the diets of traditional societies. These people typically made soups and stews from the bones, cartilage, and connective tissue of animals. This nourished the bones and joints of the people who drank this broth by providing collagen and compounds from the glucosamine/glycan family of molecules. I remember both of my grandmothers gnawing on the cartilage on the end of chicken bones. They told me that they needed that gristle for their joints. I didn't value their wisdom at the time because I thought the whole practice was a little bit disgusting. Now, I realize that they were doing what should come naturally to humans: taking advantage of a potent source of joint-healing compounds. I'm happy to say I now chew on that gristle and include those gnarly parts in soups and stews, resurrecting a proud family tradition!

Bone broth is savory, comforting, and delicious, and although we don't know exactly how it happens, the glucosamine in bone broth tends to go straight to the joints, where it is most needed.[12] Nature's magic! Bone broth is also filled with all the minerals that our skeletons need, in addition to glutamine and other amino acids that are especially healing for someone suffering from a "leaky gut." Our intestinal cells prefer to use the amino acid glutamine (instead of blood sugar or glucose) as their primary fuel for operating their cellular machinery, so when they get enough, they heal internal damage more efficiently. A daily cup or two of bone broth is an excellent start to healing a

WAHLS WARRIOR Q&A

Q: Are there specific beneficial effects of the Wahls Protocol for neuropathy?
A: I believe it is quite artificial to consider damage to the peripheral nerves as distinct from diseases that damage the spinal cord and brain. The peripheral nerves need the same important vitamins, minerals, antioxidants, and essential fats. They are also damaged by the same toxins and excessive inappropriate inflammation. In my clinics, I have seen several individuals with diabetic neuropathy and others with neuropathies in which we could not find the cause (idiopathic) respond quite favorably to adopting the Wahls Diet or Wahls Paleo Diet.

leaky gut.[13] The intestinal cells' preference for glutamine also explains why you suffer from body aches when you have the flu. Your body pulls glutamine from your muscles, leading to that deep muscle ache that accompanies many fever-related illnesses. Eating bone broth the next time you have a fever will likely reduce that achy feeling because you won't be pulling as much glutamine from your muscles. It's the secret to that old-fashioned chicken soup remedy—as long as you cook that soup broth with the chicken bones and, ideally, chicken feet. Hooves are another source of collagen. If you can get a hoof from your local butcher to add to your next soup pot, that would also contribute to an excellent broth. Our great-grandmothers were very wise! (See the recipe section at the end of the book for an easy bone broth recipe.) There is no vegetarian food substitute for bone broth. Without bone broth, you would need to take targeted supplements to obtain those key nutrients.

The Potential Harm of Vegetarianism

I hope I've convinced you that meat has a lot of great benefits for your health, but maybe you don't care. You're a vegetarian and you plan to stay that way. I understand. As I've already explained, you can be a vegetarian and still practice the Wahls Diet, but once you proceed to Wahls Paleo, vegetarianism is no longer an option.

Beyond the many benefits of animal meat, there are also many dangers that come with eating a vegetarian diet that has not been structured to ensure all the nutritional needs are met. As a physician and researcher, I do not agree that a vegetarian diet is the healthiest diet for humans—and in fact I believe it can actually be harmful, particularly if it is not practiced carefully. Furthermore, I believe that my many years as a vegetarian could have helped trigger or at a minimum accelerate my multiple sclerosis. I will not try to convince you that your religious, moral, or ethical reasons for vegetarianism are wrong, but even if you plan to continue with your plant-based diet, I believe it is important for you to understand the nutritional impact.

As my own research has led me further and further down the path of eating for health, I have become a complete convert from the vegetarian diet I used to eat. I will never be a vegetarian again. Wahls Paleo combines the most healthful aspects of vegetarianism (the 9 cups of fruits and vegetables each day) with the best aspects of the traditional Paleo diet (natural animal protein sources), and this is what I believe to be the best diet for human health.

Many people who become vegetarian stop eating meat but continue to eat a lot of highly processed foods, few vegetables, and no sources of complete protein. This leads to increasingly severe deficiencies in essential fats, protein, vitamins, minerals, and antioxidants. Such diets put them at serious risk for developing long-term health complications. But even for those vegetarians who are eating plenty of vegetables and protein, there are other compelling reasons why I believe a vegetarian diet can be harmful to health.

Vegetarian Danger 1: Skewing Your Fatty Acid Ratios

You know you need a better ratio of omega-6s to omega-3s, but what you may not know is that you probably won't get it eating only a vegetarian diet. There are many plant foods that are commonly advertised as being rich sources of omega-3 fatty acids, like flaxseeds, walnuts, and hempseeds. These foods are nutritious, and I eat them myself. However, what you may not know is that while these foods do contain omega-3 fatty acids, they also contain high levels of omega-6 fatty acids.

Also, unlike seafood and grass-fed beef, these plant sources don't actually contain omega-3 fatty acids in the form our bodies need: docosahexaenoic acid (DHA) and eicosapentaenoic acid (EPA). Instead, they contain alpha-linolenic acid (ALA), which our bodies must convert to a more usable form. ALA is a shorter chain of molecules, and your cells need to lengthen the ALA through several steps to make EPA and DHA. It is an inefficient process. Only about 5 percent (7 to 10 percent if you are pregnant) of the ALA you eat will get converted to DHA. You need to eat ten to twenty times the amount of ALA to get the equivalent amount of DHA you could get from animal sources—DHA your brain *needs*.

In studies comparing the effectiveness of high doses of olive oil, flaxseed oil, and fish oil in patients with ADHD, only those receiving the fish oil changed the ratio of omega-6 to omega-3 in the red cell membranes.[14] This is just one of many studies that show the superiority of fish oil to plant-based oils when it comes to improving the omega-6 to omega-3 ratio. There is no question that the body benefits from the omega-3s in fish oil much more than it benefits from the omega-3 ALAs in plant foods.

Vegetarian Danger 2: Vegetable Oil

As long as we're on the subject of an ideal ratio of omega-6 to omega-3, let's talk about vegetable oils, which are made by extracting the oils from seeds like corn, sunflower, or rapeseed (often using solvents like hexane, which is quite toxic—I prefer you have no exposure to these solvents, thus I recommend avoiding any refined oils and using only cold-pressed, extra virgin oils). I already told you in the last chapter that I want you to limit consumption of these oils to a few specific types and eliminate most others, but let's look more closely at why.

Vegetable oil sounds healthy, but it is one of the richest sources of omega-6 fatty acids. You need omega-6 fatty acids, but as I have already explained, they should be in balance with omega-3 fatty acids, and in this current day and age, they usually aren't. Eating vegetable oils only exacerbates the problem of excessive omega-6 intake.

But this isn't just a matter of getting a slightly better fatty acid balance. For people with autoimmune conditions, too much omega-6 can actually be dangerous. Corn oil and soybean oil are the worst offenders. They drive the ratio of omega-6 to omega-3 way out of balance, which drives inflammation. I tell my patients never to eat any corn oil or soybean oil for this reason.

Canola oil is often promoted as a source of omega-3 fatty acids, and it does contain more of these than some other vegetable oils. However, when you heat the canola oil, you break down the omega-3 fats so they become useless to your body. Furthermore, most soybean, corn, and canola oils are made from genetically modified organisms (GMOs), which I don't recommend for anyone with an autoimmune disease.

You may think olive oil is still a healthful choice, and yes, it is, on one condition: *that you never heat it!* The double bonds in olive oil are more likely to be damaged (oxidized) by heat, destroying much of the benefit. Also, the more than twenty different health-promoting polyphenols (antioxidants) that olive oil contains are destroyed when it is heated.[15] I'd rather you use it cold as part of a salad dressing or sauce so you can keep all those healthful antioxidants. Don't cook with olive oil! The best fats for cooking—the fats that remain most stable—are rendered animal fats like lard, tallow, or chicken fat. If you must use a plant-based oil, use coconut oil, which does not denature at high temperatures.

More bad news about vegetable oil: I bet you thought that trans fats were found only in processed foods, but you make them in your own kitchen and eat them unwittingly if you heat polyunsaturated oils. When vegetable oils are used for frying, especially deep-fat frying, the high heat will oxidize (damage) some of the bonds, increasing the risk of trans fat formation. The higher the heat, the more trans fats are made, and the more vitamins and antioxidants are lost in the oil (and the foods you are frying)! The more often oil is reheated, the more trans fats will be created, which is why you should never reuse frying oil. This is just one more good reason to avoid fried foods in fast-food restaurants. They certainly don't change out that french fry oil after every batch, and you can bet they use cheap vegetable oil, not lard, like they once did.

THE DANGERS OF TRANS FATS

Scientists first made trans fats back in the 1890s by adding hydrogen to fats (hydrogenation), which made them solid at room temperature. But these new fats didn't really enter the food supply until after World War II. One of the advantages of this new fat was that it was "spreadable" even under refrigeration. Also, a lot of money was spent on promoting the new cholesterol theory of heart disease, which emphasized replacing saturated fat with polyunsaturated fat (vegetable oil). The vegetable oil industry convinced the American public to replace butter with margarine (made of partially hydrogenated fats, which include trans fats) because the partially hydrogenated fats were believed healthier than the saturated fats contained in butter. How wrong they were!

Now we know trans fats are disease promoting. There is much solid research to confirm this. The trans fat molecules are inserted into our cell membranes, making the membranes stiff and interfering with the messaging between our cells. Trans fats confuse our cell chemistry as well, resulting in increased inflammation and disrupted hormone signaling in the brain.[16] The result is more rapid development of atherosclerosis (clogging of the arteries) and shrinking brains that have more difficulty communicating between the brain cells. Trans fats in the diet also increase the probability of developing obesity and diabetes. In a study by Gene L. Bowman and his colleagues[17] I've mentioned previously in which scientists measured the thinking ability and brain sizes of older adults (average age 87), they also measured brain levels of vitamins, minerals, essential fatty acids, and antioxidants, and the level of hydrogenated or trans fats in the blood. The more trans fats the study participants had, the more impaired their thinking ability and the smaller their brains.[18]

Vegetarian Danger 3: Grains and Legumes

If you are a vegetarian, you likely eat a lot of grains and legumes. It's the easiest way to get your protein. Even if you go gluten-free based on the damage gluten may do to you when you have an autoimmune disease, you will still need to combine other nongluten grains (including whole grains) with legumes to get a sufficient amount of all the essential amino acids to make a complete protein. (You may have heard that it's not true that you must combine grains and legumes at the same meal, as long as you get enough variety over the course of a few days; but the truth is that combining grains and legumes at the same meal is probably still the easiest way to be certain you get all the amino acids you need at every meal.)

But there are problems with even nongluten grains as well as with legumes. Grains and legumes contain several antinutrients that you'll get more of as a vegetarian, even if they're gluten-free. These antinutrients are phytates, lectins, and trypsin inhibitors.

- Phytate, or phytic acid, is inositol and phosphorus locked together, and it will chelate, or bind, minerals like zinc, iron, calcium, and magnesium, carrying them unused out of the body. In other words, phytates block the body's absorption of magnesium, calcium, and especially zinc, which can lead to mineral deficiencies.[19]

- Lectin is a type of sugar-protein molecule that can markedly increase inflammation in those with autoimmune problems and in genetically vulnerable individuals.[20] (Recall that you can denature most lectins by cooking grains and legumes in a pressure cooker, such as an Instant Pot.)
- Trypsin inhibitors, which primarily exist in legumes, block the digestion of the proteins crucial to maintaining your health.[21] Your efforts to eat more protein by eating legumes may be foiled by the protein source itself!

There is a way to get around some of these inhibitors, however. Germination decreases the harm from the phytates and the lectins.[22] If you soak grains, legumes, seeds, and/or nuts to begin the germination process, the plant food will produce phytase, which reduces the activity of phytates, lectins, and trypsin inhibitors. That is why I advise vegetarians to soak their grains and legumes for twenty-four hours prior to eating and wash them carefully before cooking (or use that pressure cooker on its high setting!). This also decreases the cooking time for grains and legumes. It may seem like a time-consuming or unnecessary step, but it can make a big difference in how well your body absorbs protein and hangs on to valuable minerals.

WAHLS WARRIORS SPEAK

After being diagnosed with stage 3 colon cancer and choosing radical life changes over chemotherapy, I adopted a raw vegan diet, eating only fruits, vegetables, seeds, and nuts, and I drank eight glasses of vegetable juice every day (usually carrot, celery, beet, and gingerroot). I focused on eating cancer-fighting foods every day, especially vegetables from the cruciferous and allium families: broccoli, cauliflower, cabbage, kale, onions, and garlic. I ate giant salads for lunch and dinner. I also drank fruit smoothies every day with fresh young coconut, blueberries, raspberries, blackberries, strawberries, and a banana.

However, I was not maintaining a healthy weight. After ninety days, at the recommendation of my naturopath, I added some clean meats back into my diet, including organic free-range chicken and eggs, wild-caught

Alaskan salmon, and grass-fed beef and lamb. The addition of clean meats helped me gain and maintain a healthy weight, which I was not able to do as a raw vegan. When I discovered Dr. Wahls in 2012 through her TEDx talk, I was excited to see her success in using the healing power of nutrition and her mission to share it with others. The principles of her diet are identical to the ones I followed to heal myself. I continue to follow the principles of the Wahls Diet and now I'm cancer-free. Whole foods from the earth support the body's ability to function at optimal levels: to detoxify, repair, and regenerate. They promote a healthy weight, give you energy, and make you feel good!

—Chris W., Memphis, Tennessee

Vegetarian Danger 4: Soy

Soy is one of the most popular forms of protein for people who don't eat animal products, and vegetarians, especially in the United States, tend to be heavily reliant on soy products. If you are a vegetarian, it is likely that you consume a large amount of soy because so many easy-to-make vegetarian products like veggie burgers and veggie hot dogs are made from it, and many popular vegetarian dishes contain soy foods like tofu and tempeh. Then there is soy milk, soy cheese, soy ice cream . . . Soy is one of the few vegetarian proteins considered complete by the USDA (hemp and quinoa are also, but unless they are organic, they typically contain glyphosate residue). Although some studies show some benefit to some soy products, especially for women nearing menopause, overall, soy is bad news when it is consumed in large amounts, particularly when it's not fermented.

My first concern is that 94 percent of the soy crops in the United States are genetically modified (compared to just 17 percent in 1997) and do not have to be labeled as such. These genetically modified crops are modified to be herbicide-tolerant, so they can be treated with many applications of glyphosate, a compound found in the herbicide Roundup that food giant Monsanto produces to control weeds in fields of genetically modified corn and soybeans. In fact, an increasing number of crops are now genetically modified to accommodate multiple herbicides. These include sugar beets, papaya, rapeseeds (to make canola oil), and many more. Also, many supplements are made with GMO bacteria. Many more non-GMO crops, including some legumes, grains, and hay, are finished with glyphosate to dry them more quickly for harvest. That means our dose of glyphosate (Roundup) in our food as well as in our animal feed is ever increasing, leading to greater disruption of our microbiomes in our gut as well as in the soil microbiome.

Glyphosate has been shown to be toxic to human cells grown in the lab and also to confuse hormone signaling[23] and interfere with some of the enzymes used for processing and eliminating toxins.[24] The increased use of pesticides with all GMOs and the uncertain effects of genetic modifications are reason enough for me to avoid eating them. At this point, it's a pretty good bet that anything not labeled organic or "non-GMO" is likely to be a GMO.[25] Efforts are also under way to further weaken labeling laws, prohibiting the labeling of GMO or non-GMO and the definitions for organic—this is a good reason to purchase your produce from farmers you know!

Another concern is that soy, like other legumes, also contains phytic acid, which binds to minerals, especially magnesium, calcium, and zinc, so your cells can't readily use them; lectins, which can increase inflammation in the genetically vulnerable individual;[26] and trypsin inhibitors, which can interfere with digestion. Soy also contains phytoestrogens, which are plant-based compounds that can interact with the estrogen receptors in your body. These include isoflavones, genistein, and daidzein. In traditional cultures, soy was fermented, which helped to neutralize all of these unfavorable qualities, but most of the soy we eat in this country is not fermented, so many of these antinutrients are still present in soy products like soy milk and tofu. Eating fermented soy products like tempeh and miso that are also labeled organic and/or non-GMO is the safest option. (Note that I do include some soy products in the Wahls Diet meal plan in the previous chapter, because despite their problems, they do contain nutrition that can be useful, especially for vegetarians. If you choose to use them, please do follow my recommendation for choosing organic and/or non-GMO soy products.)

Just in case that's not enough evidence for why vegetarianism is a nutritionally inferior diet, consider these additional facts relevant to what you are or are not getting if you eat a vegetarian diet:

LOVE YOUR SOY PROTEIN SMOOTHIE?

Do you make your smoothie with soy protein powder? Soy in the form of soy protein isolate is a very recent addition to the human diet. These highly processed products are often manufactured at temperatures that denature (change the shape of) the proteins, making them harder to digest.[27] We also have no historical way to predict how these fake-food meal replacement products will impact human health in the long term. Remember, scientists once told us that trans fats were better for us than butter and therefore health promoting. It took years to discover that trans fats are in fact harmful. Keep drinking those smoothies, but instead of using processed soy protein powder, just mix fresh or frozen berries and a big handful of leafy greens with some nuts or nut butter and coconut milk. Add ice or not, a little cinnamon if you like it, and enjoy—nutrient-dense but protein-powder-free. If you are going to add a protein powder to your smoothie, I suggest you use collagen from grass-fed/grass-finished animals.

- **Vitamins A and D:** Animal products are the only true sources of premade vitamins A (retinol) and D (cholecalciferol). Vegetables contain beta-carotene, which the body can convert to vitamin A, but the efficiency of this varies with the individual and some people can't do this very well.[28] Having some preformed vitamin A in the diet is helpful. Vitamin A is necessary for vision, bone health, reproductive health, and immune health.
  - Vitamin D is important to brain health, bone health, immune cell health, and the proper interpretation of DNA. The best source of vitamin D is the sun, but you can also get vitamin D from fish. Ghee (clarified butter) from organic grass-fed cows is also a good source of vitamin D as well as retinol (vitamin A), vitamin K2 MK4, and GLA. Grass-fed liver and cod-liver oil are both good sources of premade vitamin A and vitamin D as well as vitamin K2. Our wise grandmothers knew to give cod-liver oil to children each day.
- **Vitamin B$_{12}$:** To absorb cobalamin (vitamin B$_{12}$), your body will link intrinsic factor (made in the stomach) to the cobalamin molecule (obtained

through diet). Because intrinsic factor attaches well only to the animal form of cobalamin, your gut cannot readily absorb cobalamin from bacterial and algal sources. The richest source of cobalamin is liver and other organ meats. Nutritional yeast has cobalamin added to it in a form that can be absorbed, so use this liberally if you are a vegetarian. I also recommend supplementing with sublingual (under the tongue) methyl B_{12}. Methyl B_{12} is the form our brains need, and taking it sublingually means you don't need intrinsic factor in order to absorb it. Note that if you are taking folic acid or cyanocobalamin, your folate and B_{12} levels could exceed the upper level of normal, which could cause many conventional doctors to tell their patients to stop taking B-complex supplements. My approach is to check homocysteine along with B_{12}, and folate to get a better picture of whether the problem really is high homocysteine due to low B_{12} and low folate, or whether the problem is genetic SNPs that are less efficient at methylating B_{12} and folate. I suggest ongoing monitoring of homocysteine and not of folate and B_{12} (unless they were originally low), other than to monitor for good absorption. When this isn't happening, some people may need to take B_{12} by injection.

- **Stomach acid:** If you've followed a vegetarian and/or vegan diet for years, there is a greater risk of developing low stomach acid, which makes you less efficient at absorbing vitamin B_{12} (in addition to the intrinsic-factor issue mentioned above) and many minerals.[29] This can lead to a higher risk of brain and heart problems, osteoporosis, and an unhealthy balance of bacteria in the bowels, which in turn can lead to leaky gut syndrome and greater risk of autoimmune problems.

In closing this argument, I want to emphasize that I am not trying to bash vegetarians or vegans. I am only telling you what I believe is the optimal diet for those suffering from autoimmune or other chronic health conditions. You need every possible avenue to heal and maximize your health. I believe that includes a diet low in lectins and high in animal protein, with plenty of vitamin B_{12}. But you must do what best meets both your physical and your spiritual needs. See the discussion about the Wahls Elimination diet for additional guidance on strategies vegetarians can use to ensure sufficient protein and lower their exposure to lectins.

WAHLS WARRIORS SPEAK

In August 2012, I was diagnosed with multiple sclerosis. The symptoms came on suddenly: tingling and numbness in my right arm and right and left hands, bladder urgency, cognitive issues and brain fog, lower back pain, and right-foot drop. One Saturday, I was playing golf, and by the next Friday, I was using a cane to walk. I was scared and I did not know what was happening. I was started on a five-day treatment of IV steroids. I began physical and occupational therapy, and speech therapy to assist with my word-finding issues.

Desperate, I searched the Internet and read as much as I could about multiple sclerosis. I tried to discuss diet with my neurologist because I read that people with autoimmune diseases may benefit from going gluten-free.

My neurologist recommended that I stick with my "balanced" diet because gluten-free may be a fad and it was difficult to do. In October 2012, I went to a holistic practitioner who recommended that I eliminate gluten, dairy, and eggs from my diet and then take an allergy test. About that time, I discovered Dr. Wahls, whose story provided me hope. I began to incorporate the 9 cups of produce and to eat organic lean meat, lots of wild fish, seaweed, and some organ meat (though I still struggle with that). My allergy tests came back, and sure enough, I was highly sensitive to gluten, dairy, eggs, soy, and almonds. This test further validated Dr. Wahls's work.

By eliminating highly inflammatory foods and replacing them with vegetables, lean meat, and seaweed, your body can heal. It's been four months since I started the Wahls Diet, and I've increased my vitamin D levels from 17 to 52, my medicine has been reduced, and I have lost 14 pounds. I now exercise and run two miles several times per week, walk three miles a day, bike, swim, strength-train, meditate, and stretch daily. I prepare smoothies and real meals in my kitchen. Gone are the days of eating out or ordering takeout three to four times a week. By eating this way, my energy levels have increased, my brain fog and stumbling over words has been eliminated, my skin looks great, and I am more alert and present. It is not easy eating this way, and my family has also had to make some adjustments, but in the end, I choose health. I am more in tune with my body and I feed it the fuel it needs to thrive.

—Michelle M., Baltimore, Maryland

Part Three: Add Seaweed and Organ Meat

Our ancient ancestors were scavengers and hunters on African savannas millions of years ago. Food was precious, so if we killed a small animal, we ate the liver, heart, kidney, and brain, in addition to the muscle meat. We also benefited from the kills of larger predators, like lions. When lions killed their prey, they smartly ate the organ meats first. The hyenas and jackals ate the muscle meat. Our ancestors, however, were able to use early tools to break open the remaining skulls and long bones and eat the brains and marrow, which are rich sources of DHA, a key nutrient for brain growth.

We also waded in coastal waters and ate shellfish, again using our early tools to pry open the clams and mussels we found. Seaweed and sea vegetables, rich with iodine and dense concentrations of minerals, were also on the menu. These adaptations are widely believed to be what gave us the competitive advantage to survive and grow larger, more complex brains.[30] If we want to keep those big brains, we need to feed ourselves and our children more parts of the animals we eat and more vegetables from the sea, packing our diets even more full of vitamins, minerals, and antioxidants.

You: Sea Creature?

Life began more than 3 billion years ago in mineral-rich seas. Our bloodstream mineral content reflects those ancient seas: We still have a little of the ocean within us. I believe this is why the human body responds so favorably to the plant foods that grow in the oceans. Seaweed contains intense mineral nutrition as well as beneficial vitamins. Eat romaine lettuce and kale all day if you like, but adding seaweed will take your nutrition to a whole new level.

Seaweed has been used medicinally, in spas, and in food for thousands of years.[31] Traditional peoples traveled great distances or traded to ensure access to seaweed. They may not have known that seaweed provides a rich supply of minerals, but somehow they knew the value of this important food source. Traditional coastal communities in particular have naturally consumed seaweed as part of their diets, and historically Japanese and Okinawans have had 10 to 15 percent of their diet come from seaweed. These cultures have a much lower rate of heart disease, diabetes, and autoimmune problems, even though the rate of smoking and salt consumption is higher in the Japanese and Okinawans. However, as the young people abandon the traditional diets in favor of Westernized diets high in simple sugars and refined carbohydrates, we have seen the incidence of those chronic diseases steadily climb.

Sea vegetables contain nutrient profiles you can't get anywhere else. In particular, they are rich sources for iodine, which has many important functions in the body.[32] The thyroid gland, the gland that directs the metabolism and energy level of the body, is highly dependent upon iodine. In addition, the white blood cells use iodine as part of their arsenal in attacking and killing invading viruses, bacteria, and cancer cells. Iodine also helps the body properly process and then eliminate heavy metals like lead and mercury. If your diet has been low in minerals, vitamins, and antioxidants, and you or someone in your family has a history of brain or heart problems, you probably have some toxins such as lead and mercury in your fat, which includes the fat in your brain. When you are low in iodine, you are more likely to have problems with an enlarged thyroid or goiter and an underactive thyroid gland (hypothyroidism). You are also more likely to have problems clearing infections like Lyme disease.

Iodine and trace mineral intake has steadily declined in the United States over the course of the last half century, in part because physicians have been telling patients to cut back on salt. Iodized salt has been the primary source of iodine for most Americans. To make matters worse, we've been steadily adding to our diets halogen compounds that interfere with the iodine receptors in our cells, primarily through the addition of fluoride and chlorine to the water supply and bromine to the food supply. Because these halogens are chemically similar to iodine, they compete for the iodine receptors. (Some foods—including soy, flax, and the cabbage family vegetables, if consumed raw—can also slightly interfere with iodine uptake, but the benefits of these foods, as long as you also consume some seaweeds, outweigh this consideration. Cooking cabbage family vegetables can also help.)

Thus our daily requirement for iodine has increased at the same time that our intake has fallen. It is true we are taking in far more salt and that doctors advise against this trend, but the salt we tend to eat the most is the kind in processed foods, and that salt is generally not the iodized kind. Americans cook less at home, so they use less iodized salt or choose other types of salt. In response to falling iodine levels, hypothyroidism levels have steadily climbed, with some estimates putting the level of American women affected at 10 to 25 percent, all largely a result of iodine insufficiency. Fortunately for you, you needn't add more salt to your diet to get more iodine. Seaweed is a rich natural source of iodine.

WAHLS WARNING

Because of the radiation release following the Japanese earthquake and subsequent tsunami in 2011, and the continued release of radiation into the ocean that is likely to be emitted from this site for hundreds if not thousands of years, as well as the partial meltdown of the nuclear reactors that followed, many wonder about the safety of seaweed from Japan and China. These days, I am purchasing my seaweed from companies located in Canada and Maine. For convenience, I look for powdered kelp and dulse flakes that have been harvested from clean waters, are sustainably harvested and labeled organic, and have been tested for radioactivity, heavy metals, and pesticide content to provide added safety. You can also purchase dried seaweed from the companies listed in the Resources section.

Seaweed also contains many valuable minerals, including calcium, copper, chromium, iron, iodine, lithium, manganese, magnesium, potassium, selenium, silicon, sulfur, vanadium, and zinc. You'll also get vitamins in the vitamin B group (B_1, B_2, B_3, B_5, B_6, B_9) and vitamins A, C, E, and K. Other useful compounds include alginates, which are very helpful in increasing the elimination of solvents, plastics, heavy metals, and even radioactivity in the body,[33] and U-fucoidans, which improve the effectiveness of the white blood cells in fighting chronic viral infections.[34]

There are thousands of different seaweeds, which are categorized into three groups: green, brown, and red. The colors indicate which type of chlorophyll is present in the plant. The green seaweeds, such as sea lettuce, must grow in shallow water near the shore. The brown seaweeds can grow a hundred feet below the surface, and the red seaweeds can grow four hundred feet below the surface. Ideally, we should be consuming all colors of seaweed for optimal benefit.

This isn't as difficult as it sounds. You might not have noticed, but your local supermarket may carry some sea vegetables, and your natural foods store almost certainly has at least a few packaged varieties to choose from. Seaweed comes in various forms, including fresh, dried, reconstituted, flakes, and powdered. The supplement section may also include powdered versions. If you go to Asian food markets, you will be able to find large bags of a wide variety of seaweeds. However, these will have been harvested in the Pacific ocean. I prefer seaweed from a company that tests for heavy metals and radiation. (See the Resources section.)

If you are not being treated with thyroid medication, I suggest you start with a small amount. I'd also mix up the types of seaweeds you eat. The simplest is to alternate between kelp powder and dulse flakes. Start with ¼ teaspoon once a week for a month. Then twice a week for a month, then every other day. If that is going well, then you can go to the equivalent of ¼ teaspoon every day. It is best if you are adding seaweed to what you are cooking and eating. That way your taste for the food will help guide how much you are consuming. Alternatively, if you can find fresh seaweed or dried seaweed, you can add that to your cooking. The point is to gradually increase the seaweed and to use a variety of seaweeds.

Here's how much seaweed I would like you to work up to eating every day on Wahls Paleo. Choose one of the following each day:

IF YOU ARE ON THYROID MEDICATION, READ THIS FIRST

If you are being treated for an under- or overactive thyroid, adding seaweed to your diet will likely change the amount of thyroid medication that you require. Check in with your physician for guidance. Slowly add seaweed to the diet, starting with once a week, adding seaweed to the foods you are cooking. Gradually increase the frequency and amount of seaweed you are adding, and check in with your physician to monitor your thyroid levels. You may find that your medication needs to be adjusted downward (very rarely upward). Make changes very gradually and work closely with your personal physician.

- **Fresh (or soaked and reconstituted):** 2.5 ounces. One ounce of dried seaweed will reconstitute to about 1 cup of fresh seaweed.
- **Dried flakes:** 1 teaspoon in the form of flakes
- **Granules:** ½ teaspoon
- **Powdered:** ¼ teaspoon

WAHLS WARRIORS SPEAK

Just before Christmas 2011, I finally told a few dear friends that I had been diagnosed with RRMS [relapsing-remitting MS]. The next day I received an e-mail from one of them with a link to Dr. Wahls's TEDx talk, and her discussion resonated in me. I watched it over and over and was grateful to know that my craving for liver and onions once a month was exactly what I needed! Memories of gnawing on bones with my grandmother and lunching on sardines with my mother-in-law made me smile and gave me hope. The Wahls Diet made total sense to me right from the first moment I heard about it. I began to follow her diet that day, and within a week, I noticed a remarkable change in the pressure in my head, my vision, and my ability to, as I call it, "think straight." I have thanked my friend many times.
—Debra K., Accord, New York

"Organ"-ize Yourself

I get even more resistance from my patients about eating organ meats than I do about eating seaweed. I'm not sure why, because just a few generations ago, organ meats were a common part of Western diets. I have my great-grandmother's cookbook, an 1890 edition of *Compendium of Cookery and Reliable Recipes and the Book of Knowledge,* and my grandmother's 1939 *The Boston Cooking School Cook Book* by Fannie Farmer. Both cookbooks include many recipes for a wide variety of organ meats. My great-grandmother had recipes for boiled calf's head, sweetbreads, brains, tongue, tripe, heart, and liver, all of which were designed for cooking over a fire or a woodstove. I remember my mother making liver and onions at least once a week, and we kids all ate a good helping. For some reason, however, Americans have become squeamish about this healthful habit.

Weston A. Price, in his studies of the diets of traditional societies around the globe, analyzed organ meats and found them full of what he called "powerful activators" (the term *vitamins* had not yet been adopted).[35] Animal proteins, particularly the organ meats, concentrate fat-soluble and water-soluble vitamins. Liver is the richest source of the whole family of B vitamins and is the best source of vitamin B_{12}. The organ meats, liver in particular, are rich sources of vitamin A (retinol), which is critical for many functions in our cells. Liver also contains premade vitamin D (cholecalciferol). The organ meats are excellent sources of easily absorbed zinc, magnesium, phosphorus, and other minerals.

The liver, heart, kidneys, and other organ meats are potent sources of both the fat-soluble vitamins D, A, E, and K, and the B vitamins, and in an organic, grass-fed animal, good sources of the essential fatty acids, including desirable omega-3s. Organ meats are also excellent sources of creatine, carnitine, alpha-lipoic acid, and ubiquinone (which is coenzyme Q10), all of which are needed for optimal functioning of the mitochondria. Although we can manufacture coenzyme Q10 when we are young, by the time we are 50 years old, our capacity for doing so slowly declines (rapidly with some medications, especially the statin family of medications, which are used to treat elevated cholesterol).

Organ meats have a more intense taste than muscle meats, so they might take some getting used to, but there are good ways to prepare them. Here are some key points:

- **Eat organ meats several times each week, for a total of 12 ounces per week.** Leave the organ meats as rare as you are comfortable eating them. Well-done organ meats will be dry, tough, and less pleasant to eat. Gently cooked organ meats will be juicier and tastier, and retain more vitamins. Limit liver to 6 ounces per week and have the other 6 ounces be other organ meats such as shellfish, heart, or tongue. (All shellfish are technically organ meats because you are eating the entire animal, not just the muscle.)

- **Start with heart.** Heart may be the easiest to start with because you will think you are having a good steak. Note that heart is the best source of coenzyme Q10 available to us.
- **Cut up the liver into small chunks and then blend the chunks with water to make a liver slurry.** This could be added to the next soup or chili as another way to "hide" the organ meat. Or try making pâté.
- **Add ground liver to ground meat (10% liver) for your next ground-meat-based dish.** This could be used for taco or spaghetti sauce, and is a great way to "hide" the liver.
- **Add kelp or dulse to organ meat recipes to enrich your recipes with more trace minerals.** Add this to a recipe along with the liver slurry and you've got seaweed and organ meat in one dish!

For recipe ideas, see the recipe section at the end of this book.

WAHLS WARRIORS SPEAK

I was diagnosed with MS in July 2012, and honestly, I was not sure what to expect with it. Since my diagnosis, and thanks to my sister, I jumped rather quickly on trying to fix it and immediately started doing extensive research on the Wahls Diet. I have always been very active and fit, and I thought my diet was always good, but now I know I was consuming hormones and chemicals. I now eat only organic, hormone-free food. I make a smoothie every morning consisting of about 3 cups of kale; parsley; sprouted sesame, sunflower, and pumpkin seeds; sprouted walnuts; ginger; sea salt; spirulina powder; BioKefir Immunity; and a few different fruits. This makes almost 64 ounces for my breakfast and lunch smoothies. I try to eat organ meat once per week, and I also eat wild-caught fish several times a week, California sushi rolls, and seaweed salad. I stay clear of the foods tests have shown I'm allergic to, one of which is dairy, and I had all six of my fillings that had mercury in them replaced. I am working hard to follow Dr. Wahls's recommendations in full and I am happy with my health.

—DeLeia A. Indiana

Part Four: Add More Raw, Soaked, and Fermented Foods

Enzymes are catalysts that make it easier for your body to do its work. They facilitate chemical reactions like those necessary for digestion and the absorption of nutrients. As we age, our effectiveness at manufacturing enzymes declines. In the presence of a nutritionally inadequate diet, the situation gets worse. By supplying some of the digestive enzymes we need in the foods we eat, we can ensure more effective digestion and absorption of nutrients.[36] There are three good ways to do this:

1. Eat more raw foods.
2. Eat more soaked nuts and seeds.
3. Eat more fermented foods.

Let's consider these one at a time.

Raw Deal

In the beginning, our ancestors ate all of their food raw. Even when we began cooking our foods approximately 100,000 years ago, we still consumed a large proportion of it raw, including meat. Cooking foods breaks down cell walls, making some of the digestive processes easier and allowing for more absorption of the minerals and vitamins, but all raw plant- and animal-based foods are loaded with enzymes that trigger the digestion process for that food. However, once the food is heated above 117 degrees Fahrenheit, all those helpful digestive enzymes are denatured (i.e., the shapes change), which means they are no longer biologically active and have been, in essence, destroyed. Considering how much potent nutritional power animal protein has, it would be a shame not to absorb it all; yet that's what many people do when they cook— and especially when they overcook—their meat and vegetables.

Here's an interesting example of this principle in action. The first explorers of the Arctic region, who carted along their Westernized cooked rations, all died. The explorers who followed them and chose to eat according to Inuit traditions (raw meat) survived and even put on weight during their extreme experience, even though they were not native to that area or climate. Many hunter-gatherer and traditional diets include not just raw vegetables and fruits, nuts, and seeds, but raw meat, as well as fermented meat and pickled meat, which is only "cooked" via the fermentation or pickling solution rather than heat.[37]

WAHLS WARRIORS SPEAK

Since changing my eating habits, I have not had an MS symptom in more than four weeks. My skin has cleared up, I sleep better, I have stopped taking my acid reflux medicine, and my dizziness and balance issues have been significantly reduced. I am on the Wahls Paleo Diet, and I don't eat anything prepackaged unless it is grass-fed meats. I am grain-free, sugar-free, soy-free, and chemical-free; I go organic as much as possible; and I eat plenty of veggies and colors. I like that I am discovering new and colorful foods that taste good! Everything is so much fresher now, and I also thoroughly enjoy the fact that I don't have the daily muscle spasms in my chest that felt like a heart attack! I exercise three to four times a week with biking, swimming, running, calisthenics, and a weekly yoga class. Dr. Wahls has been an inspiration and a great source of encouragement. If I had not seen her video on feeding your mitochondria, I may not have even considered that what I eat could save me from pain and suffering.
—*Jodi M., Thornton, Denver, Colorado*

Today, unfortunately, there are health risks to eating raw meat, because when food is processed in massive amounts—mixing meat from hundreds of animals, as it is done at the large meat-processing plants—contamination of meat from unhealthy animals is more likely. Because of the health risk of contaminated meat, particularly in conventionally raised animals housed in massive operations, I generally don't recommend raw meat. There are times and situations where it could be appropriate: a well-prepared steak tartare from a trustworthy source, for example, or sushi from a responsible restaurant. However, one needs to be very cautious about the source of any raw meats.

WAHLS WARNING

If you choose to eat raw meats, be sure to store the meat in a deep freeze for at least two weeks before consuming, then marinate the meat in vinegar and salt for twenty-four hours prior to consumption. This will decrease the probability of bacteria and parasitic contamination but does not take it down to zero, so be aware of the very real risk of infection if you choose to do this. This risk is especially high with factory-farmed and feedlot meat.

A much safer route is to include plenty of raw fruits and vegetables in your diet and to use low-temperature cooking, for as brief a time as possible, of clean, preferably organ meat obtained directly from a farmer you trust. Order your meat rare when you can, or at least as rare as possible for you to eat it happily, and enjoy pickled meat and fish when you can get them.

Raw fruits and vegetables are, of course, easy to find and eat. I like to include raw plant food with every meal, whether a big salad or fruit for dessert, or the mixture of fruits and greens I put into my smoothie. If raw food upsets your stomach, start slowly and eat small amounts as your system adjusts. Even a little raw food is better than no raw food.

Soaking and Sprouting

One of the requirements of the Wahls Paleo level is to eat 4 ounces of nuts or seeds every day. But as you have already learned, nuts and seeds (as well as legumes and grains) contain antinutrients like phytates, lectins, and trypsin inhibitors. Not only can soaking and sprouting reduce these antinutrients enough that you will digest these foods better, but this process also generates more enzymes, further improving digestibility and nutrient absorption.

Although you will be only eating nongluten grains, legumes, and starchy vegetables twice a week at most on Wahls Paleo, soaking these foods will also increase their benefits.

But how do you do it? The first step to easy sprouting is soaking.[38]

1. Put your nuts, seeds, grains, or legumes in a glass jar or bowl. Cover them with water.

2. Soak them for twenty-four hours to initiate the germination process. This will increase the enzyme phytase, which eliminates those mineral-binding phytates, toxic lectins, and trypsin inhibitors. Nuts will also begin to manufacture other enzymes, including trypsin, which will aid in their easy digestion.

3. After the initial soaking period, you can consume your nuts, seeds, grains, or legumes, drying them in a dehydrator or oven at a low temperature (keep the heat under 177 degrees) until they are crispy again (for nuts and seeds), or cooking them (for grains and legumes).

4. For even greater benefits, you can continue the germination process by rinsing the nuts, seeds, grains, or legumes in a fine mesh strainer three times per day, then returning them to the jar with fresh water to decrease the risk of mold or harmful bacteria developing. You may not see any sprouts, but the enzymes will generate rapidly with this process over three days. Since that is what I am most interested in, I generally stop by the third day and use the food.[39]

GO NUTS!

Forget roasted nuts. Raw nuts are helpful to include in your diet because they provide some key nutrients. I advocate eating raw soaked or sprouted nuts in particular, especially almonds, walnuts, sunflower seeds, and hazelnuts. Walnuts are a good source of health-promoting omega-3 fatty acids. Almonds and sunflower seeds are excellent sources of vitamin E, a group of eight fat-soluble compounds (tocopherols and tocotrienols) that are potent antioxidants and provide key protection to myelin in the brain. They also protect cell membranes from free radical damage. I recommend eating up to 4 ounces of soaked nuts every day. Cold-pressed nut oils such as walnut and almond oil also make excellent additions to salad dressings and smoothies. (Never heat nut oils over 170 degrees or you will damage the essential oils and antioxidants.)

Some people have food allergies or sensitivities to tree nuts and will not be able to tolerate them. If you perceive that you have a problem with headache, fatigue, or any troubling symptom that is worse when eating tree nuts, stay away from them. Instead, try soaked or sprouted sunflower or pumpkin seeds as an alternative. If those both bother you, then you will need to find other sources of vitamin E, such as avocado or olive oil. Always check with your doctor for guidance if you have severe food allergies.

5. At a minimum, soak grains, legumes, nuts, and seeds for twenty-four hours, but you can continue to the sprouting phase, even beyond three days, until you see sprouts and leaves. As soon as you can actually see a sprout, eat the food right away. Sprouts are fragile and easily contaminated with bacteria that can cause diarrhea, so fresh is best. (This is another reason I generally don't sprout food for longer than three days: This minimizes the chances of bacterial contamination.)

6. After you are done soaking, do one final rinse, and your soaked, sprouted food is ready to eat.

To eat soaked nuts, seeds, grains, or legumes, you could:

1. Blend them with water.
2. Blend the nuts in a high-powered blender such as a Vitamix to make your own homemade nut milk.
3. Use the nuts combined with an avocado as a base for a pudding.
4. Put the soaked nuts or seeds in a dehydrator at the lowest temperature overnight and have a lovely crunchy snack that is packed with minerals, enzymes, and essential fatty acids. (You could also dry them in a low oven, if you can set your oven below 117 degrees.) Our family especially loves sprouted walnuts.
5. Immediately cook grains or legumes after soaking/sprouting.
6. Alternatively, cook dried gluten-free grains and legumes in a pressure cooker on high. This is what my mother and grandmother routinely did when they made soups and stews.

WAHLS WARRIORS SPEAK

After my MS diagnosis, I experienced many of the bad symptoms that come with a diagnosis of multiple sclerosis: extreme fatigue, brain fog, depression, poor balance, depth perception issues, lost sight in my right eye, MS hug, and lost use of my right hand, making it difficult to start my car, put socks on, or grab anything, really. Also, I was severely numb from the neck down, and not being able to feel my feet on the ground made it very difficult to walk or drive. After weeks of reading and research, I stumbled onto the infamous YouTube video of Dr. Terry Wahls, and that changed my life forever! That was my wake-up call. After experiencing these awful symptoms, I realized I needed to work harder on myself and decided to tackle my health issues head on. Since diagnosed, I have lost over 130 pounds, gone back to school to learn more about nutrition and how lifestyle changes support disease management, started a nutritional therapy/consulting business, and started a nonprofit called Change MS to provide support to others! It was not easy making lifestyle choices, but they can be a game changer. I was able to regain most of my function—brain fog and depression were close to nonexistent and my energy is through the roof! I am in the best shape of my life. I found for me, level 2 [Wahls Paleo] was the most beneficial, but I do jump into level 3 [Wahls Paleo Plus] a few times a year with longer periods of fasting. Looking at the end goal can be intimidating. Make each step your priority for the day, and you can climb beyond your expectations!

—Tony F., Elma, New York

Fermented Foods

Each of us is an ecosystem. We have 30 trillion body cells and about the same number of microbial cells[40] living on and in us—making us roughly half human, if you think about it on a cell-for-cell basis. However, we have about 25,000 human genes, and the microbes within and on us have 5 to 9 million genes! Every moment, trillions of chemical reactions are being driven by these microbes. As a community, they are called the microbiome, but because we have coevolved with them, I like to call them our "old friends." Many of the by-products they produce within our gastrointestinal systems (most of them live in the colon) as they ferment the food we eat are useful to us, helping build our immune systems, absorb nutrients, even influence mood (most of your mood-influencing serotonin is produced in your gastrointestinal system by the bacteria that live there).[41] The evidence is growing that the microbes in our guts speak to our immune cells, either calming the immune cells or revving up inflammation. The "old friend" microbes that keep our system running smoothly depend on the amount of soluble fiber and resistant starch in our diets. The more fiber and more vegetables patients consume, the fewer MS attacks the person has.

It is also apparent the microbes in the gut influence the level of inflammation in the brain, and the probability of acute relapse in those with brain-involved chronic diseases like MS. In fact, there are an increasing number of studies that demonstrate that the mix of microbes are different in those with MS than in those who are healthy.[42] As knowledge increases in this area, scientists and clinicians are increasingly recognizing that microbiome optimization is important for MS patients.

FIBER, RESISTANT STARCH, AND . . . POOP

To have good diversity in your microbiome, not only do you need more good bacteria coming in, but you also need soluble fiber and resistant starch because these are the foods our health-promoting microbes need to eat. You could get more sophisticated stool tests to know which microbes and microbial metabolites you have, or you could just look at your bowel movements each day and adjust your fiber intake to have a daily soft, easily passed stool (but not so much that you have fecal accidents).

In my talks, I often discuss poop. It's guaranteed to make people laugh (sometimes uncomfortably), but I could not be more serious when I say that your poop is a good indicator of your microbiome and overall health. The Bristol Stool Chart uses numbers to describe bowel movements from dry hard lumps (1) to diarrhea (7) with a variety of textures between 1 and 7. I think it is much more helpful to talk about rocks, logs, snakes, pudding, and tea.

If you are pooping tea or pudding, either you have acute diarrhea and things will quickly return to normal, or you have a chronic problem that needs to be evaluated for a chronic infection, parasites, or inflammatory bowel disease. I tell my patients who have inflammatory bowel disease or soft pudding and tea stools that they need less fiber. That means no raw vegetables or fruit. Instead, I advise more bone broth and thoroughly cooked soups and stews. Also, this kind of stool means you need to investigate to understand the root cause of the problem if it persists.

If you are pooping soft snakes, that is the ideal poop. Go for those snakes—they are your poop sweet spot! Many of us with a neurological issue have trouble with sphincter control and are at risk for accidental leakage of urine or stool if stools get too soft. As a result, you may find that snakes are hard to control and occasionally get into your pants. Simply titrate the amount of fiber in your diet to achieve soft, easily passed bowel movements without accidents.

If you are pooping rocks or dry logs (with cracks), I recommend that you increase dietary fiber. You need more raw vegetables and more soluble fiber. You can add gluten-free fibers such as inulin, green banana flour, or larch to your smoothies or tea. You could use chia seed to make chia pudding. (I make it in the morning and allow it to soak all day to begin the germination process. I eat the pudding for breakfast the next day. Sometimes I add a probiotic capsule to make a fermented chia pudding—quite delicious and another way to add more fermented foods to the diet.) Increase your fiber until your stool is soft and easy to pass.

Scientists continue to deepen our understanding of how these microbes influence our health, but we do know this much: What we eat has everything to do with that bowel population of critters. Are you creating an unruly mob in there, or a well-behaved, health-promoting population of good bacteria citizens? Are your microbes facilitating the improvement of your health and vitality, or are they worsening your health and facilitating the development of chronic symptoms and disease?[43]

What does all this have to do with fermentation? Fermented food, such as sauerkraut and other lacto-fermented vegetables, fruits, and meats, are filled with friendly, health-promoting lactobacillus bacteria (hence the term *lacto-fermentation*) that can improve your microbiome balance. Thousands of years ago, our ancestors learned how to harness the power of lacto-fermentation to help preserve the plentiful food they had available during the growing season so it would last over the long winter. They didn't know they were also improving their microbiome health and adding more vitamins and antioxidants to the foods, but they received these excellent health benefits nevertheless.

Fermentation happens when fresh food is combined with salt and sealed. The absence of oxygen encourages the growth of anaerobic bacteria, which grows in the food, transforming it into a whole new product.

The initial fermentations humans probably undertook involved fermenting honey to make mead and then eventually beer and wine. Next, they likely began to ferment roots and greens as well as meat and, in some cultures, milk.

SHOULD YOU TAKE A PROBIOTIC SUPPLEMENT?

Probiotic supplements contain beneficial bacteria and yeasts that are meant to improve the balance in the microbiome. Whether this actually happens or not is controversial. The microbes in the probiotics are generally not capable of colonizing the human gut. Probiotic supplements can add 5 billion to 15 billion live cultures per capsule to the bowels, but even these seemingly high numbers will not have much chance of making an impact in the midst of the 100 trillion bacteria and yeasts living in and on your body, especially if you keep feeding the more pathogenic microbes with a diet of processed food and sugar. Spore-based probiotics are more likely than non-spore-based probiotics to persist after the probiotics are stopped. Higher doses of probiotics are also more likely to persist for longer, but if you really want your microbe mix to change, you have to change what you eat. Adding more fiber and more fermented foods—especially those you make yourself—is a much more effective way to add (and keep) the friendly, health-promoting bacteria back in your system.[44]

You also need to feed that good bacteria with soluble fiber (from vegetables, seeds, and fruits, especially psyllium seed husks, ground flax or chia seeds, inulin, green banana flour, larch, prunes, berries, almonds, legumes, cabbages, onions, and mushrooms).

Probiotic supplements have a better chance of making an impact in a friendly environment, so once your gut is doing better (such as after you have been on any level of the Wahls Protocol for a while and following it diligently), they could be beneficial for you. If you do use probiotics, rotate the kinds you use, to increase the variety of species you are introducing into your system.

But we don't eat the way our ancestors ate, and our dietary changes have also affected our "old friends." Over the past hundred years our diet has shifted, containing many more carbohydrate-rich foods like sugar, white flour (including gluten-free white flours), white rice, and white potatoes. As a result, unfamiliar species are thriving in our microbiome and our old reliable friends are dying off. With each round of antibiotics, we kill off many more beneficial bacteria, encouraging an overgrowth of sugar-loving yeasts (*Candida*) and giving the bad guys an even greater advantage.

By removing processed foods and replacing them with greens, sulfur, and color (the 9 cups), you will provide the good bacteria in your bowels with the fiber they need to thrive, but eating more fermented foods with live cultures will help return your bowels to a healthier condition. Traditional cultures would have a live-culture fermented food with every meal. You can, too. (I do.)

Fermented Choices

Not sure what fermented foods to eat? These are the ones I recommend:

- **Yogurt and kefir.** Yogurt is probably the most common fermented food in the American diet. Kefir is a similar food, but thinner, more like a beverage. However, because I have instructed you to avoid dairy, you should still avoid milk-based yogurt and kefir. Instead, there are lacto-fermented almond and coconut milk yogurts and kefir products that are delicious served with fresh berries or blended into smoothies—or all by themselves, if you enjoy the tart flavor. Choose unsweetened varieties.

- **Kombucha tea.** This is a delicious combination of yeast and bacteria. Kombucha is made by adding a kombucha mother (a pancake-shaped symbiotic colony of bacteria and yeast) to green or black tea along with some sugar, which is digested by the bacteria. You can buy it in health food stores or possibly in your regular supermarket. You can also make it at home. (See the recipe at the back of this book.) If you are diabetic or pre-diabetic, you want to lower your sugar intake. In that case, dilute kombucha with water, or allow it to ferment on the counter for another week to reduce the sugar content.

- **Lacto-fermented cabbage, sauerkraut, kimchi, and pickles.** See the recipes and Resources section at the back of this book. You can also buy these, but note that the lacto-fermented varieties do not contain vinegar. Use several different brands (especially those made locally) of fermented foods, as each company has a unique mix of bacterial species in their products. Be sure the food label says "live culture." You will find these in the refrigerated section.

- **Nutritional yeast** (*Saccharomyces cerevisiae*). This food product is grown on sugarcane or beet molasses for several days and is then killed by heat and dried, typically forming into light yellow flakes. It is rich in B vitamins, RNA (ribonucleic acid), minerals, and protein. Additional B vitamins, including cobalamin (vitamin B_{12}), are often added, making it a very useful foodstuff for vegetarians. However, nutritional yeast has naturally occurring free glutamate, which may act as an excitotoxin for some, leading to headache and irritability. Note that people with inflammatory bowel disease and systemic lupus are more likely not to be able to tolerate nutritional yeast. If you have either of these conditions, I don't recommend nutritional yeast.

- Nutritional yeast is not the same as *Candida* yeasts, which are potentially harmful yeasts common in the human gut, and nutritional yeast will not increase or affect the growth of *Candida*. It has a rich, cheese-like flavor that can make the transition to dairy-free easier, so if it agrees with you, then by all means enjoy it. If you have any sense that it is causing you headaches or that you have any other problems with it, do not use it. (Note that brewer's yeast is also made from *Saccharomyces cerevisiae*, but it does not have the B$_{12}$ added and does not have that rich cheese-like taste that many enjoy in nutritional yeast. This is why most people prefer nutritional yeast.)

Non-grain-based spirits. Because beer and many distilled spirits are made from grain, I suggest avoiding those unless they are specifically labeled gluten-free. However, non-grain-based spirits such as rum, wine, and gluten-free beer are permissible . . . and they are fermented. (For best health outcomes—lowest risk of cancer, stroke, heart disase, and all-cause mortality—I recommend

WHY SOME FERMENTED FOODS MIGHT GIVE YOU TROUBLE (AND WHAT TO DO ABOUT IT)

Some people with MS have evidence of an overgrowth of *Candida albicans*, a harmful yeast, in their bowels.[45] The *Candida* species releases by-products that diffuse into the bloodstream and can be toxic to brain cells and mitochondria, leading to severe fatigue and brain fog.[46] This can occur because of antibiotic use as a child or an adult and/or because of a sugar/carb-intensive diet. It could also occur because of acid-lowering medication.[47]

Some people who have trouble with *Candida* may find that they cannot tolerate nutritional yeast or even any kind of mushroom. Some with MS and autoimmune problems cannot tolerate products made through yeast fermentation, either, like kombucha, vinegar, and wine. I did not eliminate such foods from my diet, and most of my clinic patients and study patients have done well with nutritional yeast, but I do acknowledge that the occasional person will do better removing all yeast products and mushrooms. There will be some MS patients who do better if they avoid all products of yeast fermentation, including wine and vinegars. This is an individual matter, so if you eat these foods, pay attention to how well you tolerate them.

alcohol not be consumed daily. Women should have no more than one small glass of wine or beer or one shot of spirits no more than a few times a week. Men should have no more than two.)

This is the essence of Wahls Paleo: Cut back on your carbs, eat more meat, gradually add seaweed and organ meat as your taste buds adjust, and eat more raw, soaked, and fermented foods every day. It won't take long before you'll be noticing a distinct and wonderful difference in your health. You're eating more like your ancestors now, and that ancient, natural, healthy glow is going to creep back in. Keep going, stay strong, and if you make a mistake or eat something you shouldn't, forgive yourself and get back on track. Wahls Paleo is your path to healing, so why not get on that path as soon as possible?

Below is a box containing all the basic rules for Wahls Paleo, followed by one week of Wahls Paleo meals.

CALL TO ACTION

To get a colorful free printable one-page summary of the foods on Wahls Paleo, go to terrywahls.com/bonus.

WAHLS PALEO AT A GLANCE

For Wahls Paleo, you will follow all the rules for the Wahls Diet (the 9 cups, gluten-free, dairy-free, and all other foods and processes forbidden or limited, including eggs, nonorganic soy, refined sweeteners, and microwaving). You will also add these additional rules. Continue to eat to satiety. You may increase or decrease the amount of vegetables, fruit, and meat you eat according to your size, but make sure to do so in proportion:

- Increase grass-fed, wild-caught meat and fish intake to 9 to 21 ounces per day, according to your size and gender. Include 16 ounces per week of wild-caught cold-water fish (herring, sardines, salmon) as part of your total animal protein allowance.

- Work up to 2.5 ounces of fresh or reconstituted seaweed, 1 teaspoon dried flakes, or ¼ teaspoon powdered seaweed daily.
- Eat 12 ounces of organ meat per week as part of your total animal protein allowance.
- Have lacto-fermented food daily.
- Have up to 4 ounces of nuts and seeds daily, either raw or soaked for twenty-four hours.
- Limit white potatoes, gluten-free grains, and legumes to two servings per week. (This is a maximum—even better, eliminate these foods completely.)
- Fats permissible for heating are ghee, coconut oil, lard, and other rendered animal fats, such as duck fat and chicken fat. Do not cook with any vegetable oils other than coconut oil.
- Eliminate all nonfermented soy products. (Tempeh and miso are still okay, but tempeh is often made with grain, so be sure it is gluten-free—and it counts as one of your two weekly grain servings.)

Wahls Paleo Meal Plan

I hope you are excited about ramping up this new, slightly more challenging, but so much more therapeutic level of the Wahls Protocol. Here is a sample seven-day meal plan to help you transition successfully into Wahls Paleo.

Wahls Paleo Week

All foods that have corresponding recipes at the end of this book are marked with an asterisk (*). These are just suggestions—once you are comfortable with Wahls Paleo, you can construct your own meals. Just remember that it is always a good idea to rotate your food, rather than eating the same thing every day. Rotate your greens, your organ meats, your sea vegetables, even your nuts and seeds, and enjoy the bounty and wonderful variety that nature has provided.

	Breakfast	**Lunch**	**Dinner**
Day 1	Smoothie: • 1 cup bok choy • 1 cup orange sections (2 small) • 1 cup pineapple • 1 tablespoon nutritional yeast • water/ice 2 medium chicken breasts without skin (6 ounces is the amount we used in our recipe analysis)	1 serving Basic Skillet Recipe* (Pork Chops and Red Cabbage) Salad: • 3 cups bok choy • 1 small tomato (½ cup) • ½ cup sweet red pepper • ½ cup daikon radish • 1 tablespoon sliced almonds • 1 tablespoon extra virgin olive oil • balsamic vinegar to taste Fruit cup: • 1½ cups strawberries • 1 kiwi ½ cup Kombucha Tea*	1 serving Liver, Onions, and Mushrooms* 1 cup cooked carrots Salad: • 2 cups bok choy • 1 tablespoon sunflower seeds • ½ cup summer squash • ½ cup raw celery • dried basil to taste • 1 tablespoon extra virgin olive oil • balsamic vinegar to taste ¼ cup fermented beets 1½ cups fresh pineapple Throat Coat herbal tea or licorice or other herbal tea
Day 2	Smoothie: • 1 cup parsley • 2 cups green grapes • 1 tablespoon nutritional yeast • water/ice 1 serving Liver Pâté* 2 ounces raw turnip slices (about ½ cup) 1 medium stalk celery	1½ servings Salmon or Chicken Salad* 2 cups raw collards (wrap) 4 scallions or spring onions 4 medium radishes ½ cup cubed cantaloupe ½ cup Beet Kvass* mixed with ½ cup water	2 medium chicken breasts without skin (about 6 ounces) 1 cup chopped sweet potato 2 teaspoons extra virgin olive oil ⅛ teaspoon cinnamon Salad: • 3 cups spinach • ¼ cup sliced onion • 1 clove garlic • 1 tablespoon sunflower seed butter • lime juice to taste ¼ cup fermented red cabbage ¾ cup fresh blueberries Tension Tamer herbal tea

	Breakfast	*Lunch*	*Dinner*
Day 3	Smoothie: • 1 cup bok choy • 1 cup kiwi • 1 cup strawberries • 1 tablespoon nutritional yeast • water/ice 3–4 ounces canned sardines in tomato sauce 1 medium celery stalk ½ cup raw turnip slices	2 servings Basic Skillet Recipe* (Pork Chops and Red Cabbage) Salad: • 3 cups romaine lettuce • 2 cups spinach • ½ cup red peppers • 2 teaspoons flax oil • balsamic vinegar to taste 1 cup raw kiwi ½ cup Kombucha Tea*	6 ounces beef rump roast 1 medium potato with skin 1 teaspoon extra virgin olive oil 1 medium cooked carrot ½ cup lacto-fermented okra 1 cup strawberries chamomile vanilla herbal tea
Day 4	Smoothie: • 1 cup cilantro • 1 small orange (~½ cup) • 1 cup pineapple • 1 tablespoon nutritional yeast • water/ice 7 ounces turkey breast without skin 6 medium spears asparagus 1 teaspoon extra virgin olive oil	1 serving Basic Skillet Recipe* (Collards and Ham Skillet) 1 cup chopped baked sweet potato 2 teaspoons extra virgin olive oil Fruit Cup: • 1 cup pineapple • 1 cup raspberries • 2 tablespoons raw almonds ½ cup Beet Kvass* plus ½ cup water	2 servings Salmon or Chicken Salad* Salad: • 2 cups bok choy • 2 cups spinach • lime juice to taste • 1 tablespoon flax oil • ½ cup tomato • 2 tablespoons soaked sunflower seeds ¼ cup lacto-fermented carrots 1 cup grapes mint herbal tea
Day 5	Smoothie: • 1 cup spinach • 1 cup strawberries • 1 cup peaches (~1 medium) • 1 tablespoon nutritional yeast • water/ice 1 serving Basic Skillet Recipe* (Salmon and Kale Skillet)	2 servings Basic Skillet Recipe* (Lamb Chops with Broccoli) 1 cup cooked beets Salad: • 3 cups bok choy • 2 cloves garlic • ½ cup cilantro • ½ cup green pepper • ½ cup fresh grapes • 1 tablespoon sunflower butter • lime juice to taste ½ cup Kombucha Tea*	2 servings Algerian Chicken with Asparagus* ¼ cup kimchi 1 medium peach herbal tea

	Breakfast	**Lunch**	**Dinner**
Day 6	Smoothie: • ½ cup raw beets • 1 small orange (~½ cup) • 1 cup cherries • ¼-inch piece fresh gingerroot, grated • 1 tablespoon nutritional yeast • water/ice 1 serving Basic Skillet Recipe* (Heart and Mustard Greens) 1 cup cantaloupe	4 ounces sardines in tomato sauce ½ cup daikon radishes 1 medium celery stalk ½ cup zucchini 1 cup chopped baked sweet potato Salad: • 2 cups spinach • 2 cups kale • ½ cup strawberries • 4 medium spears asparagus • 2 teaspoons extra virgin olive oil • lime juice to taste 1 medium orange ½ cup Beet Kvass* plus ½ cup water	1 medium turkey drumstick with skin removed (~6.6 ounces) 1 serving Mashed Turnips* 2 teaspoons extra virgin olive oil ½ cup parsley 1 cup cooked carrots ¼ cup lacto-fermented pickles 1½ cups cherries chamomile herbal tea
Day 7	Smoothie: • 1 cup parsley • 1 cup green grapes • 1 kiwi (about ⅓ cup) • 1 tablespoon nutritional yeast • water/ice 6 ounces beefsteak, topped with the following (to be cooked together): • ¼ cup onions • ¼ cup mushrooms • ¼ cup green peppers • 2 teaspoons ghee	2 servings Rosemary Chicken* 1 cup acorn squash 2 teaspoons extra virgin olive oil 6 medium asparagus spears, topped with 1 teaspoon extra virgin olive oil ½ cup Beet Kvass* plus ½ cup water	1 serving Seafood Stew (Paleo version)* Salad: • 3 cups bok choy • 2 cups spinach • ½ cup cilantro • ½ cup tomato • 1 tablespoon extra virgin olive oil • lime juice to taste ½ cup organic raw cultured carrots Fruit Cup: • ½ cup muskmelon • ½ cup watermelon • ½ cup blueberries herbal tea

Chapter 7

WAHLS PALEO PLUS

YOU MAY NEVER need to do Wahls Paleo Plus, but I hope you will read this chapter anyway. I bounce between ketogenic eating (high fat, moderate protein, low carbohydrate) during the winter months and a low-glycemic version of Wahls Paleo during the spring and summer. I did do the Wahls Elimination version of Wahls Paleo for six months and reintroduced food items one by one. I found that I tolerated occasional consumption of high lectin foods (a couple times a month). I enjoy fresh heirloom tomoatoes with basil from my garden occasionally during the summer as a treat, but daily consumption of high lectin foods triggers my face pain on the third day. Knowing this allows me to have occasional legumes and nightshades in a social gathering, as long as I don't keep having them. After progressing through every level of the Wahls Protocol and experimenting with every aspect of the nutrition program, I settled here because I have the most mental and physical energy eating this way. Some will enjoy so much improvement at the Wahls Paleo level that they don't feel the need to move on to Wahls Paleo Plus. If you are still having more symptoms with Wahls Paleo, then I recommend following the Wahls Elimination Diet (page 122) for 10 days before deciding whether you need to adopt the ketogenic version of my program: Wahls Paleo Plus.

Wahls Paleo Plus includes everything you were doing at Wahls Paleo, with a few additional considerations:

- **Eat more fat!** I want you to add more fat to your diet. If you tolerate coconut oil, use at least 5 tablespoons of oil (coconut oil or ¼ can or more of full-fat coconut milk) every day. You may also use ghee or unheated olive oil to get your fat calories. If your cholesterol is high, or becomes high on coconut oil, then you will need to use olive oil for your fat.
- **Reduce the daily 9 cups of fruits and vegetables to 6 to 9 cups, depending on your gender and size (or even 4 to 6 cups for very petite women).** Fruit is limited to 1 cup per day or less for berries. All dried fruits are excluded, as are canned fruits and commercial fruit juices.
- **Eliminate all grains, legumes, and white potatoes.** This includes rice milk (use coconut milk instead) and all forms of soy, including organic and fermented.
- **Limit starchy vegetables, like beets or winter squash, to raw only, always with at least 1 tablespoon of fat and some animal protein to lower their glycemic index.** I'll talk more about what this is later in this chapter.

WAHLS PALEO PLUS

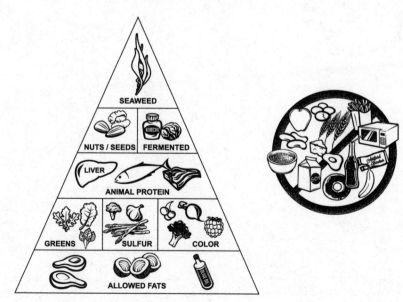

If you want more starchy vegetables, you may eat them raw, but also with at least 1 tablespoon of fat.

- **Reduce your meat intake back to 6 to 12 ounces.**
- **Monitor your fasting lipids while following Wahls Paleo Plus.** You will want to confirm that you tolerate a high fat diet. See page 235 for a discussion on lipid monitoring and management.

This diet sounds crazy to a lot of people, and I understand why. How can you possibly eat that much fat for health? That little fruit? No grains or potatoes at all? I have very good reasons for prescribing this diet, and as I mentioned, it is the diet I follow myself, with great results. I believe you will be more likely to get behind the diet if you understand how it evolved.

Once again I have laid out the comparison of the average diet compared to my program, this time the Wahls Paleo Plus. What is noteworthy is that

Wahls Paleo Plus		
Nutrient*†	U.S. Diet (%)	Wahls Paleo Plus (%)
Vitamin D	31	59
Vitamin E	55	97
Calcium	74	54
Magnesium	88	122
Vitamin A	100	411
Pyridoxine	121	226
Folate	122	191
Zinc	123	200
Thiamine	128	215
Vitamin C	133	393
Niacin	154	239
Iron	164	238
Riboflavin	175	301
Cobolamin	201	524

* Compared to dietary reference intakes, recommended dietary allowances (RDA) for females 51–70 years; Wahls Paleo Plus Diet adjusted for 1,759 calories. (National Academies of Science, Engineering, and Medicine; Institute of Medicine; Food and Nutrition Board)

† Average nutrient intake from food for females 50–59 years. (What We Eat in America, NHANES 2009–2010, ars.usda.gov/SP2UserFiles/Place/12355000/pdf/0910/Table_1_NIN_GEN_09.pdf, accessed May 25, 2013.)

Wahls Paleo Plus is still much more nutrient-dense than the standard American diet, even though I have increased the fat consumption so drastically. Most ketogenic diets require the addition of vitamins and other supplements because the nutrient density becomes so poor due to the severe restriction on carbohydrates. Wahls Paleo Plus is much more balanced than the traditional ketogenic diets in use because it still requires such a diversity of plant foods, increasing the vitamins and minerals in the diet.

CALL TO ACTION

Go to terrywahls.com/bonus to download a color pyramid for your refrigerator summarizing the key elements of Wahls Paleo Plus.

My Version of "Keto"

Wahls Paleo Plus is a modified version of what doctors call a *ketogenic diet*. In a ketogenic diet, fat is high and carbohydrates are low, so that the body switches from burning glucose from carbohydrates to burning fat as fuel (I'll explain how later in this chapter). The ketogenic diet isn't new, although it is new as a fad for healthy people. Traditionally, the ketogenic diet was prescribed for people with certain very specific health issues like seizure disorders, but in my research I have found it to be of extreme benefit to people with other types of brain problems, not just seizures—in the modified form you will find in this chapter.

Now that more people know about them and want to try them, ketogenic diets continue to evolve. In order for you to accept the unconventional dietary characteristics of Wahls Paleo Plus, I want you to understand what a ketogenic diet is and why it is so good for your brain, especially if you have an autoimmune disease with neurological symptoms.

THE ORIGIN OF
THE THERAPEUTIC KETOGENIC DIET

In 1911, a clinical study showed that water diets, also called fasting, increased the effectiveness of treatments for epilepsy.[1]

The insights into how ketosis protects the brain have continued to deepen. Ketosis inproves the efficiency and number of mitochondria throughout the body and brain. It stabilizes the cell membranes, making them resistant to the repeated misfiring that occurs when seizures cause rhythmic jerking of arms and legs.[2] In addition, ketosis changes the pathways that make neurotransmitters in our brains and reduces the production of free radicals (biochemical "trash") and the expression of our genes.[3] In 1921, Dr. R. M. Wilder at the Mayo Clinic developed a diet that would allow patients to eat some food but have the same benefits as they would enjoy from fasting. This diet was very high in fat, included some protein, and had almost zero carbohydrates. He reported success with his epilepsy patients.[4] Dr. M. G. Peterman, also at Mayo, described the first ketogenic diet to be used with children suffering from epilepsy.[5]

Some of this research fell out of favor when Dilantin, the first effective anticonvulsant drug, became available in 1938. (Anticonvulsants continue to be a popular treatment for epilepsy, even though these drugs are not effective for up to 30 percent of individuals with seizures.) But scientists continued to explore the notion that a diet that promoted fat burning instead of sugar burning could improve seizure disorders.

In 1971, it was discovered that consuming medium-chain triglyceride (MCT) oil, extracted from coconut oil and palm kernel oil, generated more ketones per calorie than other fats.[6] Because a ketogenic diet depends on the manufacture of a certain level of ketones, this meant that diets using MCT oil as the sole fat source could include carbohydrates at a slightly higher level than was used in the 1920s and still generate ketones. That discovery made it possible to modify the original ketogenic diet to create what became known as an MCT ketogenic diet, which is much easier to follow because it allows a wider variety of food. Wahls Paleo Plus is actually a modified MCT ketogenic diet, because it relies heavily on coconut oil and full-fat coconut milk, both foods with high levels of medium-chain triglycerides.

The public interest in ketogenic diets increased when, in 1993, two-year-old Charlie Abrahams, son of Hollywood director and writer Jim Abrahams, became seizure-free on a ketogenic diet after previously having uncontrolled seizures. This led to the development of the Charlie Foundation to promote the diet and fund research. In 2011, there were more than seventy-five centers that used a ketogenic diet to treat refractory epilepsy. Additionally, physicians are now studying whether ketogenic diets can treat a much wider array of health problems: Parkinson's disease, dementia, ALS (these studies were stopped because people lost too much weight), chronic migraine, autism, stroke, and psychiatric diseases.[7] There is also exciting research indicating that ketogenic diets are an excellent way to fight an active, even advanced cancer.[8]

The Ketogenic Diet 101

In the simplest terms, the ketogenic diet is a diet that puts you into ketosis. Ketosis is a state of burning fat, rather than sugar, as a primary fuel source. The human body defaults to using glucose from food as an energy source, but when you eat a high-fat, very low-carbohydrate diet, glucose won't be available for fuel. If you eat a low-carbohydrate, high-protein diet, your body will burn amino acids and make sugar from them. You will still have a high insulin level (as protein also elevates insulin through this process). If you eat a low-carbohydrate and low-protein diet, you can still survive because the body is creative and has evolved to survive even in the absence of carbohydrates and protein. When deprived of both carbohydrates and protein, the body switches into a state of nutritional ketosis, in which the liver begins producing ketone bodies—acetoacetate, acetone, and beta-hydroxybutyrate. These provide fuel in the absence of glucose, and it is actually a superior fuel, especially for the brain.

Brains cannot burn long-chain fatty acids because they can't cross the blood-brain barrier. Ketones *can* cross the blood-brain barrier, so as your liver

KETOSIS AND CANCER

Our bodies are very good at burning fat, but our cells do not choose to burn fat when they have an easy supply of simple sugars. It's easier to burn glucose because the splitting of the sugar molecule (glycolysis) occurs outside of the mitochondria, in the cell cytoplasm. Cancer cells typically rely on glycolysis because they cannot burn fat. That is one of the reasons why ketogenic diets make cancer cells more vulnerable to chemotherapy.

burns fat and produces these small molecules known as ketone bodies (which are a by-product of fat burning), they proceed to cross the blood-brain barrier to be burned as fuel in your brain cells' mitochondria. The longer you are in nutritional ketosis, the more enzymes for burning the ketones will be upregulated—that is, increased—making it increasingly easy for your body to utilize the ketones. In other words, you get used to this alternative fuel source.

You may have heard that ketosis is dangerous. There are forms of ketosis that can be damaging to you, but this is not one of them. Nutritional ketosis is *not harmful*. In fact, it is healing, and has long been a mechanism for human survival.

In human history, fat was often an easier fuel source to find than carbohydrates or protein. When we did not have food to eat, we could always rely on our body fat (unless severely underweight) as a source of fuel for our mitochondria! In cold climates during the winter, carbohydrate-rich foods (fruits and vegetables) weren't available, but animal foods were, which is why our bodies adapted to switch to protein-burning. If there was no food available, we could burn our own stored calories—our fat. That is when we switch to fat-burning mode, giving us the the ability to survive winter and starvation.

When starchy foods became plentiful with the advent of agriculture, and even more so with industrialization and modernization, humans became less likely to spend much time in ketosis. There were usually sources of carbohydrates available all year long. Modern industrialized societies have diets packed with carbohydrates, so most people are sugar-burning all the time.

But we still have the ability to switch into ketosis, whether we ever choose

WAHLS WORDS

Fatty acids are considered long-chain if they have more than twelve carbon atoms, medium-chain if they have between twelve and six carbon atoms, and short-chain if they have fewer than six carbon atoms. The medium-chain fats found in coconut oil and short-chain fats found in ghee can enter the bloodstream directly from the small bowel. The long-chain fats, by contrast, are absorbed into the bloodstream through a longer, more complex process. That difference is just one of the reasons why consuming coconut oil and ghee (or medium-chain fatty acids, sometimes called MCTs or MCT oil) is more desirable while practicing Wahls Paleo Plus.

to do it or not. This is useful because ketosis has the added benefit of decreasing inflammation (while sugary, starchy foods promote inflammation). This is especially important for brain health.

My own research, as well as self-experimentation, has centered on an exploration of how a diet rich in MCT fats and low in carbohydrates might impact multiple sclerosis and other neurological conditions (remember that some people's cholesterol elevates while on coconut oil and they may need an alternative approach—see page 235 for specifics). This is how Wahls Paleo Plus evolved. This diet, if followed strictly, will put you into a mild state of nutritional ketosis, but it contains more carbohydrates than the traditional ketogenic diets because of the importance of including a rich supply of nonstarchy vegetables for nutrient density. Vegetables contain carbohydrates, but these and a small amount of berries (a relatively low-carb fruit) are the only carbohydrate sources. To me, this is the best of both worlds: The diet has the benefits of ketosis and high fat for brain health and low carbohydrates to reduce inflammation and stabilize blood sugar, but it is also nutrient-dense beyond other ketogenic diets. To some, Wahls Paleo Plus may seem extreme, but I want you to understand that it is far less extreme than standard ketogenic diets that require supplementation because they are so nutrient-poor. Wahls Paleo Plus is designed to be workable in the real world. It's challenging, but it's certainly not impossible. I do it, and so do many other Wahls Warriors, with great results.

WAHLS WORDS

Wahls Paleo Plus prioritizes foods with a low *glycemic index* because in order to encourage ketosis (fat burning), the body cannot have easy access to glucose for sugar burning. Glycemic index is a measure of how much a food causes a rise in blood sugar. The highest number on the glycemic index is 100, which indicates the effect of pure glucose on blood sugar over a two-hour period. A food with no carbohydrates at all (which consequently will not introduce any sugar to the bloodstream), such as pure fat, will have a glycemic index of 0. Coconut oil is an example of a food with a glycemic index of 0. All other foods with any carbohydrate or sugar content will have a glycemic index number based on how quickly it raises blood sugar—most foods will not raise blood sugar as quickly or as high as pure glucose, but will raise it higher and more quickly than pure fat, which would not raise it at all. Low glycemic foods are those with a glycemic index number of 55 or lower. (Glycemic index values for foods can be found via a search function on this website, from the University of Sydney: glycemicindex.com.)

The glycemic index varies depending on many different food factors, such as amount and types of sugars and starches, fat, protein, and fiber content of food; physical structure; food processing; and type and amount of cooking. Other factors, such as how well the food is chewed and what foods were eaten at prior meals, can also impact blood sugar levels, so the number isn't always as simple as a list may lead you to believe. Vegetables and fruits vary dramatically, depending on variety as well as other factors, such as whether they are cooked or raw, ripe or unripe. You can also lower the glycemic index of a food by combining it with fiber, fat, and protein, which slows down the absorption rate of the carbohydrate.

Glycemic load predicts the blood sugar response when a specific amount of a particular food is consumed. It considers both the glycemic index of a food and the amount of available carbohydrate in the portion eaten. A high glycemic index food could potentially have a low glycemic load if the amount of carbohydrate in the food is low and/or if the amount eaten is small. This can also be influenced by ripeness (in the case of fruit) and how long the food was cooked.

KETOSIS WITHOUT MCTS:
LIPID MONITORING
AND THE OLIVE OIL SOLUTION

If your physician has instructed you to follow a diet low in saturated fat because of concerns about heart disease or an elevated blood cholesterol, or if you have the ApoE4 gene (page 242), you can still do a ketogenic diet. Under normal circumstances, I recommend eating coconut oil to get into ketosis. Coconut oil has the benefit of being rich in medium-chain triglycerides (MCT). The benefits of MCT oil is that it allows you to consume more carbohydrates—good for you and your microbiome—while still achieving nutritional ketosis.

The downside of MCT is that some people, due to their genetics and their microbiomes, do not do well with a diet high in saturated fat. Coconut oil and MCT oil cause their cholesterol to shoot up when they consume the amount of coconut oil that is part of an MCT-fueled ketogenic diet. If you are doing Wahls Paleo Plus and you don't know whether you are tolerant, you should monitor your lipids six weeks after you begin Wahls Paleo Plus. If your cholesterol goes too high (your doctor can advise you), then you may be one of those people who should not take MCT oil or use coconut oil. You could also do some more advanced testing of your genes. The genetic tests will give you guidance for your tolerance of saturated fat and whether you would do better to use olive oil for your fat source. If your cholesterol does not go too high after six weeks on Wahls Paleo Plus, you are fine to proceed with MCT oil and coconut oil usage.

If you do switch to olive oil (or start with olive oil, if you already know you must limit saturated fats), know that you can't make as many ketones from olive oil as you can with MCT oil, so you will likely need to further restrict your carbohydrates down from the 50 to 80 grams you can use on a coconut oil diet down to 25 to 35 grams or less. Keeping carb intake that low is much more challenging to do. You could make it easier to get into low-level ketosis by practicing time-restricted eating, or eating for only a short period during each day, such as during an eight-, six-, or four-hour window of time (see page 252 for more information about time-restricted feeding).

Are You in Ketosis?

When you embark upon Wahls Paleo Plus, adding fats and reducing carbohydrates further, you may want to know whether you are actually in nutritional ketosis. When I developed Wahls Paleo Plus, I began by choosing low glycemic foods and eating them in a way that would give them a low glycemic load, replacing cooked starchy vegetables like sweet potatoes with raw versions of starchy vegetables, or using nonstarchy vegetables instead, and reducing fruit to 1 cup (or ½ cup) of berries only. I also consumed an entire can of full-fat coconut milk every day. (For those using olive oil, I recommend consuming 4 to 6 tablespoons of olive oil every day.)

To see how well this was all working, I began checking my urine for the presence of ketones using a blood meter. However, I no longer recommend using urine strips to monitor if you are in ketosis. That is not a reliable method. If you wish to follow a ketogenic diet, the most effective way to know if you are in ketosis is to monitor your ketones in your blood or breath.

If your cells are still burning sugar (carbohydrates), you will have zero ketones in your blood. My goal was to have some ketones in the blood—not a high number, just some. More than 0.4 mmol/L means you are in ketosis, and more isn't necessarily better. I didn't need the level to be high, but I wanted to see if I could induce at least a low level of ketosis while still consuming my green, colorful, and sulfur-rich vegetables.

I was eating 3 cups of greens, 1 or 2 cups of sulfur vegetables, and 1 to 2 cups of color. I kept the greens higher because I knew Wahls Paleo Plus is relatively lower in calcium, and greens are a good source of both calcium and magnesium. Furthermore, since I was cutting down on vegetable intake, I needed to stress the most nutrient-dense vegetable group of all, which is leafy green vegetables. I was not eating as many berries. My blood ketones ranged from 0.4 mmol/L to 3.0 mmol/L. Nutritional ketosis begins at level 0.5 mmol/L. I was often, though not always, in nutritional ketosis. I was ecstatic. I could still eat a very nutrient-dense diet that would give me the nutrition my brain cells needed while maintaining nutritional ketosis! Now, with more time and experience, I am consistently in ketosis (during the winter months).

Because I consumed 500 to 700 calories either as coconut oil, full-fat coconut milk, or olive oil, I was consuming only around 6 ounces of meat per

WAHLS WARNING

In some studies, medium-chain triglyceride diets, upon which Wahls Paleo Plus is based, have been associated with side effects such as diarrhea, vomiting, bloating, and cramps. Other studies have found that these side effects can be reduced by more slowly increasing the amount of medium-chain triglycerides (like coconut oil) in the diet. This means you may want to ease gradually into Wahls Paleo Plus rather than leaping in with both feet.

There is also the risk of having a significantly higher cholesterol value. Diets high in coconut fat and low in carbohydrates may increase the total cholesterol and your HDL (high-density lipoprotein), or "good cholesterol," but would also likely at the same time reduce the number of oxidized cholesterols that are the most damaging of all the cholesterol particles.

You can assess your fasting lipids with advanced lipid testing to specifically measure the oxidized cholesterol values, to know if you tolerate coconut oil (see page 348 for more on advanced testing). Or you can obtain genetic testing to see if you have the genes in your DNA or your microbiome's DNA that increase the probability that you will have an elevated cholesterol if you try to use coconut oil to get into ketosis. (The oxidized cholesterol is a different number from the LDL, or low-density lipoprotein. See the Resources section at the end of the book for advanced lipid testing labs available through a functional medicine practitioner.) Another danger for children and young adults up into the early 20s: Neither the medium-chain-triglyceride diet nor Wahls Paleo Plus should be used by people in this age group who take valproate (a seizure medication also used for other diagnoses such as migraine headaches), as there have been some reports that the combination causes liver failure.

day instead of my usual 9 to 12 ounces, and 6 to 9 cups of vegetables and berries, but it was working and I was still getting plenty of antioxidants. When we did an analysis of the micronutrient content of my diet, I was still well over the RDAs for vitamins and most minerals, but I was low on calcium. Therefore, I knew I would have to pay special attention to eating high-calcium foods to be sure I was still getting sufficient calcium and plenty of vitamin D—hence all those leafy greens! Again, this is why I have you skew your proportions somewhat, reducing sulfur-rich and colorful vegetables while keeping the greens at 3 cups.

Whether you are using coconut oil or olive oil as your main fat, monitor your blood ketones to get feedback on whether you are in ketosis. If you are above 0.4 mmol/L of ketones, you are in nutritional ketosis. If you are not, you need to reduce the carbohydrates further, increase the fat, and/or lengthen the time you are not eating each day, until your blood ketones are greater than 0.4 mmol/L. You may have to eliminate the berries and starchy vegetables

WAHLS WARRIORS SPEAK

I learned about Dr. Wahls from my dentist, who told me that someone close to him was using diet to turn around their MS and having significant results. I have primary progressive MS, spine and hip arthritis, ankylosing spondylitis, mitral valve prolapse, situational depression, epilepsy, and neuropathy. When PPMS spread to my speech centers, it was a shock, more so than the physical limits.

Over the initial three months on this diet, and on targeted supplements, my speech gradually made gains from severe disfluency; my tremors lessened; and I went from unintelligible speech attempts and gasping for breath to speaking coherently again. I still need to use a wheelchair to travel any distances, but I am doing more of the tasks that I had given up for more than a decade, such as cooking once or twice a week. I can clean and chop vegetables, something that used to wear me out, and I don't fall asleep in the midst of tasks anymore. My husband and daughter used to tell me that they'd shared things with me in conversation and I wouldn't remember what they'd said. Those days are over. I used to have days, even weeks, where I slept for hours after very little activity. Now I have much more energy and am able to engage in life more. I seldom nap these days, and my family is so touched by how far I have come, as am I! Thanks to Dr. Wahls, I have hope and fight in me!

—Yolanda M., Hercules, California

entirely—even the raw ones—or you may be able to tolerate small amounts now and then. If you pay attention to your blood ketones, it will help guide how you structure your diet.

I want you to be able to have a chance at getting the benefits of this diet right now, however. Do work with your personal physician if you elect to try Wahls Paleo Plus, to monitor how both you and your blood work respond to this new way of eating. It is necessary to work closely with your medical team to monitor the effects of a ketogenic diet long term if you decide to do this for more than one year.

THE RISKS OF LONG-TERM KETOSIS

For most people with chronic diseases, especially those that are autoimmune in nature, ketosis can be incredibly therapeutic. However, this is generally not a diet that I recommend for the long term (years) or permanently, unless there are compelling medical reasons. Throughout human history, ketosis was a state that typically occurred during winter or during periods of famine, not all year round. When the weather warms and vegetables and fruits begin to grow again, it is natural to eat more of these foods and move back out of ketosis. Over the long term, ketosis can make the body think that it is not getting enough nutrients, and it can divert valuable resources to survival, when that is not necessary for you. Some of the undesirable changes that can happen to your biochemistry with long-term ketosis include:

- **Shifts in sex hormones**. If the body thinks you are starving, it may hinder reproduction. *Do not get pregnant while on Wahls Paleo Plus*. A ketogenic diet during pregnancy could result in alterations in embryonic organ and skeletal growth that could be associated with organ dysfunction and/or potential behavior changes in postnatal life. If you find out you are pregnant, I advise switching to the Wahls Diet or Wahls Paleo.
- **Increased cortisol**. If the body thinks you are starving, it will go into stress mode, increasing stress hormone levels, which can have a cascade of negative effects.

- **Suppressed thyroid function**. To conserve energy, the body may hinder the production of thyroid hormones.
- **Reduced immunity.** While autoimmune conditions can mean overactive immunity, long-term ketosis could suppress immunity too much, resulting in the increased risk of infections and serious consequences from infections.

WAHLS WARRIORS SPEAK

My diagnosis with multiple sclerosis was a true wake-up call. Seeing my own decline at a prime time in my life altered me. At the time of my diagnosis in November 2006, I weighed more than 280 pounds. By the end of the year, I needed to use a walker. That's when I started my quest to research MS and how various factors, like nutrition and exercise, affect it. I started slowly incorporating my various findings into my daily life and progressed to only using a cane for my instability issues. In spring 2011, I gave up the cane, was more than 130 pounds lighter, and have been going strong ever since! I was determined not to be in a nursing home at 50 years old without any future. I could not bear that, so I made a decision and I continue to fight my battle with MS every day. I strongly believe in moving forward! I have had to learn to do some things differently, but that is okay. MS is not a death sentence—it just means that you will have struggles and challenges, but you can also have some wonderful rewards if you allow them into your life.
    —Pam J., Pecatonica, Illinois

If you decide to try Wahls Paleo Plus, it's okay to ease into it. In fact, I prefer that you do. In our clinical trial, we ease people in over a three-week period. I find that it's easier for people to adapt if they allow their fat-burning enzymes to gradually upregulate (increase) so it is easier for their mitochondria to burn more fat. I suggest you do the same and come to this over one to three weeks (or longer) if you are coming from the standard American diet. If you have been practicing Wahls Paleo, you will likely be able to transition more quickly.

Remember that I have evolved my eating patterns over the last seventeen years, adapting how I ate as I learned more about the needs of my brain and understood more and more about nutrition. I suggest you work with your family and begin making the changes at a pace your family accepts. No diet works if you don't stick to it, and it is much easier to adopt these big changes if you implement them gradually and the entire family joins you on the journey, or is at least supportive of your efforts and willing to help you.

What to Do

Now that you understand what Wahls Paleo Plus is, let's look more closely at how to follow the guidelines. This version of the diet takes the principles all the way. You will be incorporating every aspect of the Wahls Diet and Wahls Paleo unless they contradict the rules of Wahls Paleo Plus, which supersedes the others:

- You will maximize the vitamins, minerals, antioxidants, and fatty acids that are so critical for your brain while minimizing the sugars that can cause problems in your gut.
- You will still eat a lot of greens, sulfur-rich vegetables, and brightly colored produce, though it may be closer to 6 cups (or maybe 4 if you are a petite woman or unable to use coconut oil/milk because it elevates your cholesterol) than the 9 cups recommended at the Wahls Diet and Wahls Paleo levels.
- You will still eat organic and/or wild-caught meat, including organ meat.
- You will still incorporate seaweed and fermented foods.
- You will monitor your fasting lipids to assess your tolerance to a high-fat diet and to coconut oil/coconut milk.

The difference is that you'll tweak your ratios to add more fat and fewer carbs and you'll eat less often. As you get into nutritional ketosis, your body will begin to efficiently burn fat. I predict that you won't be as hungry on Wahls Paleo Plus, and you'll find eating just twice a day not so difficult. Here are your specifics.

IF YOU HAVE THE APOE4 GENE

Everyone is born with two copies of a gene called ApoE, and those two copies can be any combination of three types: ApoE2, ApoE3, and ApoE4. The most common version is ApoE3, and this gene is not associated with any particular health risk. However, the ApoE4 gene impairs fat metabolism and increases inflammation in many of the inflammatory pathways. This gene has been associated with an increased risk of Alzheimer's disease, as well as an increased risk of cardiovascular disease, rapid aging, stroke, and autoimmune disease. (The ApoE2 variant is the rarest, and seems to be associated with a decreased risk.) Anyone could have two copies of any of these, or one copy of any and one copy of any other. For example, you could be ApoE⅔ or ApoE¾, or ApoE⅔ (or any other combination).

If you have a family history of dementia, you may want to get tested to see if you have one or two copies of the ApoE4 gene (one copy increases your risk slightly, two copies increases your risk more). Some people don't want to know, even though having the ApoE4 gene (even two copies) is *not* a guarantee that you will develop Alzheimer's disease. Some people do want to know, so they have more motivation to make lifestyle changes that could decrease their risks.

There are many recommendations for those who have one or two copies of the ApoE4 gene, such as the importance of cardiovascular exercise (there is evidence that regular exercise can completely eliminate this risk factor). Less certain are dietary recommendations. Some people believe that a high-fat diet is dangerous for ApoE4 due to impaired fat metabolism, while others believe that a high-carb diet is dangerous due to the increased inflammation risk.

If you know you have the ApoE4 gene, you may be wondering if Wahls Paleo Plus is safe for you, considering the high fat content. This is controversial, but the current thinking is that it is saturated fat in particular that is inflammatory for ApoE4. For this reason, for ApoE4-positive people only, I recommend avoiding MCT oil, coconut oil, coconut milk, ghee (clarified butter without the milk solids), and fatty red meat on any level of the Wahls Protocol. You can still do a version of Wahls Paleo Plus, if you get your fat from seafood and olive oil and use intermittent fasting rather than MCT oil to get into ketosis (see page 235). I also recommend avoiding bacon and animal fats. Some people with the ApoE4 gene have success eating every other day, which is a good option for those people who can handle it. (It's not for everyone.) For more about intermittent fasting, including options for time-restricted feeding and fasting-mimicking diets, see page 252.

Part One: Add More Fat, Especially Coconut Oil and Full-Fat Coconut Milk

Now it's time to really ramp up your fat intake, mostly through coconut oil or full-fat coconut milk if you tolerate it (both, as I explained before, have properties that will keep you in ketosis even with vegetables and some berries in your diet). I want the majority of your calories to come from fat. Your goal is to have a source of medium-chain fats at each eating occasion.

On a 2,000-calorie diet, aim for 144 grams of fat for approximately 1,300 calories. For the average woman eating 1,790 calories, that would be 129 grams of fat at 1,160 calories. Remember, if you are still not showing ketones in your blood after fully committing to Wahls Paleo Plus for one week, you need to increase your fat intake and further reduce the carbohydrates.

You might think it will be hard to include this much fat in your diet, but coconut milk or olive oil can be added to smoothies and used in salad dressing and for cooking meats (coconut oil only) and vegetables. Coconut milk can be added to smoothies, soups, and other recipes, used in coffee and tea, or consumed plain. The amount of medium-chain fats in 1 tablespoon of coconut oil is equivalent to about 5 tablespoons (approximately ⅓ cup) of coconut milk. Take care not to confuse coconut water with coconut milk. Coconut water is the clear liquid from inside a coconut, and it is fat-free. Also be sure you have the full-fat milk, not the "light" variety. Full-fat coconut milk provides 11 grams total fat per ⅓ cup serving compared to 4.5 grams total fat for the light version. Other coconut products that could be included in the diet include coconut cream and coconut butter. Coconut cream contains more medium-chain fat than coconut milk and is thicker. Coconut butter, sometimes called coconut cream concentrate, is finely ground dried coconut meat. Avoid "cream of coconut," because it is sweetened with sugar.

FAT FACTS

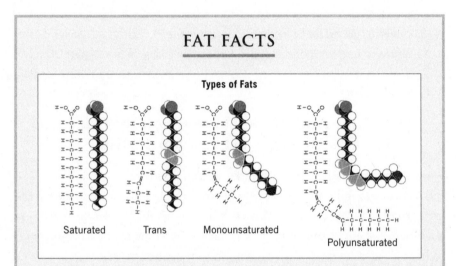

Types of Fats

Saturated   Trans   Monounsaturated

Polyunsaturated

Let's learn a little more about fats, because they are so important at this level.

Fats are chains of carbon and hydrogen atoms with two oxygen atoms at one end. In three dimensions, the carbon backbone makes a gentle zigzag pattern. In the drawings above, you see the long line of *C*s. These are the carbon atoms, or the black line with the zigzag white line in the drawings. The hydrogen atoms are the *H*s and are represented by the white balls. The dark gray balls are the oxygen atoms. The light gray balls represent the double bonds. A double bond is when a carbon atom does not have two hydrogen atoms attached to it, instead having only one attached. Those double bonds are fragile, and are more at risk of being oxidized and converted to a toxic fat that is damaging to blood vessels. Those double bonds change the shape of the fat that cells use to conduct the biology of life. Remember, fats can be long-chain, medium-chain, or short-chain, depending on how many carbons have been strung together.

Saturated fat. Saturated fat has a hydrogen atom at every available spot on the fat. It is very stable when heated and does not convert to dangerous oxidized fats, which can be damaging. Animal fats and coconut oil are primarily saturated fats. Their stability makes them the best choice for cooking.

Trans fat. Usually the double bonds in mono- and polyunsaturated fats have the single hydrogen atom on the same side of the chain. When they are on opposite sides of the carbon chain, it is in the "trans" position and is a trans saturated fat, often shortened to *trans fat*. The trans position puts a kink in the fat, changing its shape and increasing the likelihood that it will be oxidized and therefore become extremely damaging to blood vessels.

Monounsaturated fat (MUFA). A monounsaturated fat is a fat with one double bond with the *H*s on the same side of the carbon chain. This changes the shape of the fat and is a useful fat to cells. However, the double bond is more vulnerable to being oxidized by heat and becoming a damaging trans fat. Examples of foods rich with MUFAs include olive oil and walnuts, but both also contain PUFAs. Don't cook with these—use only cold extra virgin varieties.

Polyunsaturated fat (PUFA). A polyunsaturated fat (PUFA) has more than one double bond and has more kinks and turns in its shape. As the number of double bonds increases, the fat becomes more vulnerable to heat, which will break the double bonds, creating oxidized fats, including damaging trans fats. This is why I recommend you not heat or cook with any plant oil. Heating these oils will increase the likelihood that the double bonds will be broken and oxidized, creating damaging molecules. Instead, use olive and nut oils cold on your salads, and avoid plant oils completely if they contain primarily omega-6 PUFAs (corn, soybean, sunflower, most commercial "vegetable" oils, etc.) so that you can improve your ratio of omega-6 to omega-3 fats.

Also avoid refined oils, which use solvents to extract more oil from the plant. Always use cold-pressed extra virgin olive oils.

Omega-3 fatty acids. I introduced you to the concept of essential fatty acids in the last chapter, but perhaps you would like to see how they look. As you can see from the illustration, there are three types of omega-3 fatty

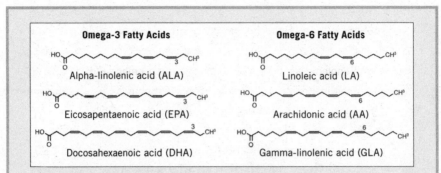

acids: ALA, EPA, and DHA. All the omega-3 fatty acids have a 3 on the chain on the right side; this refers to the third carbon from the distal end. As you may remember, ALA must be converted in the body to EPA and DHA, making it a less efficient source for omega-3 fatty acids. (This is in plant foods like flaxseeds and walnuts.)

If you have an autoimmune problem, heart problem, and/or brain problems, it will likely be harder for you to manufacture sufficient EPA and DHA from ALA. For this reason, you are better off getting your EPA and DHA straight from animal sources like grass-fed wild game and other grass-fed meats, wild fish especially from cold-water climates, and eggs from grass-eating chickens (but only if you are able to confirm that you do not have a food sensitivity to eggs). (Remember that this is one of the reasons why I do not recommend vegetarianism.)

Omega-6 fatty acids. You need omega-6 fatty acids, but most people get far too many. Ideally, you should get a ratio of omega-6 to omega-3 fatty acids of between 1:1 and 3:1, but most people get far more omega-6s. The number 6 in the term *omega-6* refers to the double bond at the sixth carbon from the end.

Linoleic acid (LA) is an essential omega-6 fatty acid, meaning your body cannot make it, and it is an important precursor to arachidonic acid (AA), which is used to make many signaling molecules in the body. Food sources for LA are nut and seed oils. Our bodies can easily make AA from LA, though animal fats are a good direct source of AA. When the ratio of AA to DHA is shifted too strongly toward AA, the body begins producing too many inflammation molecules, leading to excessive inflammation. The typical American diet is strongly tilted toward LA because of the high seed oil content.

Gamma-linolenic acid (GLA) is unusual for an omega-6 fatty acid in that it reduces inappropriate inflammation. Food sources include borage oil, primrose oil, black currant oil, and hemp oil.

WAHLS WARRIORS SPEAK

I was diagnosed in 2013 after experiencing sudden pain and numbness that spread from my toes all the way up to my chest. I had never had previous symptoms and the diagnosis was a complete shock. Upon leaving the hospital, I was given an appointment with the chief neurologist in three months. In that time, I began exhaustive research while my symptoms persisted. I was experiencing "pins and needles" feelings on a good day and severe pain on other days. I had the "MS hug" constricting feelings around my waist and an electric shock that shot through my body when bending my head down. Any weight on my body caused pain, even clothing or sleeping with a light sheet. In my research, I was lucky enough to find Dr. Wahls and her protocol. My partner, Chuck, and I started it right away. My symptoms began subsiding after a few months. I felt confident walking and driving on my own again, and I was finally able to return to my beloved yoga practice. During this time, Chuck's high blood pressure dropped to very normal levels and he felt energized. Eventually, by the end of the year, I was left with numbness in only one big toe. I did not start any disease-modifying drugs. I had an MRI exactly one year after my diagnosis, which showed no new lesions, and the existing ones had diminished. It has now been six years since that diagnosis and we've strictly stuck to levels 2 or 3 of the Wahls Protocol. The feeling in my big toe returned and I've never felt better. It was a journey, but we have proof that it works. We are forever grateful for Dr. Wahls and her protocol.

—Rene Putz, Chicago, Illinois

Part Two: Cut Back to 6 Cups (or Even 4)

With the limits on higher-carb plant foods in Wahls Paleo Plus, go ahead and reduce your 9 cups of vegetables and fruits down to 6, or even 4. When I was eating Wahls Paleo, I was eating 9 to 12 cups of vegetables and fruits per day (I can go higher because I am very tall). Now that I am on Wahls Paleo Plus, depending on the day, I actually eat closer to 6 to 9 cups per day (of which 3 cups are still greens because leafy green vegetables are the most nutrient-dense of the vegetable food group, and they are high in calcium and magnesium). If you are a petite woman, you may be down to just 4 cups. If that's the case, eat 2 cups of greens, 1 cup of sulfur-rich vegetables, and 1 cup of colorful vegetables.

Part Three: Eliminate All Grains, Legumes, and Potatoes

On Wahls Paleo, you cut down your nongluten grains, legumes, and potato servings to twice per week. Now it's time to eliminate them completely (including all soy products, as well as rice milk and soy milk—your new favorite milk is full-fat coconut milk!). If your symptoms are severe and you want to create the most healing environment for your brain cells and your mitochondria, it is extremely important to drastically lower your carbohydrate intake, and these foods simply contain too many carbs. It will be difficult or even impossible to get into even mild ketosis eating these foods, so they are off your list for now. There are many other nutrient-dense plant foods to choose from on Wahls Paleo Plus. You might be eliminating the ones you are more accustomed to eating, but this is your chance to branch out and explore new foods. See the food lists at the end of this book and the menu ideas at the end of this chapter for help.

Your new focus is on animal protein and nonstarchy vegetables.

Part Four: Limit Starchy Vegetables to Raw Only

Starchy vegetables have a lot of carbs, but not as many as grains, legumes, and potatoes. Still, it's time to limit these foods—like winter squash, carrots, and beets—to raw only. When you do have raw starchy vegetables, you will need to eat them in a particular way: with more added fat and some protein. Adding a generous amount of fat—coconut oil or ghee (clarified butter without the milk solids) or olive oil—to your raw starchy vegetable will help keep your body in a state of mild ketosis. Also, the fat actually helps your body absorb more of the nutrients. Don't forget to have some protein with that raw vegetable as well.

Try a raw beet salad with cold-pressed olive oil and freshly squeezed lemon juice, or get a kitchen tool (called a spiralizer) that can cut raw winter squash or carrots into thin "spaghetti noodles" and enjoy those with a raw marinara sauce (blending fresh tomatoes, herbs, and olive oil). Be sure there is fat such as olive oil with those raw salads or raw "noodles." The carbohydrates are not so readily absorbed, so you'll be able to maintain the nutritional ketosis. However, if you don't show blood ketones after one to two weeks, you may need to increase the coconut milk (or lengthen the time you are not eating each day—see page 252). If you're still not showing ketones, then you may need to cut out even raw starchy vegetables entirely.

Part Five: Reduce Protein

You'll also have to cut your protein back down to 6 to 12 ounces per day, according to your size and gender. Your cells can take amino acids from protein and convert them into sugar to burn in your mitochondria. (The scientific/ technical term for this is gluconeogenesis.) For this reason, if you eat too much protein, you will not get into nutritional ketosis. You need enough protein to do the work of living, but not so much that you are converting protein into sugar!

Part Six: Limit Fruit to One Serving per Day of Berries

Fruit has a lot of carbohydrates, but the lowest-carb fruits are also the most nutritionally dense. It's time to cut out the apples, bananas, and pears because of their high carb content. For now, eat only berries. You'll still get your "color," but you won't get all the carbs. If you eat your berries with a couple of tablespoons of full-fat coconut milk, you will slow down the release of sugar into your bloodstream even more, which will be more helpful for keeping you in nutritional ketosis. (This also tastes great!)

WHAT IF YOU ARE
LOSING TOO MUCH WEIGHT?

Some people on the Wahls Diet, Wahls Paleo, or Wahls Paleo Plus, while enjoying great benefits, lose too much weight. Doing a ketogenic diet is never recommended for anyone with a body mass index (BMI) of 19.5 or lower. If you are really thin, ketogenic eating is not appropriate. You can use an online calculator using metric or nonmetric measures to determine your BMI here: nhlbi.nih.gov/health/educational/lose_wt/BMI/bmicalc.htm. If your body mass index drops below 19.5, I recommend you go out of ketosis and ramp up your fruit and carbohydrate intake. In addition, I have patients consume Wahls Fudge (recipe on page 463) if they are losing too much weight. The advice is to eat as much of it as you like until you get back up to a healthy weight. Continue to eat it at the quantity you need to maintain your weight (likely you will not be able to do a ketogenic diet long term). Our patients who have lost more weight than we wanted have all found this to be a very effective and tasty way to maintain a desired weight. This fudge is delicious and energy-dense, but still fits into the parameters of the Wahls Protocol. It is also a terrific end-of-the-meal treat to serve to your guests and still be completely compliant with the Wahls Protocol. Eat fudge! (How's that for a prescription?)

WAHLS WARRIORS SPEAK

I was first diagnosed with endometriosis (I was told it was autoimmune) when I was 15 years old and landed in the hospital with intense abdominal pain. I was diagnosed with my second and third autoimmune diseases in my 20s: narcolepsy and two movement disorders—restless leg disorder and periodic leg movement disorder. Also in my 20s, I was diagnosed with in-flammatory bowel disease, severe ischemic colitis, severe gastroparesis, and severe gastritis. I took drugs for Parkinson's as well as psychiatric drugs, stimulants, and sedatives to control the symptoms of exhaustion, hallucinations, and unwanted movements. I had constant stomach pain, alternating bouts of diarrhea and constipation, bouts of stomach paralysis, and two occasions of colon ulceration and hemorrhage. In my late 20s, I was bitten by a tick, developed a rash and lymph nodes the size of golf balls, and an infectious disease doctor confirmed Lyme disease. In my late 30s, I developed asthma. In 2014 alone, I landed in the emergency room three times and owned seven rescue inhalers. I was diagnosed with my fourth and fifth autoimmune diseases in my 30s: autoimmune thyroiditis and psoriasis. At age 40, I developed pericarditis and landed in the hospital, which led to my sixth and seventh autoimmune diagnoses of fibromyalgia and systemic lupus. My lupus symptoms were mouth ulcerations, malar rash, constant fever, arthritis, joint and body pain, pericarditis, pleuritis, hair loss, exhaustion, hematologic abnormalities, and extreme photosensitivity. During one Texas summer, I did not leave my house for three months unless the sun had gone down. By age 43, I had lost my career and was disabled. I looked 20 years older than I was, I was overweight, and my hair was falling out. I could not imagine a boyfriend still being able to love someone so sick. I could no longer take care of myself or my house. I was a recluse. I had no meaning or purpose.

In August 2014, my boyfriend bought me a copy of The Wahls Protocol. I started at Level 1 of the diet for two weeks, then moved straight to Wahls Paleo Plus. I started a Wahls Diary and vowed to give the protocol a three-year trial. I have now been a dedicated Wahls Warrior for over four years. Using food and functional medicine along with faith, meditation, muscle restoration, and biohacking, I was in remission from every disease listed above except thyroiditis after 18 months. After 24 months, I discontinued all my prescription medications except my thyroid medication. Now, four years later, I am still only on thyroid medication and LDN [low-dose naltrexone]. I still deal with fatigue, but it gets better every year. In 2014, I was convinced I would die from lupus, but I am now convinced that I am disease-free and will live a long and vibrantly healthy life!

—Shannon P., Austin, Texas

Part Seven: Eat Just Once or Twice a Day, and Fast Every Night for at Least Fourteen Hours

Another new component of this level of the Wahls Protocol is the introduction of intermittent fasting or time-restricted feeding. Intermittent fasting is another practice that mimics how our ancestors normally ate. Food was not available 24/7 for our ancestors. In fact, eating was an occasional activity, depending entirely on the success of the hunting and gathering efforts of our ancestral mothers and fathers. Having a steady constant source of high-calorie food is a very recent development in human history. Our bodies were made to eat when we had food, but also to stop eating when there was no food or food was scarce. You may recall earlier in this chapter that the first time doctors recognized ketosis was with water fasting. They then figured out how to mimic the effects with a high-fat diet. But fasting does put you into ketosis, just as a ketogenic diet does, and your mitochondria love this. It is helpful to extend the time between your meals at this level of the diet, because when your body isn't digesting, it can focus its energy on cellular repair and maintenance, cleaning up dead cells, detoxifying waste more efficiently, and generally giving all the parts of your body that work to digest food constantly a much-needed rest.

Intermittent fasting, also called time-restricted feeding (some people distinguish these two terms, but for our purposes, they are the same), is a less extreme way to fast, involving shorter periods of fasting. This might mean fasting for 14 or 16 hours per day (eating only within a window of 8 or 10 hours), or eating every other day. Your mitochondria will thrive if you eat just once or twice a day and fast every evening for at least fourteen hours between your evening meal and your morning meal. Or you can be even stricter, eating during only an eight-, six-, four-, or even one- or two-hour window during the day, fasting the rest of the time. The most common way to do this is to wait until lunch, or early afternoon, to eat anything. Some people aren't hungry right away anyway. Some prefer to eat only breakfast and lunch, and skip dinner. Some more experienced intermittent fasters may eat just one meal a day, which is my routine.

Daily fasting, like the long fasting associated with winter, leads to increased efficiency in your mitochondria and encourages your cells to produce more mitochondria per cell.[9] Our bodies are primed to expect long periods of nutritional ketosis—every winter, in fact!

Although fasting is controversial and I don't recommend long fasting periods (you are not a hibernating bear) without careful, direct supervision by a medical professional who is monitoring you daily, there is growing evidence that intermittent fasting reverses age-related decline in animal models and may also reverse progressive brain disorders. This likely occurs through improved efficiency in the mitochondria, the increase in the number of mitochondria in each cell, and the additional nerve growth hormones generated by fasting, which stimulate brain cell growth and additional brain cell connections.[10] Some people do enjoy longer fasting periods—you can achieve this effect by fasting every other day, but you don't have to go that far. Instead, just fast fourteen or more hours every day, which can include overnight while you are sleeping.

Eating only twice or even just once a day is not that difficult once you adjust to Wahls Paleo Plus, because nutritional ketosis diets tend to suppress the appetite (whereas high-carb diets tend to stimulate the appetite). When blood sugar is kept very stable, you will likely find that you are hungry only when your body genuinely needs food, and that is probably only twice per day for most people who adhere strictly to Wahls Paleo Plus. Calorie restriction (cutting daily calories to approximately 65 percent of normal intake for certain periods of time), has also proven to be an effective intervention for obesity, diabetes, insulin resistance, and reduction of cardiovascular disease risk factors, but it leaves one chronically hungry. Eating every other day without increasing your calorie consumption on the days you do eat is also very effective, but these methods may be more difficult for many people.

For those who want to embrace this method of getting or staying in ketosis, I recommend starting with longer feeding windows, such as a ten-hour feeding window and a fourteen-hour fasting window. Gradually lengthen the fasting time to between sixteen and twenty-two hours (meaning you would eat during an eight- to two-hour window). This will gradually increase your exposure to ketones, lower your insulin levels, give you improved insulin sensitivity, and even increase energy and improve many other measures of health.

It's not for everyone—not everyone can handle prolonged periods without eating—but Wahls Paleo Plus tends to suppress appetite, so after you have been practicing this level of the Wahls Protocol, you may find that you naturally begin to practice intermittent fasting. (This is how people who use olive oil as their fat source can achieve ketosis without MCT oil—see page 235.)

Even if longer fasting or shorter windows of eating aren't comfortable for you at first, keep working toward fasting at least fourteen hours between dinner and breakfast. With a fourteen-hour fast, your body can much more effectively accomplish the important work of cellular repair. If you find it uncomfortable to eat only twice a day, go ahead and keep having three meals until you feel ready to make this change. If you do eat three meals, try making one of your three meals a smoothie only, which is easier for your body to digest quickly. This is also a good way to pack in a good portion of your vegetables and fruit. (Don't forget to add full-fat coconut milk or olive oil!)

Note: I would prefer you completely eliminate alcohol at this stage, or at least reserve it for very special occasions only. If you do have a drink, choose a low-carb drink like vodka or very dry wine. The main reason to minimize alcohol is that your body will metabolize the calories in the alcohol first, before any other energy sources, including fat. Also, your liver has to work hard to process alcohol, and you don't want to tax your liver needlessly when you are trying to heal.

The longer you stick with Wahls Paleo Plus, the easier it gets. I find it's not difficult to follow at all anymore. I do suggest that you continue to monitor your blood ketones. It will give you feedback on your dietary choices and help keep you on track. Results will also keep you motivated, so as you progress with Wahls Paleo Plus, pay attention to how you feel and write down your physical and emotional reactions to the diet in your Wahls Diary. If you feel great and notice improvement in your symptoms, keep going! If it's too difficult for you at this stage in your life because of family or personal reasons, it's okay to go back to Wahls Paleo or Wahls Elimination for now. This is a much preferable alternative to giving up completely. Stay strong so that your Wahls Protocol, at whichever level you choose to practice it, can work for you.

THE RISKS AND BENEFITS OF LONGER-TERM FASTING

Fasting for long periods isn't for everyone, but there is some evidence that it can be beneficial. Going sixteen to forty-eight hours without any food is a kind of extended form of intermittent fasting, or what is sometimes called periodic fasting. In animal studies, periodic fasting has shown great benefits on many different health measures and may be particulary useful in slowing, stopping, or even reversing disease progression. Extended or periodic fasting from two to as many as twenty-one days has resulted in documented improvement in diabetes, cardiovascular disease, cancer, neurological disorders like Alzheimer's disease and Parkinson's disease, and stroke, with interesting regenerative effects all over the body. Don't do extended fasting without direct, daily supervision by a medical team experienced with extended fasting.

In order to get stem-cell-boosting effects in your pancreas, heart, liver, and blood vessels, you need to fast for at least five days, or up to seven days. Periodic fasting promotes stem-cell-based regeneration and long-lasting metabolic effects. Dr. Valter Longo's team at the University of Southern California Longevity Institute has done extensive research on the benefits of periodic fasting in animal models of aging, heart disease, cancer, and multiple sclerosis, working out the details of the favorable changes that are achieved by water fasting. In addition, he has worked out how to do this using a fasting-mimicking diet, so the beneficial effects can be achieved without doing a water fast. He has also developed a fasting-mimicking diet kit (prolonfmd.com) that mimics the physiologic benefits of the periodic fast while still allowing for the consumption of a small amount of food.

I used to do water-only periodic fasting as part of my anti-aging strategy, but I have switched to using the fasting-mimicking diet kit for my fasting days. See the Resources for more information.

Periodic fasting may be the safest way to boost your own stem cells and improve your body's ability to self-repair. I believe periodic fasting could have tremendous potential for health benefits, if it works in your life.

But if you do any kind of fasting, you must be medically supervised by your personal medical team. They should look over your medication list, your blood pressure, your blood sugar, and kidney and liver blood tests to confirm they are functioning normally and confirm you would be expected to tolerate fasting. Also, no saunas or vigorous workouts during the fast! If you elect to do periodic fasting, it is important to continue sipping on bone broth or clear vegetable broth with sea salt to prevent electrolyte imbalance and lower the risk of fainting during the fast. I do suggest taking a resistant starch such as inulin to provide food for your microbiome. Both these strategies can make fasting more tolerable.

This is a potent strategy to give your native stem cells a boost. But you must work with your personal medical team if you wish to add fasting to your routine.

Caution: As with Wahls Paleo Plus, you should not practice any form of fasting if you are pregnant, beyond a twelve-hour window while sleeping. Also, do not practice fasting if you do not have your medical team's approval. Fasting is contraindicated if you are underweight, are fighting an infection, are taking insulin, or are suffering from a hormonal imbalance such as with your thyroid or with estrogen or testosterone.

WAHLS PALEO PLUS AT A GLANCE

At the Wahls Paleo Plus level, you will continue to follow all the parameters of Wahls Paleo, with the exceptions below. Eat to satiety, but remember that the goal is to consume few carbohydrates, low to moderate protein, and plenty of fat. Eating a diet that is approximately 65 percent fat with liberal use of medium-chain fat sources like coconut oil and full-fat coconut milk will maintain nutritional ketosis. (If you are relying on olive oil to get into ketosis, keep in mind that time-restricted feeding will probably be required in order for you to achieve low-level ketosis and that a further restriction of carbohydrates will be required—see page 235.)

Eat at least 68 grams or more of fat, either through 4 to 6 tablespoons of coconut oil, ¾ to 1 can (about 1¾ cups) or even more of full-fat coconut milk, or 4 to 6 tablespoons olive oil. At each meal or snack throughout the day, you may use both coconut oil and full-fat coconut milk, as well as unheated olive oil or ghee, as desired. If you weigh more than 150 pounds, you will probably need 700 or more calories of fat. If you are not in nutritional ketosis after one to two weeks, you may need to increase the fat intake, decrease carbohydrate intake, or lengthen your intermittent fasting window. (You may also need to add another resistant starch such as inulin to feed your microbiome sufficient fiber—your goal is still to have one soft bowel movement per day.)

NOTE: You can now buy "coconut milk" in cartons in the store, but this is *not* the same as canned coconut milk. It is much lower in fat and contains fillers and additives, and often sugar. This is not the kind of coconut milk I recommend. Look for the full-fat kind in cans. There are also a few brands in cartons at Indian or Asian groceries, but the coconut milk you buy shouldn't have more than two to three ingredients. Unsweetened varieties in cartons are okay for a dairy substitute at the Wahls Diet and Wahls Paleo levels, but not for Wahls Paleo Plus.

- The 9 cups of vegetables and fruits daily may be reduced to 6 cups (even 4 cups for petite women). No white potatoes, legumes (including any soy, such as soy milk), or grains (including gluten-free grains and rice milk). If you still need some milk, stick to unsweetened full-fat coconut milk.
- Limit starchy vegetables, like beets and winter squash, to raw, always accompanied by at least 1 tablespoon of fat and some protein. If you are not in nutritional ketosis after two weeks, you may need to eliminate starchy vegetables.
- Limit fruit to 1 cup per day, only berries. Always eat these with fat, such as coconut milk. Do not consume other types of fruit, dried fruit, canned fruit, or fruit juices, all of which are higher in sugar. If you are not in ketosis in two weeks, you may need to eliminate berries entirely.
- Reduce protein to 6 to 12 ounces according to size and gender.

- Reduce meals to one or two per day, with fourteen to sixteen hours between dinner and breakfast. If you must eat three meals, be sure to maintain that twelve- to sixteen-hour fast.
- Save alcohol for rare special-occasion events.
- Use resistant starch, such as inulin, as needed to maintain one soft, easily passed bowel movement daily.
- Monitor your fasting lipids six weeks after starting Wahls Paleo Plus.

Wahls Paleo Plus Meal Plan

Congratulations on making it to this most advanced level of the Wahls Protocol! You are about to experience profound changes in your health. Try this sample meal plan and monitor your reactions to every change carefully, so you can customize your plan based on what foods work for you and what changes don't agree with you.

Wahls Paleo Plus Week		
All foods that have corresponding recipes at the end of this book are marked with an asterisk (*).		
Day	*Breakfast*	*Dinner*
Day 1	Smoothie: • 1 cup spinach • 1 cup blueberries • 1 cup full-fat coconut milk • 1 teaspoon ground cinnamon • 1 tablespoon nutritional yeast • ½ cup ice 1 serving Salmon or Chicken Salad* wrapped in collard leaf (1 cup) 1 serving Beet and Cranberry Mixture* ¼ cup fermented pickles	1 serving Liver, Onions, and Mushrooms* ½ cup cooked broccoli 1 teaspoon extra virgin olive oil Salad: • 2 cups romaine lettuce • 2 cups bok choy • ½ cup tomatoes • ½ cup green pepper • 2 cloves garlic • 1 tablespoon extra virgin olive oil • balsamic vinegar to taste • dried basil to taste • 1 tablespoon sunflower seeds ¼ cup kimchi Licorice or other herbal tea ½ cup full-fat coconut milk (add to tea if desired)

Day	Breakfast	Dinner
Day 2	Smoothie: • 1 cup kale • 1 teaspoon green tea powder • 1 teaspoon ground cardamom • ¾ cup full-fat coconut milk • ½ cup ice 1 serving Liver Pâté* ½ cup raw turnip slices 1 medium stalk celery ½ cup Kombucha Tea*	1 serving Basic Skillet Recipe* (Lamb Chops and Broccoli) 1 tablespoon horseradish Salad: • 3 cups spinach • 2 cups kale • 5 medium radishes • ¼ cup sliced carrots • ¼ cup cucumber slices with peel • dried basil to taste • 1½ tablespoons chopped walnuts • 2 tablespoons extra virgin olive oil • balsamic vinegar to taste ¼ cup fermented sauerkraut ¾ cup strawberry halves with 1 tablespoon full-fat coconut milk 2 cups chamomile or other herbal tea with ½ cup coconut milk
Day 3	1½ servings Turmeric Tea* 3¾ ounces canned sardines in tomato sauce ½ cup raw carrot slices ½ cup parsley ½ cup daikon radish 1 serving Beet and Red Cabbage Mixture* plus 2 tablespoons coconut oil ½ cup Kombucha Tea*	1 serving Basic Skillet Recipe* (Heart and Mustard Greens) 1 serving Brussels Sprouts, Bacon, and Cranberries* Salad: • 4 cups romaine lettuce • 2 cloves garlic • 1 tablespoon gingerroot • dried oregano, to taste • 1 tablespoon extra-virgin olive oil • balsamic vinegar to taste • 1 tablespoon sunflower seeds ¼ cup lacto-fermented okra pickles 1 cup cherries chamomile herbal tea ½ cup full-fat coconut milk

Day	Breakfast	Dinner
Day 4	1 serving Bone Broth–Carrot Soup* 1 serving Rosemary Chicken* 1 serving Beet Greens and Bacon* 1½ ounces raw almonds (soaked) ½ cup Beet Kvass* plus ½ cup water	1 serving Seafood Stew* (Paleo Plus version) 1 cup raw spiralized butternut squash (add to stew just before serving) 1 tablespoon extra virgin olive oil Salad: • 4 cups bok choy • ¼ cup celery • 1 tablespoon sunflower seeds • 5 medium black olives • 1 tablespoon gingerroot • dried oregano to taste • 1 tablespoon extra virgin olive oil • lime juice to taste 1 cup raspberries herbal tea ½ cup full-fat coconut milk
Day 5	1 serving Bone Broth–Pepper Soup* 1 serving Basic Skillet Recipe* (Collards and Ham) 1 serving Fruit Pudding* ½ cup Kombucha Tea*	1 serving Algerian Chicken with Asparagus* 1 cup Cauliflower Rice* 1 tablespoon extra virgin olive oil ¼ cup fermented sauerkraut Salad: • 4½ cups bok choy • ½ cup cilantro • ½ cup fresh orange sections • ¼ cup sliced cucumber with peel • 4 teaspoons extra virgin olive oil • lime juice to taste herbal tea ½ cup full-fat coconut milk

Day	Breakfast	Dinner
Day 6	1½ servings Bone Broth–Cauliflower Turmeric Soup* Salad: • 3 cups kale • ½ cup radish • ½ cup sweet yellow peppers • ½ cup tomato • ¼ cup chopped onion • 1 tablespoon extra virgin olive oil • 1½ tablespoons chopped almonds (soaked) • balsamic vinegar to taste 3.5 ounces canned salmon ½ cup Beet Kvass* plus ½ cup water	1 serving Basic Skillet Recipe* (Pork Chops and Red Cabbage) ¼ cup kimchi 6 medium asparagus spears Salad: • 2 cups spinach • ½ cup sweet red peppers • ½ cup sliced cucumbers • ½ cup sliced mushrooms • 1 tablespoon extra virgin olive oil • lemon juice to taste 1 cup cantaloupe 1 serving Hot Cocoa*
Day 7	1 serving Bone Broth–Avocado Soup* ¾ serving Basic Skillet Recipe* (Steak and Mustard Greens) 1 serving Beet and Cranberry Mixture* 1 tablespoon extra virgin olive oil ½ cup Kombucha Tea*	1 serving Coconut Milk–Fish Soup* 1 tablespoon jalapeño pepper ¼ cup kimchi Salad: • 3½ cups romaine lettuce • dried basil to taste • ¼ cup sliced carrots • 1 teaspoon sesame seeds (raw, soaked) • 1 teaspoon extra virgin olive oil • lime juice to taste Mixed berries: • ¼ cup strawberries • ¼ cup blackberries • ¼ cup raspberries • ¼ cup full-fat coconut milk 1 cup chamomile tea 2.5 fluid ounces full-fat coconut milk (add to tea if desired)

Part Three

GOING BEYOND FOOD

Chapter 8

REDUCING TOXIC LOAD

Y OU'VE COME A long way. You've worked through the Wahls Diet, perhaps staying there, or you've progressed to Wahls Paleo, or perhaps
you've even moved on to Wahls Paleo Plus or Wahls Elimination. If
you are staying strong with the dietary changes, you are almost certainly noticing some improvements, but the Wahls Protocol isn't just about food. You
can do more. You can go further. In this section of the book, I will give you
some non-food-related prescriptions that are all part of the Wahls Protocol.
First and foremost, let's talk about toxins.

We no longer live in the world inhabited by our grandparents. Since
World War II, we have relied on chemistry to lessen our work and enrich our
lives in many ways. Unfortunately, due to pollution of the air and water, pesticides and other chemicals used on agricultural products, chemical preservatives and colors used in drinks and processed foods, and food itself that has
been chemically manipulated (like hydrogenated oils and high-fructose corn
syrup), many of those chemicals end up inside us because we eat them, drink
them, inhale them, or touch them.

When substances enter the body that do not naturally occur within the
body or are not expected to enter the body (for example, the body expects food,

water, and oxygen, but not pesticides, food coloring, or drugs), they are called xenobiotics or exotoxins (*exo* means outer, so this word means toxins that come from outside the body). Some xenobiotics or exotoxins won't have any effect, but many can confuse the signaling that goes on within and between our cells. A great and decades-long experiment is being conducted, and we, the unsuspecting public, are the guinea pigs. Our living, working, and recreational environments are now loaded with toxins, more than ninety thousand of which are registered with the Environmental Protection Agency (EPA).

Many of these toxins come from food additives and toxic residues from industrial food production (the main reason I recommend organic and home-grown food), but food is not the only source of chemicals in our environment. Let's look beyond our dinner plates for a moment, at the vast pollution and contamination in every aspect of our lives: arsenic-treated wood on play structures; off-gassing from the paint, carpets, and furniture in our own homes; residue from plastics; heavy metals in the water supply; air pollution from factory emissions, vehicle emissions, power plant emissions; even possibly electromagnetic waves, microwaves, and Wi-Fi radiation (which may have biologic effects on our cells). We fill our mouths with mercury through our dental fillings; we wash our clothes and slather our skins with products that contain endocrine disrupters that can affect hormonal signaling in our bodies; and on top of that (back to that dinner plate), we don't eat sufficient nutrients to help our bodies efficiently dispose of the toxins we ingest, breathe, absorb, and apply. It's a wonder our mitochondria work at all!

In her seminal environmental book *Silent Spring*, published in 1962, Rachel Carson wrote:

> For the first time in the history of the world, every human being is now subjected to contact with dangerous chemicals, from the moment of conception until death. In the less than two decades of their use, the synthetic pesticides have been so thoroughly distributed throughout the animate and inanimate world that they occur virtually everywhere.[1]

Many studies have linked various environmental chemicals with a wide variety of health issues, like neurodegeneration, mood disorders, diabetes, chronic heart disease, and cancer.[2]

WAHLS DIARY ALERT

Answer any of these questions in your Wahls Diary:

- What toxins do you think (or know) you've been exposed to over your lifetime? Anything in particular beyond the average person living in the developed world? Do you have a job working with chemicals? Do you work on or live near a farm? Do you live near a factory?
- After you finish this chapter, list some of the ways you think you will be able to reduce your toxic exposure.

To confuse the matter further, in addition to all these environmental chemicals, toxins come from our own bodies. These are called endotoxins, because they are from our own chemical processes (*endo* means within). They can be bacteria or the waste products from chemical reactions. Healthy people without susceptible genes who regularly receive complete nutrition should ideally be able to eliminate these efficiently, but if you are missing any of the nutritional elements necessary to keep the engine of detoxification running smoothly, you may have more trouble eliminating endotoxins as well as xenobiotics. Depending on your genetic susceptibility as well as your health and past exposures, you may be particularly sensitive to the toxins inherent in our environment. The result is that the finely tuned symphony of life that should be making its music of robust health inside you begins to get out of sync.

If you have MS or another autoimmune disease, chances are good that you *are* sensitive to these toxic influences. The good news is that while it is not possible to live a completely toxin-free existence, there are ways to drastically minimize your exposure to toxins, as well as increase your body's ability to process them and eliminate them efficiently and effectively. Most important, you must do two things:

1. Maximize your body's natural detoxification process
2. Minimize your toxic exposure

FOOD ADDITIVES AND OBESITY

Food additives, such as food colorings and preservatives, may have many negative health effects, including increasing intestinal permeability and the probability of proteins inappropriately entering the bloodstream. Another risk is obesity. Many food additives are what are called excitotoxins. These substances drive overconsumption because they (1) alter the microbiome balance to favor more pathogenic microbes that may influence food cravings, and (2) change the taste and consistency of food to make it more irresistible. Both these factors can encourage overeating that has nothing to do with natural hunger. This is just one more reason why it is a good idea to cook at home with real whole-food ingredients that don't contain additives.

Promote Natural Toxin Elimination

Many of my patients test positive for heavy metals, and I was no exception. My lab tests showed I had toxic levels of multiple heavy metals, so I detoxed naturally through my dietary protocol as well as other gentle methods, including regular sessions in an infrared sauna, clay masks, supplemental algae and kelp, and some other supplements that specifically target the body's detoxification systems, until my body eliminated the toxic metals and my health was remarkably improved. Two years later, the follow-up labs showed that I had cleared out the excess heavy metals.

Many people have a name for the process of encouraging toxin elimination: cleansing. Trendy as cleansing may be, it's an ancient practice, and cleansing rituals are a part of many traditions. Often these cleansing rituals were associated with spiritual purification or healing: cold and hot springs, sweat lodges, mud baths, fasting—all are ways to help the body cleanse itself of impurities so it can work better.

Now we know more about the human body than our ancestors did. We know which organs specifically work to process and eliminate toxins. The main workers are:

- The liver
- The kidneys
- The sweat glands
- The lymphatic drainage system

Before we can understand how to promote the important work of detoxification, it's important to understand how detoxification happens in the body.

Most toxins are fat-soluble, so they must be converted to water-soluble substances in order to be excreted in the bile (through the liver), the urine (through the kidneys), sweat (from the sweat glands and through the skin), breath (through the lungs), and lymph (through the lymphatic system). This process happens in two parts:

1. In phase one, the toxins are converted to reactive metabolites using chemical processes like oxidation, reduction, hydrolysis, and dehalogenation. In other words, they are released from the fat and set free in the body. The toxins are then more active and actually more toxic because they are no longer trapped in the fat cells. But the body has a plan.
2. In phase two, your cells attach a side chain to the newly active toxin. This could be another chemical structure, such as a sulfur group, a methyl group, or a specific amino acid. This makes the toxin water-soluble so it can be flushed out of the body.

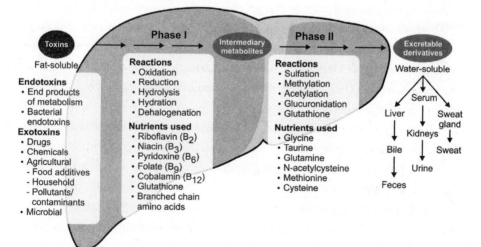

Toxins enter and exit your body in many ways. Of course, many toxins come from the food you eat, but that is not the only way. Your lungs will move toxins into your body if you are smoking or exposed to air pollution, but can move toxins out through exhalation. Your skin will move toxins into your body if toxins come into contact with your skin (such as through personal care products or chlorine from a pool), but can move toxins out through sweating. The lymphatics transport the biologic wastes of cellular metabolism as well as bacteria and viruses into the lymph nodes and then back to the heart, where they will be mixed with the blood and transported to the liver and kidneys for removal.

Every part of this process must work correctly in order to release the toxins from the body. If the toxin is converted to the reactive metabolite (phase one) but is not converted to a water-soluble state (phase two), it can actually be more damaging to the body. If digestion is not working, toxins can remain in the body for too long and may be reabsorbed. If the lymphatics are not draining well, the fluid will back up, leading to swelling in the involved leg or arm. If the backup is severe, skin ulcerations develop.

Acne-like rashes can develop with some toxin exposures, such as bromine poisoning, which is associated with an acne-like rash. Bromine exposure is increased as iodine-based preservatives are replaced by bromine-based preservatives in the food supply. The additional chlorine and fluoride in the water treatment further increases the halogen load, which increases toxicity from the bromine and makes us at greater risk for developing insufficiency of the thyroid. As one clears excess bromine, acne may appear around the mouth.

These are just some of the reasons why people sometimes have negative experiences with detoxification. Once the toxins are ready to exit, we need to help them exit so they don't continue to circulate in the body freed from the fat, where they can do more damage.

There are important ways to do this, and fortunately not only are they easy but you are probably already doing them. The best way to do this is to eat your 9 cups of greens, color, and sulfur-rich vegetables, plus seaweed and organ meat, to facilitate this two-phase process and effectively eliminate the toxins. This will provide your body with all the substances it requires to effectively process the toxins to a state where they can be released. Specifically, be sure to get plenty of:

- Selenium and iodine (from seaweed)
- Zinc and coenzyme Q10 (from organ meat)
- Thiols (from sulfur-rich vegetables and greens)
- Flavonoids (from bright colors)
- Minerals (from iodized sea salt and seaweed)
- Complete amino acids (from animal protein or balanced vegetarian proteins combined to include all the necessary amino acids, as I talked about in chapter 6, "Wahls Paleo")

BRAIN DETOXIFICATION

Did you know the brain has a lymph system that is involved in clearing out the trash from the brain? Scientists didn't know this until recently, when these "hidden" lymphatic structures were discovered. As you sleep at night, the brain processes the trash (amyloid in particular) and removes it via the glymphatic system (this is the name for the lymphatic system in the brain). The brain generates amyloid proteins (plaques) to bind up the infectious particles and toxins that made it past the blood-brain barrier so they are less harmful to the individual. Every night, some of these amyloid plaques are cleared . . . *if* you have a well-functioning detoxification system *and a* sufficient number of hours of deep high-quality sleep. If the amyloid plaques accumulate due to impaired functioning of the glymphatic system, the brain is more likely to develop tangles that damage the brain. This process begins in our 20s. If you have amyloid plaques and tangles, you are at greater risk of developing cognitive problems. If your brain is inflamed *and* you have amyloid plaques and tangles, you are much more likely to have more severe problems with memory decline and dementia. The strategies to reduce the damage from amyloid are to improve clearance by improving the quantity and quality of sleep (see pages 380 to 387). In addition, ashwagandha, an Indian herb that has been used for memory and brain support for hundreds of years, can help to reduce inflammation and improve clearance of amyloid plaques. I recommend taking 500 to 600 milligrams per day. Other natural substances that have been tested and found to increase clearance of these plaques incude turmeric, brahmi (also called *Bacopa monnieri*), and L-serine.[3]

Adding spices with a favorable impact on detoxification can support your body's efforts even further by improving the efficiency of the detoxification enzymes in the liver, kidneys, and sweat glands (in part by impacting which genes in our DNA are turned on and turned off). The spices will help ensure the proper balance of the detoxification enzymes that are on hand to process and eliminate the toxins you encounter each day. Liberally add these herbs and spices to your food:

- Aloe
- Burdock
- Cayenne
- Dandelion root
- Dill
- Ginger
- Horseradish
- Parsley
- Peppermint
- Rosemary
- Saffron
- Turmeric

Other substances that can be valuable for detoxification include silymarin (from milk thistle seeds used for teas or supplements) and Pycnogenol (from maritime pine bark as a supplement; I'll talk more about supplements in chapter 10).

Nutrition is important, but there are some other great detox strategies I'd also like you to consider. Here are my favorites:

- **Poop better.** Our gut bacteria are responsible for clearing approximately 25 percent of the xenobiotics (foreign substances or toxins) we encounter. Being constipated decreases this clearance, so it is important to stay regular. Eat fiber to have a soft, easily passed bowel movement each day and you will improve your toxin clearance.
- **Sweat.** Many societies have sweating rituals as part of the purification process. The sweat glands are very effective at removing heavy metals, plastics,

and solvents. A sauna is an excellent way to sweat on purpose—it causes the blood vessels to dilate (the body's internal cooling mechanism), increasing the heart's output. This actually accomplishes an effect similar to aerobic exercise! (I discuss this further in the next chapter, "Moving for Healing.") However, saunas are not for everyone. Do not use saunas if you are or could be pregnant. Many people with MS and other chronic health issues can be severely intolerant to elevations in body temperature. Do not use a sauna until you can tolerate it well. I needed to recover remarkably before I was able to tolerate taking a sauna—this didn't happen until six months into my recovery. When I was finally able to stand the heat, I purchased an infrared sauna for my home. It sits next to the Endless Pool I swim in each day. I began taking a sauna four days a week as part of my detox protocol.

- **Use mud/clay and activated charcoal.** Clays have been used for thousands of years to rejuvenate skin and health. Clay baths for the body or face will extract heavy metals, solvents, and other toxins stored in the fatty tissues of the skin, and activated charcoal can be incorporated into these baths and masks.

WAHLS WARNING

If people adopt my diet overnight, as the people who are entering our clinical trials often do, it is common to experience "detox symptoms." Even a gradual introduction to the Wahls Diet at any level can result in detox symptoms, especially if you have a particularly large burden of toxins stored in your body, but a sudden dietary change can make these symptoms more noticeable and uncomfortable. But in most cases, the old adage applies: Better out than in! If you are prepared for the symptoms of detox, you will know what they are and not mistake them for a flare-up of your illness. They may include the following:

- Acne-like reactions in the skin (likely from bromine that is being excreted via skin)
- Headache

- Body aches
- Malaise
- Temporarily worsening fatigue
- Marked craving for sugar and carbs (by-products of dying sugar-loving yeasts and bacteria that are trying very hard to keep you eating a lot of carbs)
- Bad-smelling breath, sweat, or stool

The good news is that these detox symptoms typically begin tapering within a couple of weeks for our clinical trial participants. In my clinical practice, I tell people to wind down the bad food as they wind up the good food over a week. When it is done that way, the detox symptoms are generally somewhat less bothersome. And remember what's happening when you feel them: The bad stuff is coming out!

WAHLS WARNING

Note that activated charcoal, edible clay, kelp, and chlorella will not only absorb toxins, they may also absorb medicines from your bloodstream, including those you take by mouth. If you are on any medication, let your doctor know if you plan to work to improve your detoxification and what methods you plan to employ, and follow your doctor's directions regarding the best way to do this so as not to interfere with your medication.

- You can also make these masks yourself. A wide variety of clays can be found in health food stores or through online stores. Mix the clay or activated charcoal with chlorella (see the next bullet) and sea salt to make a paste, apply to your skin, and allow it to dry. Leave it on for thirty minutes, then rinse it off. Another way to use clay is to make a diluted clay bath in a bucket for soaking the feet. It's quite relaxing to mix this with magnesium salts. (Afterward, dump the muddy water in the yard so it doesn't clog your plumbing!) Or make a very diluted clay/water mixture and soak in the bathtub for thirty to sixty minutes. If you ever get the opportunity to go to a spa that offers mud baths, take advantage of this effective detoxifying therapy.

- **Use chlorella and kelp.** Algae and kelp absorb released toxins so they cannot be reabsorbed back into the bloodstream. Not only are they good for your diet but they can be useful applied to the skin, with clay (as explained above) or in a seaweed mask. However, a warning: If you are going to use algae, I suggest you use only chlorella. Wild algae and spirulina are more likely to be contaminated with harmful cyanotoxins that can cause neurologic damage.[4] These algae cyanotoxins are a variation of the noxious toxins produced by algae in the red tide algae blooms associated with fish die-offs and beach closures in polluted coastal waters.[5]

- **Improve lymphatic return.** The purpose of the lymphatic system is to carry away waste that the body generates and accumulates from daily living. Sometimes, however, lymphatic flow and drainage can slow down and waste can back up in the lymphatic system. A very simple way to improve lymphatic drainage is to practice simple inversions. If you invert yourself using an inversion table or lie on the floor with your hips next to the wall and your legs elevated vertically along the wall, you will increase the return of blood and lymph from your legs, where it can pool, back into your circulation. Inversion is an excellent way to reduce swelling in the legs if you are experiencing swelling related to decreasing physical activity (or airline travel). Start with brief amounts of time and very gradually increase the time with the legs elevated. If you experience swelling in the arms due to decreasing activity of the arm(s), elevating the involved arm(s) overhead can also be quite helpful. Another way to improve lymphatic return is dry brushing.

- **Dry brushing.** This is a technique that increases detoxification through the skin, removes old skin cells, and helps improve lymphatic flow since the lymphatic vessels are just beneath the skin. The technique is simple. Use a gentle brush or a clean, dry washcloth to stroke your skin, starting with your feet, in a gentle circular fashion up toward your heart. Do each leg, then your abdomen. Next, do each arm. The whole process typically takes just five to ten minutes. You can do this daily if you wish. Many people like to do this just before showering or bathing.

Minimize Your Toxic Exposure

We encounter toxins in the environment all the time, but one of the most intense—and most easily controlled—is what touches your skin. As your largest organ, the skin is important for toxin elimination, but what people don't always realize is that it also absorbs toxins from the environment. Think about all the soaps, lotions, sunscreens, and medicines you've applied to your skin. You soak those up and they enter your system. Read the labels: All of the chemicals named in the ingredient list will need to be processed and eliminated by your liver and kidneys.

For this reason, one effective way to minimize your toxic exposure is to choose organic personal hygiene products—those that are as natural as possible. Also consider how many products you really need to use. If you are bathing daily, washing your armpits and groin with soap, and eating a clean diet, you probably aren't going to need a lot of other personal care products. You're going to look and smell great naturally. For instance, you may be able to skip an antiperspirant, which often contains aluminum, a heavy metal that has been implicated in dementia, Parkinson's disease, and neurodegeneration. If you do still want to use some sort of deodorant, look for a natural brand that doesn't contain aluminum. Or you can use a light dusting of baking soda instead.

The furnishings, building materials, cleaning products, cookware, food

WAHLS WARNING

The low-grade estrogen effect from the plastics, perfumes, solvents, and hormones in our foods and personal care products has been linked to early menstruation in girls as young as 7, falling sperm counts worldwide, increased problems with erectile dysfunction in men in their 20s (a common complaint in primary care clinics), and infertility in women due to polycystic ovary syndrome. They are also implicated as contributing to the development of obesity, metabolic syndrome, and diabetes. This is why they are sometimes referred to as endocrine disrupters. These compounds disrupt and confuse the hormone signals of our endocrine glands.

storage containers, and even the water coming out of your faucets can also expose you to hundreds of synthetic compounds that interfere with your cells' chemical operations, often by gently nudging your hormonal system out of balance. If you detoxify your indoor environment—all at once or a little at a time as manageable—you can minimize toxic exposure where you live, and that can make a big difference in your internal toxin load. Here are some strategies:

- Filter your air. Unfortunately in the last year, due in part to increased emissions into the air in the U.S. and increased burning of coal in Asia, the air quality has declined in many American cities. Some of my patients have experienced improved energy and reduced symptoms by adding high quality air filtration into their homes—you might consider this. See Resources for additional information.

- Gradually replace synthetic carpets, curtains, and bedding with natural fabrics. These synthetic materials can release or off-gas chemicals that you breathe in for years. Good fabric choices for the home include wool, organic cotton, hemp, and bamboo fabric.

- Gradually replace all particleboard, plywood, fiberglass, fiberboard, and paneling in your furniture, cabinets, walls, and floors. These materials can also off-gas toxic compounds into your indoor air. Replace them with natural hardwoods and bamboo.

- Paint only with low-VOC (volatile organic compounds) paint for indoor surfaces.

- Open your windows as often as possible to ventilate your indoor spaces, and place a few green plants around the house. Plants help detoxify your air. If you have allergies, consider a high-quality air cleaner for your bedroom, where you spend many hours of your life breathing deeply.

- Switch to natural or "green" household cleaners. Vinegar, baking soda, and hydrogen peroxide can take care of most jobs, or purchase natural cleaners. Clean your house at least every week to keep dust particles, bacteria, and mold in check.

- Replace all the plastic food storage containers in your home with glass ones. An economical way to do this is to save glass jars from foods like pickles and salsa, and use those to store leftovers.

- Replace coated nonstick pans with stainless steel or enameled cast iron.

- Filter your water. There are many levels of filtering available; even a pitcher with a filter can reduce toxins in your tap water. Whole-house charcoal filtration systems in which the filter is replaced annually is the most effective. A reverse osmosis system is also a superior option because it is the only way to remove the various drugs that have likely entered your water supply. However, the downside of reverse osmosis is that it also removes minerals.

And what about in your mouth? If your mouth is full of "silver" fillings that contain mercury, a small amount of mercury vapor is released every time you chew food, and this can be absorbed into your body. There is a relationship between the number of mercury fillings in the mouth and the amount of mercury in the brain. Many people decide to have their mercury fillings removed, but I do not advise this without proper research and consideration. Removing mercury fillings can actually release more mercury into your body if it is done incorrectly. As the dentist removes the fillings, the drilling will vaporize some of the mercury, which can then be inhaled and reabsorbed by

---

WAHLS WARRIOR Q&A

Q: Will the Wahls Protocol help with PCOS (polycystic ovary syndrome), endometriosis, infertility, or other hormonal issues like PMS and hot flashes?
A: Once our endocrine glands begin to get out of sync, the chemistry of our cells begins to falter. These changes can make adult women hormonally much more like men, and adult men hormonally much more like women (think polycystic ovary syndrome, infertility, erectile dysfunction, obesity, mood problems, and insulin resistance). The ovaries and testicles make the most potent sex hormones, which activate and develop the secondary sex characteristics like breast growth, menstrual cycles, body hair, and lower voices, beginning in adolescence. The adrenal glands also make sex hormones to a lesser extent, and fat makes sex hormones, too. In addition, there is an increasing amount of evidence that many synthetic compounds (e.g., plastics, solvents, fragrances, etc.) can fit into the sex hormone receptors and confuse our biology.[6]

> Hormonal issues can feel like a huge problem, but in many cases the answer is relatively simple. Diet can make a huge difference for women suffering from PCOS and infertility as well as other hormonal issues like PMS and the symptoms of menopause. Also consider whether hormone disruption from plastics, solvents, fragrances, and pesticides could be contributing to hormone imbalance. Furthermore, unrecognized gluten sensitivity can be a factor in endometriosis, polycystic ovary syndrome, erectile dysfunction, and infertility problems. Many of these conditions are also related to insulin resistance. Stabilizing blood sugar and lowering insulin levels by decreasing carbohydrates and reducing the body's toxin load is the prescription. The more completely you can embrace Wahls Paleo or Wahls Paleo Plus, the more quickly insulin will normalize, and likely so will sex hormone ratios. Also, go meticulously organic and do what you can to improve the detoxification pathways in order to reduce hormone disruption.

your body. It is important to work with a dentist who has been specifically trained in the safe handling of mercury fillings to minimize the risk of increasing the mercury load released in the process. Look for someone who has been specifically trained by the International Academy of Oral Medicine and Toxicology (IAOMT).

Note that it has become increasingly popular for dentists to call themselves holistic, mercury-free, or biologic dentists because they no longer use mercury/silver fillings. However, many of these dentists have not received advanced training in the safe removal of mercury. Do your research!

Another dental problem is the use of fluoride as a strategy to reduce dental decay and as an addition to city water. Fluoride is toxic to bone and brain cells and is associated with reductions in IQ of children.[7] Better to not use fluoride to prevent dental cavities; instead, eliminate white flour and sugar from the diet and stick with the Wahls Protocol, which will give you the intensive nutrition you need to fight dental decay.

Finally, consider your EMF exposure. This is a controversial subject—that EMFs, or electromagnetic frequencies—pose a danger to human health. However, the fact is that we are bombarded with EMFs from Wi-Fi routers, cell

WAHLS WARRIORS SPEAK

Knowing that I had numerous "silver" fillings and a "silver" cap that needed oral surgery to be removed, as well as a "mercury tattoo" [a tattoo with mercury in the ink], I took Dr. Wahls's advice and began the process of investigating my mercury levels. I had my urine, blood, and hair tested for mercury, and needless to say, I had high levels of it in my body. Because I'd experienced such marked improvements in my MS symptoms after following the Wahls Diet for a short period of time, I began the process of mercury detoxification immediately. I had all of the mercury removed from my mouth and I detoxify regularly in other ways. I continue to do dry body brushing. I take supplements, which include bentonite clay and additional B vitamins. I eat plenty of algae and cilantro; and of course I treat myself to a weekly clay (Aztec bentonite clay) footbath and facial. I loved learning about all the beneficial properties of herbs, spices, and teas from Dr. Wahls. Every day, I put a dash of cardamom in my tea, and I add turmeric to my bone broth.
—Debra K., Accord, New York

THE NEW TOOTHBRUSH

Ditch the fluoride-based toothpastes. In fact, ditch all commercial toothpastes. Instead, try this. Keep a jar of cold-pressed coconut oil in the bathroom, and when you are ready to brush your teeth, draw the toothbrush across the coconut oil and brush with that. Or you could use a few drops of olive oil, oregano oil, or tea tree oil, which will suppress the bacteria contributing to plaque development. The other thing you could do is to use baking soda. Although it is a bit abrasive for ongoing daily use, brushing a couple of times a week with baking soda or potassium bicarbonate will also help improve detoxification by increasing the alkalinity of your urine. You can also mix potassium bicarbonate and liquid emu oil or coconut oil as another great option for brushing your teeth.

phone towers, smartphones and -watches, computers, and more, in ways unlike any previous period in history. Morever, "dirty electricity" refers to electrical currents that have entered the alternating current, adding more high-frequency oscillations. Additional oscillations occur when a current is converted between DC and AC—this happens with devices powered by lithium batteries (like computers and cell phones) as well as solar panels and coiled fluorescent lights.

Do these EMFs have biological effects? Many believe they do, and there is even a condition called electromagnetic hypersensitivity (EHS) that, although not yet proven to be directly related to EMFs, seems to cause mild to severe health issues (such as headaches, nausea, anxiety, depression, and fatigue) related to EMF exposure.[8] There is much to learn on this topic, but I for one do not want to wait around for this condition to be proven before I take precautions. If you are having difficulty with persistent symptoms, you don't have to eliminate all technology from your house. But you might consider turning off routers at night, keeping computers out of the bedroom, and keeping clocks away from the head of the bed. You can also buy radiation blocking sleeves for your cell phone, and even silver shirts and hoods made of EMF-blocking fabric. You can also buy meters that can show you where there is excess EMF activity in your home environment.

See the Resources appendix at the back of this book for more information and sources for protective products.

All in all, detoxing isn't particularly hard, but it does require vigilance. Implement these concepts as best you can given your time and financial constraints: pure organic food, a clean home, natural materials on and around you as much as possible, and a systematic nurturing of the body to help it eliminate toxins the way it is designed to do. It is the perfect complement to the Wahls food plan and an essential part of the Wahls Protocol.

Chapter 9

MOVING FOR HEALING

I F YOU AREN'T mobile now and you change nothing about what you are doing, you're not going to become mobile in the future. This sounds obvious, but people don't often see it this way. They believe that rest will allow them to move more later, but as *later* gets further and further away, muscles begin to degenerate and your whole physical system degrades. What happens when you don't start a car engine for years? At some point, it's going to seize up, and then it's going to take a lot more to start it than turning a key.

Because people with MS experience fatigue as the disease progresses, many physicians have been telling MS patients not to exercise. The belief was that this would reduce fatigue, leaving more energy for everyday life. Now we know how wrong this is. Numerous studies have shown that a wide variety of exercise programs, such as yoga,[1] strength training,[2] aerobic training,[3] and high intensity interval training[4] are very helpful for reducing fatigue and improving the quality of life for the person with MS.

I'm not going to tell you that you have to run a 5K or even walk around the block. Each person is different. You may be able to do things that someone else with MS can no longer do; yet another person with MS may be able to do things you can't do anymore. You can do only what is possible for you. What you must *not* do is neglect what is still possible for you. A downward spiral into immobility does not have to be your fate. Movement begets movement, and energy expenditure can, if done correctly, result in more energy, not less. Lack of mobility leads only to immobility.

You Were Designed to Move

Exercise has been essential for our species from the very beginning. For countless years, our ancestors traveled six to twelve miles a day on average, intermittently running as fast as they could to capture our food or, even more critical, to get away from predators or enemies. Our brains are hardwired to expect that level of activity.

Not only that, but brains depend on exercise for growth and maintenance. You might think that only your muscles, heart, and lungs benefit from exercise, but exercise directly impacts both your brain and spinal cord. Your brain literally depends on exercise for the growth factors it needs to thrive. Exercise stimulates the release of particular hormones in the brain that nourish brain cells (namely, nerve growth factor, or NGF), brain-derived neurotrophic factor (BDNF), and other growth factors that all stimulate the growth of brain cells and more synapses or connections between brain cells.[5] If you don't exercise, your brain won't get this all-important growth-hormone "bath" and your body will react by pruning the unused neural connections and making fewer new connections. Your body will also spend less time repairing those areas, and the result will be atrophy and brain shrinkage. You are more and

WAHLS WARNING

Before starting a new physical exercise program, particularly for those who are not doing any physical activity at all, you should speak with your physician and get clearance. This will give you a chance to ask for a physical and/or occupational therapy evaluation, with the purpose of designing an exercise program appropriate for you at your current state of health and mobility.

more likely to have early memory loss, declining social skills, and increased irritability and mood troubles.

The damage that results from a lack of exercise is cumulative. The amount of exercise that you do over your lifetime will impact your risk of developing Alzheimer's disease. Those with less exercise over a lifetime have a higher risk of dementia, and the theory is that the brain growth hormones you don't get when you don't exercise may actually contribute to the progression of Alzheimer's. And speaking of mood disorders, regular exercise, either aerobic or strength training, is as effective or even more effective than the Prozac family of medications for treating mood disorders like depression.[6] On a system-wide basis, exercise also lowers the excretion of cytokines that cause excessive inflammation.[7] In short, little or no physical activity is very bad for your well-being.

If you're not already on an exercise program, it is essential to start one, and this is an important part of the Wahls Protocol. Your exercise program should include stretching for shortened muscles, balance training, strengthening to build muscles, and aerobic conditioning to improve endurance. Strength training generates the largest gains in nerve growth factors,[8] so do not neglect this important element! You don't have to be a power lifter. Start where you are. I urge you to begin a program of stretching and conditioning now, whatever your health status is. It will help protect your brain, improve your mood, and lessen the risk of heart disease, dementia, diabetes, obesity, and other chronic health problems.

WAHLS DIARY ALERT

In your Wahls Diary, track how often you exercise, for how long, and what you do. Also write down when you don't exercise and why. Your Wahls Diary can help hold you accountable—writing it down could increase your chances of getting up and doing it. Remember, no matter how small your movements or how short your exercise session, it still counts, and it's still better than nothing. The more you do, the easier it will become. Write it all down, and you'll also be able to track your progress as you get stronger in the months to come.

Getting Started

Most people do better with exercise when they are held accountable. There are many ways to do this. Although I've always been active, for years I kept an exercise calendar. I wrote down what I did every day—a quick summary of my workout in just a few lines in my weekly planner. You can use your Wahls Diary to do this. It's a way to be accountable to yourself. You might also consider exercising with a friend or reporting your exercise to a friend, who will ask you about it if you don't report back.

Or maybe you need something more. You may be more motivated to exercise if you work with a professional coach or a physical therapist. The advantage to working with a professional is that you have someone who can evaluate your progress and adjust your training program as you progress. If you have any impairment in your gait or balance, I urge you to see a physical therapist for a clinical evaluation. You can ask your physician for a referral. A physical therapist can evaluate precisely which muscles are strong and weak, how flexible you are, how good your balance is, how much endurance you have, and whether there are any corrections you can work on with your gait. If you don't have visible impairments, try an exercise therapist or athletic trainer for an assessment, personalized exercise program, and subsequent coaching. A good physical therapist and/or athletic trainer can design a specific exercise program for you and help you set and track specific goals. You will probably work with the therapist or trainer in the clinic or gym, and you will also likely get "homework"—exercises you can and should do on your own at home between sessions.

Even if you don't have access to a professional, you can design your own exercise program. There are many simple exercises you can do on your own that specifically target some of the issues that MS presents. These are primarily in four categories:

1. Stretching and lengthening
2. Balance
3. Strengthening
4. Cardiovascular fitness

OCCUPATIONAL THERAPY FOR HAND FUNCTION

Some individuals with autoimmune disease have challenges with hand function. We depend on fine motor coordination to sign our names, dress, eat, and bathe, so losing hand function can create considerable dependence on others. If you have an impairment in hand function, you can ask your physician for a referral to an occupational therapist, who can assist you with improving the function, strength, and coordination in your hands. Occupational therapists can assist with identifying adaptive tools and designing an exercise program for your hands, wrists, and arms to keep your hands and arms fully functional. Using squeeze balls and grip-strengthening barbells will improve grip strength. It is also important to practice spreading and extending the fingers to prevent the development of hand contractions. If you are beginning to have hand symptoms, I urge you to begin working with an occupational therapist. Hands are critical—get help right away if you notice any weakness or clumsiness developing.

I recommend doing a few exercises out of each category every day when possible. Or rotate through the days: stretching one day, balance the next day, strengthening the next day, cardio the following day. Do all four regularly at your own level for the most balanced program, to the extent that you are able. Let's look at each category separately.

Stretching

Dancers and martial artists are all focused on maintaining good flexibility. As a tae kwon do practitioner, I should have known to spend as much time on stretching as I did on strengthening, but I didn't do this as I became disabled. As a result, my calf muscles and hamstrings became shortened. I have spent years now working on stretching them back out.

Nearly everyone with MS develops shortened muscles, especially the calf muscles, hamstrings, and gluteal muscles. Muscle spasms and muscle stiffness are also common problems with MS patients, often because of decreasing activity. Doing regular stretching will help reduce the spasticity and stiffness greatly, but even if you aren't experiencing this problem, stretching and lengthening will benefit you. For anyone with MS, a regular stretching regimen can reduce spasms and muscle stiffness and help improve mobility. Stretching is also key for restoring or maintaining a normal range of motion, which is essential for mobility. It can also help reduce the trouble with leg cramps and spasms at night.

If your doctor has prescribed baclofen, which increases the neurotransmitter gamma-aminobutyric acid (GABA), it may be to help reduce MS-related spasticity and stiffness in your muscles. This can be helpful to many people but should be combined with a stretching program. With a good exercise program, medication may eventually become unnecessary. Research has shown that the combination of baclofen with a program of stretching is the most effective strategy to treat and prevent shortening of muscles, muscle spasms, and muscle stiffness.[9]

The following stretches are those I do and recommend. The images and summaries for the stretches that follow (and the neuromuscular reeducation exercises later in this chapter) are adapted from exercise education materials provided in the Toolkit from the Institute for Functional Medicine. Your therapist may have different or additional suggestions for you.

1. *Soleus/Achilles Stretch*

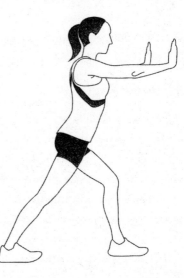

Stand about three feet from a wall with both feet flat on the ground. Place your hands against the wall. Step forward with your right foot, keeping both heels flat on the floor. Lean your hips toward the wall while keeping your left leg straight, to stretch your calf. Hold 10 seconds. Repeat with the other leg. Do a total of 10 times each leg.

2. Hamstring Stretch

Sit with your legs straight out in front of you, feet against a wall. Hold your hands behind your back if you can. (If you cannot, rest your hands on the floor beside your hips.) Bend at the hips and lean your trunk forward until you feel a stretch in your hamstrings, along the backs of your thighs. Hold 10 seconds. Return upright. Do 10 stretches.

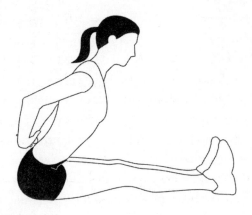

3. Gluteal Stretch

For your gluteal (buttocks) muscles, lie on your back on the floor and pull your knees up across your chest. Do one leg at a time for a more intense stretch. Hold 10 seconds. Do 10 stretches on each side.

4. Psoas Stretch

Your psoas runs along the front of your hip and can get tight, especially if you sit frequently. Here's how to stretch it back out. Place your right knee on a chair. Your left leg should be straight, with your foot flat on the floor next to the front of the chair. Slowly bend your left knee until you feel a stretch along the front of your right hip. Do not arch your back. Hold for 10 seconds. Repeat on the other side. Do 10 stretches on each side.

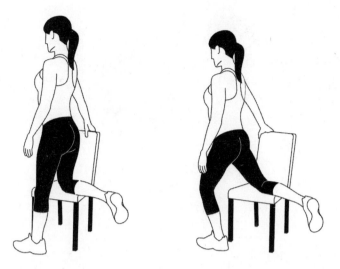

5. Quadriceps Stretch

Your quadriceps are four muscles on the front of your thigh. To stretch them, lie facedown on the floor. Bend your right knee. Reach your right arm back and grab your toe or ankle. Pull your foot into your backside until you feel the front of your thigh stretch. If you can't quite reach your foot, loop a scarf or towel around your foot and pull on that. Hold for 10 seconds. Repeat with the other leg. Do 10 stretches on each leg.

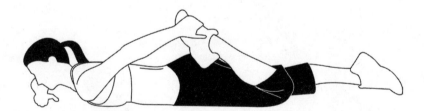

6. Erector Spinae 1

The next two stretches are for your erector spinae muscles, which are the muscles in your back around your spine. For this first one, sit in a chair and bend forward. Reach down to grasp your calves with both hands. Pull your body toward the floor. Hold for 10 seconds. Relax. Repeat 10 times.

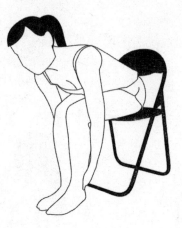

7. *Erector Spinae 2*

For this back-stretching exercise, get down on your hands and knees. If this is painful, you may do this on a padded exercise mat or even on your bed. Place your hands under your shoulders and your knees under your hips. Slowly let your back sag down and raise your head up. Don't push your back down; just let it hang. Hold for 10 seconds. Then let your head hang down. Pull your stomach in and arch your back up. Hold 10 seconds and return to a flat-backed position. Repeat 10 times.

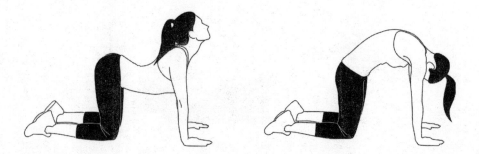

Balancing

Balance often becomes a problem for people with mobility issues. People with MS and other autoimmune conditions may also have a loss of sensation in the legs or feet, and/or issues with dizziness and impaired proprioception (not having a good idea of where things are in space, like not realizing where your foot is exactly). As we age, our ability to sense where we are in space diminishes, even in the best of circumstances. MS or any disease affecting the brain and muscles can speed the decline of this particular kind of awareness.

You can prevent or slow this loss by doing balance training. Your physical therapist can give you specific exercises, but an easy way to start is to simply stand on one foot for as long as you can. When I first started doing balance training, I did this in the hallway so I could easily touch the wall to regain my balance. I would lift one foot and start counting. My goal was to lengthen the amount of time I could stand on one leg. I can now do thirty seconds on either leg and have moved on to some Pilates and yoga poses.

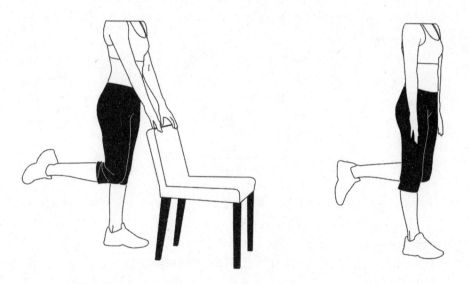

This is an excellent beginning exercise for anyone with balance issues. Start in the hallway or next to the kitchen counter so you can catch yourself when your balance falters. I suggest making it your goal to be able to stand straight up on one leg for thirty seconds or even one minute. Once you have achieved that goal, you can get more advanced placing one foot ahead of the other like you are on a balance beam. When that is easy, you can try balancing on one foot while leaning forward with your arm reaching forward. You can also try this with your eyes closed, but be sure you have something to grab if you start to fall! Always stay safe when working on your balance.

WAHLS WARRIOR Q&A

Q: Why do MS feet turn purple, swell, and feel so disgusting, and what can I do about it?

A: The blood returns to the heart through the veins. The flow of blood from the legs and arms depends on the contraction of the muscles of the arms and legs. When the arms or legs become weak, there is less muscle pumping on the veins. The blood tends to back up, causing the swelling and the purplish discoloration. This is made worse by having more inflammation molecules in the blood. To help reduce the purple discoloration and swelling, two things are helpful. First, increase the contraction of muscles in the arms or legs. Doing more exercise and/or electrical stimulation of the calf muscles or arm muscles is helpful. Spending time with the arms or legs elevated above the heart would also help drain the extra blood back to the heart. Second, reduce the inflammation molecules and improve blood fluidity by eating more sulfur-rich vegetables. More bright colors and greens would also be helpful. I have observed these improvements in both our clinical trial and in my clinical practice.

Regular balance training can make a big difference in regaining your sense of where things are in space, and it can also help to prevent falls, which can lead to serious injury. If you would like more guidance and structure in your balance training, consider a beginning yoga class or a yoga class for people with health issues, including "chair yoga." Yoga has many poses that are excellent balance training—at all levels.

Strengthening

Strength training is your next priority. Declining strength is a primary factor in falls and injuries, not to mention accelerated loss of mobility. Strength training combats this effect by utilizing the body's natural ability to adapt to whatever you do with it.

If you were already exercising regularly, you may also notice your strength decreasing slowly over time (although with the Wahls Protocol, you should be able to reverse this trend). I had been doing a daily workout for decades before I was diagnosed. After the diagnosis, I thought that my strength training and swimming were going to keep me mobile, but despite my daily workout, my strength slowly declined. I had to change my ten-pound dumbbells for eight-pound dumbbells, and then eventually I had to drop to five pounds. Still, I didn't let this stop me. I kept strength training to fight the decline.

Every patient is different, but there are a few strength issues that seem to plague MS patients. One particular strength issue we often see is weakness in the leg muscles that pick up the toes while walking. This was one of my first clear signs, when my wife, Jackie, noticed I was dragging my foot on a long walk. This often causes people to trip over their toes as they swing the leg forward and is a common cause of falls and injury. Strengthening the muscles that flex your ankle and toes upward can make a big difference in your stability. There are some easy ways to build this strength on your own:

1. Simply lift your toes and point your foot to the ceiling as high as possible. Count to 10. Repeat 10 times. This is a simple place to start.
2. When that is easy, stand on your heels with your toes pointed up off the ground, your hand on the wall for balance. Hold for 10 seconds. Repeat 10 times, or do this throughout the day when you think about it.
3. When that is easier to do, then you can walk down the hallway on your heels with your toes in the air, again hanging on to the wall for balance.

You likely have other weak muscles that need training—most people do. Work on those, too. Having a therapist or trainer give you a specific strengthening program is important, because your program can be tailored to your individual needs. If you are still relatively mobile, I urge you to look for a group exercise class that would fit your interests and your schedule. Talk to the instructor, explain your health issues, and then discuss how he or she would approach having you in class. Tai chi, yoga, and Pilates are particularly good because of the strength and balance training involved.

If you never strength train, your body will think your muscle cells aren't important and won't devote resources to them. If you do strength train, then you are working the muscle cells to exhaustion, actually damaging them slightly—but in a useful way. Your body, being adept at cellular repair, will repair the cells over the next twenty-four hours, rebuilding them to tolerate slightly more work, in response to the new strength needs. That is why you want to do strength training every other day: You need a day to recover and let your body make you stronger in response to your efforts.

Recovery time may not be necessary for your training at first. If you are very weak, your exercises in the beginning will likely be more aerobic than strengthening. If you don't work hard enough to break down the muscle cells, you won't need twenty-four hours for repair. However, as you get stronger, you can do more strength work. Your therapist or trainer will let you know when you are actually working your muscles hard enough that you need to do your strength training every other day.

There are also many strengthening exercises you can do at home, in addition to the ones I listed above to help keep your feet from dragging, such as those that involve weights or resistance bands. I strongly recommend you get guidance from a physical therapist or a qualified trainer, who can customize your program to exactly what you need.

Neuromuscular Reeducation

Before we move on to cardiovascular training, I want to tell you about a type of exercise that combines both balance training and strength training. It's called neuromuscular reeducation. Because these exercises help coordinate your brain and body, neuromuscular reeducation exercises are very useful for people with mobility issues as well as proprioception issues.

As you do these exercises, your endurance will slowly improve, too, which will be good for your heart and can help you work up to a point where you are able to do cardiovascular exercise. They involve balancing on an exercise ball while smoothly and carefully doing certain movements. If you don't have an exercise ball, your local gym may have them available for gym use by members. They are also inexpensive to purchase at athletic stores or discount stores like Walmart, Target, or athletic resale shops such as Play It Again Sports.

For every exercise on the following pages, keep a slight tilt in your pelvis to stabilize your lower back before doing any movement.

1. Flexion

Kneel behind the ball and grasp it with your arms, lacing your fingers together in front of the ball. Slowly roll your body forward on the ball and gently rock forward and backward. Work on maintaining your balance while smoothly performing this movement. (Stop if you feel any pain. Go only as far as you can comfortably while maintaining your balance.)

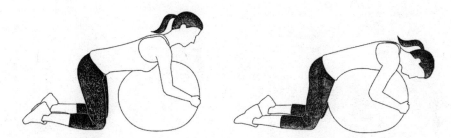

2. Extension

Squat with the ball behind you and place your back on the ball. Slowly roll your body backward on the ball. Reach above your head with your arms, gently rocking forward and backward. If you can, lean all the way back on the ball. (Stop if you feel any pain. Go only as far as you can comfortably while maintaining your balance.)

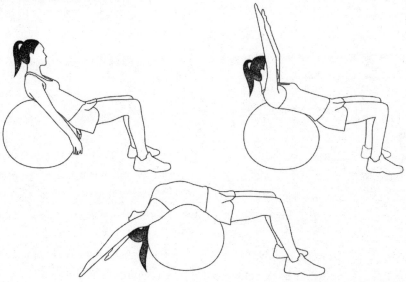

3. Lateral Flexion

Kneel with the ball on your right side and put your right arm on the ball for balance. Extend your left leg out to the left. Slowly roll your body on top of the ball. Reach above your head with your free arm. Repeat on the other side. (Stop if you feel any pain. Go only as far as you can comfortably while maintaining your balance.)

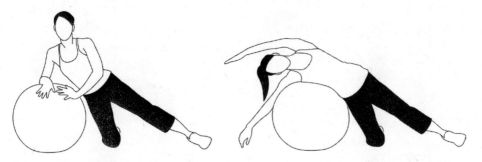

4. Seated Leg Lift

Sit on the ball with your knees bent at a right angle. Bounce up and down easily at first, then more energetically while maintaining your balance. Then lift one foot at a time, carefully maintaining your balance. When this becomes easy, lift one leg at a time and extend it parallel to the ground. Do not slouch!

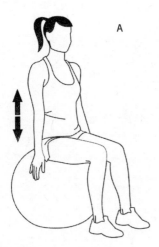

A

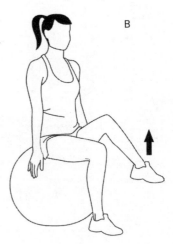

B

5. *Downward-Facing Bridge*

Kneel on the floor in front of the ball. Roll over the ball so it is under your stomach. Place your hands on the floor in front of the ball. Keep both sets of toes on the floor, feet about two feet apart. Extend one arm parallel to the floor, keeping the other hand on the floor. Lower the outstretched hand and then extend the other arm out parallel to the floor. Next extend one leg out parallel to the floor, then return and extend the other leg out parallel to the floor. Once this becomes relatively easy, try extending one arm and the opposite leg parallel to the floor. Hold each position for a count of 10.

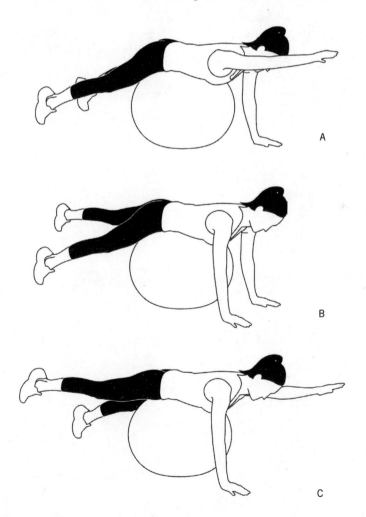

A

B

C

6. Upward-Facing Bridge

Sit on the ball. Walk out and roll down over the ball until the ball is between your shoulder blades, and your body is parallel to the floor. Lift one foot at a time, performing a small march. Then lift and extend overhead one arm at a time, parallel to the floor, while continuing to march. When this is easier, try extending one leg and the opposite arm and holding for a count of 10. Repeat on the other side.

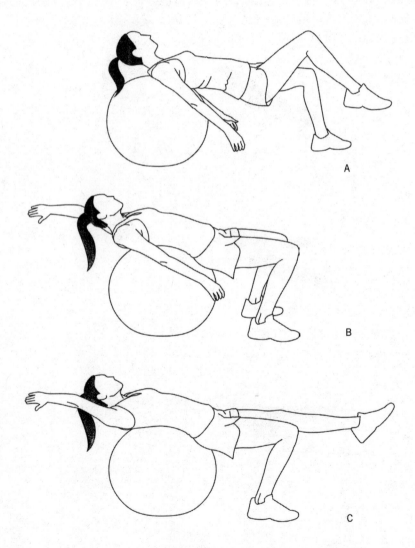

A

B

C

7. Curl-Ups

Solidify your core with this ab-strengthening version of sit-ups. Sit on a ball and roll forward so the back of your rib cage rests on the ball. Curl up and reach toward your knees with arms extended in front of you. If this is too difficult, place more of your back on the ball. When you can do this, try curling up with your arms folded across your chest. The most advanced level is to curl up with your arms behind your head, as pictured below. Be careful not to strain your neck during this exercise. Try to keep your neck relaxed so all the effort comes from your abdominal muscles. If you still feel a strain on your back, roll back so even more of your back is placed on the ball.

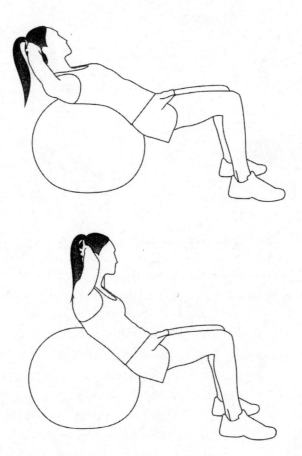

8. *Superman*

Place the soles of your feet against the wall and your knees on the ground (or on a mat). Rest your belly over the ball. Keep your chin tucked in. Slowly push off the wall and align your trunk and legs in a straight line. Hold for 10 seconds. Roll back. Try it again, reaching your arms out in front of your body like Superman, forming a straight line from feet to hands. Hold for 10 seconds and roll back. For the most advanced level, add a swimming motion, like you are doing the crawl stroke, alternating your arms as they reach overhead. Another advanced way to do this is simply lie on your stomach with a ball (or several pillows under your belly) and hold your arms and legs out.

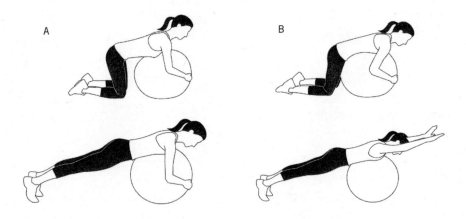

Cardiovascular Conditioning

When people think of exercise, they often think of cardiovascular conditioning (often simply called *cardio*) first. Cardio is the kind of exercise that gets your heart rate up: walking, jogging, using an elliptical trainer or treadmill, or doing an aerobic exercise class. Cardio is important, but I want to emphasize that stretching, balance, and strengthening, as well as some targeted neuromuscular reeducation, are equally important for people with mobility issues.

Cardiovascular conditioning benefits the body in a different way from other exercises because it involves the heart and lungs. However, what constitutes a vigorous cardiovascular workout for one person might be effortless for another person, so it's hard to say exactly what you should be doing other than doing something that doesn't hurt but still gets your heart rate up, has you breathing more quickly than you do at rest, and maybe even gets you to break a sweat.

For me, aerobic workouts were always a part of life. I used to run until I had to slow down because of mysterious hip pain. I got into biking and then cross-country skiing. I picked up roller skis and started skiing on blacktops. I often took my children with me, pulling them behind me in a trailer either with wheels or skis. Jackie and I took them on easy biking trails through the woods and taught them to cross-country ski when they were old enough.

Soon, however, I found I wasn't able to cross-country ski using the faster skating technique. I was annoyed with myself, thinking I was getting old and out of shape, despite the fact that I had gotten up every day since college to work out before starting work. I hadn't missed a day in years. When I was finally diagnosed with MS, part of me felt relieved: I hadn't been a slug after all. There was a reason for my declining exercise ability.

However, I kept up because I knew daily exercise was important if I wanted to continue walking. For a while, I walked uphill slowly on a treadmill for twenty minutes, but then that became impossible. That's when I discovered swimming.

Swimming is an excellent form of aerobic conditioning for people with MS and other mobility issues. I put an Endless Pool into my home in 2002, and I have to thank my mom for encouraging me to spend the money to do this. She reminded me that my health and stamina were incredibly important to maintain. If the pool helped me do that, it was worth getting. The Endless Pool is a pool with a current generator. It is a swimmer's treadmill. (For more information, see the Resources section at the back of this book.) I swam every day. I have come to like swimming in cold water, particularly in the evening, so I do not heat my pool. I will swim in 65-degree water and ease myself into the water gradually, allowing my body to get used to the cold. (This isn't for everyone. Most people need warm water, or at least warmer than 65 degrees!) The cold water lowers my core body temperature, which—at least for me— seems to help me have a deeper, more restful sleep. I begin by doing the crawl stroke with my goggles and snorkel on so I don't have to worry about breathing technique or craning my neck. I'll swim for fifteen to thirty minutes in the evening and then spend time stretching.

You may not be able to put a pool into your house, but most communities have a recreation center with a pool, and many private gyms have pools. Even if you don't know how to swim, you can try walking in the water. The water provides resistance but also cushions joints for a potentially less injurious workout. I know many patients who "water walk" and get quite a good aerobic workout doing it.

Other options include water aerobics classes, which are generally easier on the body than regular aerobics classes. Or if water really isn't your thing, do something different:

- Walk on a treadmill with bars to hold on to if you have balance issues. You could also try treadmill training with partial weight support, which can be a useful adjunct to physical and/or occupational therapy. Partial body weight treadmill training is being studied in those with MS and results suggest it is helpful.[10] Your physical therapist may have the right kind of treadmill to do this.
- Try an elliptical trainer, which is a no-impact machine that approximates a running movement.
- A stationary bicycle simulates bicycling without the balance requirements or weather considerations. Reclining bikes offer an alternative position and are good for those who may need back support.
- Rowing machines offer a good all-over workout, no water required.
- Many of my patients do gentle yoga classes and Pilates classes, which can be adapted to different levels and abilities but provide stretching, strengthening, and an aerobic component, and use body weight and balance.
- Ballroom dancing improves balance and coordination, and any form of dancing has benefits. Dancing is increasingly recognized as a useful tool to improve function in Parkinson's patients and for neuro rehab. Some dance studios offer dancing specifically for Parkinson's patients or are adapted to people who have mild to severe mobility impairment.
- High-intensity interval training (HIIT) is a method of exercise that gets the maximum benefit out of a short period of time. There are different ways to do HIIT, but essentially it involves short periods of high-intensity exercise (such as 20 to 90 seconds) followed by short periods of moderate-

or low-intensity exercise, repeated over the course of 15 to 30 minutes. The advantage of this workout is more rapid growth of muscles and more rapid positive changes to inflammation molecules, all occurring in about half the time it would take doing regular physical therapy training. The disadvantage is that it is more intense and requires a medical clearance and a therapist or trainer with which to work.

- A workout appropriate for people experiencing deficits in one limb is constrained limb therapy. In this exercise, the good limb is constrained and only the affected limb is exercised. The training starts with intensive rehabilitation exercises that are progressively more challenging. This approach is used for stroke patients to improve hand function and is beginning to be applied to MS patients as well. If you have hand weakness, finding a therapist who is skilled with constrained limb therapy may be very helpful. It is certainly an intense program requiring significant commitment over several months and is a very new concept, but it shows great promise as an exciting new therapy.

- The 7-Minute Workout[11] is a good option for those who worry they won't have enough time to work out—it's a full-body workout in just seven minutes created for those who are healthy enough for a high-intensity interval training routine. There are many different versions online, some more intense than others. I recommend this workout for those who are young and healthy enough to do high intensity interval training. In my clinics, I have people start with just one or two repetitions of just half the excercises listed. As they get stronger, they may add additional exercises or repetitions gradually. The key is to start moving, but at the level of effort you can manage! There are many different versions online with varying levels of difficulty, as well as apps for smartphones and tablets that take you through the exercises.

- Martial arts and CrossFit-type classes also improve strength, endurance, and balance but require a higher level of strength and conditioning.

Work with where you are right now. If you can only walk down the driveway and back, that's a starting point. If you can ride a stationary bicycle for five minutes, that's a starting point. Anything is better than nothing. If possible, again, I want to emphasize the importance of working with a physical or occupational therapist or personal trainer to evaluate your muscle strength, flexibility, balance, and gait and to create a personalized exercise program that covers all the exercise bases. However, you can get started today, even before you book your first appointment. You can start engaging your muscles again right now. All you have to do is move. Why waste any more time?

If you do some kind of cardiovascular conditioning on most days, or at least three days per week for as long as you can tolerate, you will be making good progress.

Vibration

Another workout I have come to enjoy that combines strengthening with balance and also has an aerobic component is whole-body vibration. I discovered whole-body vibration after reviewing a study on this therapy by Dr. Richard Shields.

The principle of whole-body vibration is that by standing on a vibrating platform, your muscles make hundreds of constant tiny corrections in response to the changing position. Your body is also required to sense where you are in space, so it sends a flow of messages to your brain to compensate for the motion. This is great for your proprioception. All of the messages to and from your brain stimulate the release of hormones in the brain (the nerve-growth hormone family that stimulates repair and building connections, which I talked about at the beginning of this chapter). Your body is also stimulated to release hormones in the muscle, which in turn promotes muscular growth and repair in the muscles, tendons, and bones.

Dr. Shields is studying the impact of whole-body vibration for maintaining muscle and bone strength in paralyzed individuals. In the research literature, whole-body vibration has helped those who are deconditioned or have thinned bones to improve both bone and muscle strength.[12] It has also been used by American astronauts and Russian cosmonauts to stimulate more bone and muscle strength, in order to increase the tolerance for space travel, and many athletes have also embraced whole-body vibration.

WAHLS WARRIORS SPEAK

I've been in a wheelchair for seven years. I was diagnosed with RRMS in 1995, but that changed somewhere around 2002–2003 to secondary progressive MS. Along with MS, I've had three surgeries for trigeminal neuralgia. I started the Wahls Diet about thirteen months ago but have been very strict on it for about six months.

Since I've been on the diet, my right hand, which had been totally clenched into a fist since 2001, has started to relax and I've been able to cut down on my pain medications to less than half of what I used to take. Before the diet, I could stand up for only one minute while holding on to something and walk using a hemi-walker for about twenty feet. Now I can stand up for seven minutes and walk 160 feet. I used to do e-stim, but now use a full-body vibration machine twice per day, which is great for massage and my circulation. I continue to hope and pray that I will be able to walk and drive again someday, and I thank God every day that I was introduced to this diet.

—*Patricia O., Gainesville, Florida*

The research on the benefits of whole body training continues to grow. Many different conditions have been shown to improve after regular vibration training:

- **Aging:** Geriatric patients showed decreases in muscle loss,[13] improved motor function, strength, balance control,[14] improved EEG function, improved heart rate variability,[15] and higher scores on the Mini-Mental State Exam (MMSE—a structured test of mental status used for dementia patients).[16]
- **Blood sugar:** Vibration training improved glucose control in diabetic patients.[17]
- **Bone density:** Clinical studies have shown that whole-body vibration can have modest benefits for improving bone density and strength in those who have low bone-mineral density or who are deconditioned.

Menopausal women also showed improved bone density with regular training.[18]

- **COPD:** Whole-body vibration training is associated with improved lung function and exercise tolerance in COPD patients.[19]
- **Leg Strength:** A meta-analysis of 24 studies demonstrated that vibration improved muscle strength and performance of the legs in healthy adults.
- **Multiple Sclerosis:** An 8-week study using whole-body vibration training three times a week in people with MS demonstrated increased bone density, better ankle range of motion, and decreased fear of falling.[20]
- **Stroke:** Stroke patients showed improved function with vibration training.[21]

The evidence continues to grow that the increased sensory input from the changes in position that occur during whole-body vibration sessions and the changes in muscles to maintain posture during the whole-body vibration session improve the connection between the brain and the body, leading to improved cognition and motor performance. In addition, the increased force on the skeleton and tendons improve bone mineral density and tendon strength. Multiple studies have shown improved bone density, better balance, and better walking and sit-to-stand function and even better blood sugar levels! If you can get access to a vibration training, it may be a useful adjunct to your physical training—the evidence is certainly there to support its benefits.

Ideally, you will find a clinic or a gym that has a whole-body vibration machine so you can test this out for yourself and have your physical therapist or trainer assist you in designing a program specifically for whole-body vibration that matches what your body needs. I do not recommend doing this on your own, at least until you fully understand how to use the machine and you have a plan that has been designed specifically for you. These machines aren't cheap, either: Costs range from a few hundred dollars to $15,000 or more. See the Resources section for more information.

E-Stim

As you may remember from the introduction to this book, I discovered e-stim while reviewing a research protocol and was interested in how this therapy was being used on people who had lost mobility. I convinced my therapist to let me try a test session and found it to be of great benefit in restoring my strength and mobility. I have since incorporated it into the Wahls Protocol, and I believe it is a useful tool for reversing muscle atrophy and loss of mobility.

E-stim isn't the most comfortable experience in the world. Some people are more sensitive to it than others, and some people think that it is actually quite painful. The greater the level of inflammation in your muscle cells, the more painful e-stim is likely to be for you. It must be done *in addition* to exercise, not instead of exercise, and furthermore, it must be done *at the same time as volitional* (purposeful) *exercise*, so that it can reinforce the brain/muscle connection. Otherwise, building muscle won't be as useful to improving your

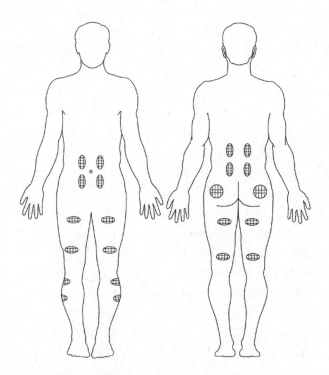

These are the motor points where I placed electrodes to stimulate the muscles that my therapist had identified as weak. Note that my physical therapist worked with me in placing the electrodes and testing which muscle was in fact being stimulated to confirm that the location was correct to stimulate the intended muscle group. Because we are all unique, each individual will often need adjustment of the location of the electrodes to get the desired muscle group. Your muscle weaknesses may be different than mine.

walking and hand function. Despite these inconveniences, it is heartening to know that you can grow more muscle with e-stim and exercise than you would by exercise alone. Here's how it works.

Officially called neuromuscular electrical stimulation (NMES), e-stim is the application of tiny pulses of electrical current over the nerves that normally give your muscles the instructions to contract. In order to deliver this current, a therapist places electrodes over the skin in particular areas and hooks them to the machine with wires that deliver the electric pulses. A physical therapist has access to this equipment, although you can purchase e-stim machines online and use them at home to reduce pain. (Always work with a physical therapist, occupational therapist, or athletic trainer first to see where you need to apply the electrodes and to design a program that specifically addresses your unique needs. You may then be able to use a machine on your own.)

Functional electrical stimulation (FES) is an alternative way to use e-stim, in which the electrical current is timed to create a functional movement, such as how your muscles would react when riding a bicycle. This is a good way to improve any exercise or activity you want to be able to do in your life. E-stim was initially used by athletes to help them recover from injuries and surgeries more quickly, and many choose to continue e-stim after recovery. Although the research into NMES continues to expand, no one has yet conducted a long-term study over many years, so the safety of long-term use has not yet been clinically established. Still, the benefits of NMES and FES for helping maximize the benefits of exercise are noteworthy, and long-term use may indeed be beneficial, especially for those with limited mobility.

Electrical stimulation can be of great benefit to anyone who has experienced deconditioning for any health-related reason. E-stim has been studied and found to improve quality of life and function in people with advanced heart failure,[22] chronic lung disease including COPD,[23] osteoarthritis including pain relief in the knee,[24] rheumatoid arthritis,[25] and dysphagia related to brain injury. It has been used to prevent muscle wasting in comatose patients, to reduce spastic muscles after stroke, and to help stroke victims recover function more quickly (even five years after the injury)[26] and has improved function in people with cerebral palsy, including improved use of affected legs, arms, and hands.[27] It has even proven useful for incontinence—specifically, bladder and bowel control issues in people with MS.[28] Poor control of the bladder and bowels can occur with MS as well as with many other autoimmune and neurological conditions, and even with simple aging. Doing Kegel exercises (practice squeezing the muscle to stop the flow of urine) can help, but it is now possible to use a vaginal or rectal probe to add electrical stimulation of the appropriate muscles. If you have problems with accidents, doing Kegels augmented by electricity may be quite helpful to you. The good news is that this treatment does have FDA approval and is covered by many insurance companies, unlike many other uses for e-stim.

E-stim is useful for many aspects of MS and other chronic health problems or age-related declines that have resulted in declining strength and endurance. (We are the first to publish results of using exercise augmented by neuromuscular electrical stimulation in the setting of multiple sclerosis.[29]) It can be used for overall fitness, but it is particularly useful to target specific areas of weakness as well as walking. For example, e-stim devices such as the WalkAide and Bioness deliver an electrical current to the nerve going to the muscle that lifts the foot upward at the ankle, making it easier to walk without catching one's toes. Research has shown these devices to be helpful in improving walking speed and endurance.[30] Bioness also has devices to stimulate the thigh muscles and improve hand function.

E-stim tackles weakness by triggering the generation of nerve growth factors that are important in nourishing and maintaining brain cells. Without physical activity, levels of nerve growth factors, including brain-derived neurotrophic factors (BDNF), fall. Brain health suffers as a result. E-stim is associated with increased BDNF and other nerve growth factors as well as endorphins, all of which are good for reducing brain inflammation and risk of brain atrophy. In addition, NMES has been associated with improving cytokine profiles (indicating it has anti-inflammatory action) and improved insulin sensitivity in diabetes patients.

The research on the benefits of FES and NMES to help manage a wide variety of conditions of severe disability and multiple diseases has grown rapidly. For more details about the latest research on the benefits of FES and NMES, please check out the e-stim course that I host on my website; see terrywahls.com/estimcourse/.

I certainly noticed improved mood, mental clarity, and steadily improving energy when I added e-stim to my regimen. I still use NMES while I do my strength-training workout to get the most effective challenge to my muscles and the most favorable metabolic effects from muscle training. I still check in with my physical therapist every 4 to 6 weeks and plan to do so for the rest of my life (presumably another 60 years or so!).

I am growing steadily more enthusiastic and much more bullish on the benefits of adding NMEs and FES to augment workout intensity, so I highly recommend it, if you can find a way to access it. Even if you are using only OTC devices to add a little more intensity to your workout, your muscle strength, hormones, cytokine profile, and metabolism may benefit. The Resources section at the end of the book contains more information on the devices that I have personally used. Your therapist may have experience using other devices.

E-STIM AND PARALYSIS

If you are paralyzed or have severe mobility impairment, e-stim may still be beneficial. Patients who are paralyzed experience metabolic changes when their muscles are less active. Their inflammation levels increase, central obesity increases, insulin sensitivity declines, blood lipids worsen, and the risks of obesity, diabetes, and heart disease increase.[31] The person is more likely to have constipation and spontaneous bone fractures. There are devices now that allow paralyzed individuals to use functional electrical stimulation to cycle their legs or arms. The electricity drives the muscles to contract and do work and reduces the metabolic harms of inactivity. Those who have some volitional use of the arms and legs report regular cycling with these devices has also led to improved motor function. In addition, those with severe mobiity impairment who did FES cycling experienced gains in strength, fitness, quality of life, and reduce fatigue. However, such use is not FDA approved and is unlikely to be covered by your health insurance.

WAHLS TOOLS

E-stim electrodes are attached with sticky pads that are reusable and disposable. The reusable electrodes are self-adhesive and work for ten to thirty applications, depending on how thoroughly you clean your skin and how well you care for the electrodes. You can also use CarbonFlex electrodes that do not have an adhesive gel but instead use elastic compression straps or compression shorts and socks to hold the electrodes in place. The CarbonFlex electrodes can be reused for over a year. You need to moisten the CarbonFlex electrodes with water to make them conduct electricity without excessive resistance (pain). I used the CarbonFlex electrodes for years quite successfully. The larger the electrode, the more comfortable the current. I used three- and four-inch-diameter electrodes for the greater comfort larger electrodes provide. The supplies will range from $25 to $100 per month, depending on how many sessions you use it for each day.

GETTING E-STIM TREATMENT

Getting e-stim treatment may not be simple for you. Here's why: The FDA approval for the use of e-stim is not for specific disease states. That is because device makers would have to conduct clinical trials for every disease state for which they wish to have an FDA-approved indication. That would cost millions for each disease state and be cost-prohibitive.

Instead, the medical device makers sought and obtained FDA approval for electrical stimulation of muscles for more general muscle-related issues like muscle spasms (see the on the next page). The FDA has approved electrical therapy devices as either over-the-counter (OTC) or prescription-only devices. The OTC devices have less power and can be used only for muscle toning. The prescription devices can be used only under the direct supervision of an authorized practitioner, such as a physical therapist, and are approved for the following indications:

1. Muscle spasm
2. The prevention of disuse atrophy
3. Relaxation of muscle spasms
4. Muscle reeducation
5. Postsurgical stimulation of calf muscles to prevent blood clots
6. Improving range of motion

If your condition doesn't specifically sound like what e-stim is supposed to help, you may have trouble getting your doctor or physical therapist to refer you for this treatment. What many physicians and treating physical therapists don't realize is that there is a growing body of research that supports the use of e-stim to help people improve their strength and endurance.

Print out these two papers and take them with you to your appointment (Note these two papers are also in the bonus materials at terrywahls.com /bonus):

1. *Neuromuscular electrical stimulation and dietary interventions to reduce oxidative stress in a secondary progressive multiple sclerosis patient leads to marked gains in function: a case report (ncbi.nlm.nih.gov/pmc /articles/PMC2769364/)*
2. *Rehabilitation with neuromuscular electrical stimulation leads to functional gains in ambulation in patients with secondary progressive and primary progressive multiple sclerosis: a case series report (ncbi.nlm .nih.gov/pmc/articles/PMC2769364/).*

It may be helpful to show these peer-reviewed publications to your treating therapist to justify giving you a test session. You can also remind your therapist that NMES is approved for muscle atrophy. If you are deconditioned and have muscle spasms and/or muscle pain, your muscles have likely atrophied. However, you will likely still have to pay out of pocket for NMES, as it likely won't be covered by your medical insurance. It will however be very helpful to accelerate your rehabilitation. You can learn more about this from the e-stim course.

CALL TO ACTION

You can get copies of relevant articles from my website, terrywahls.com /bonus.

Using E-Stim

If you want to investigate using electrical stimulation to assist your exercise training, here are some things to consider:

- **You still have to exercise.** E-stim is not a replacement for exercise. It is a way of supercharging the workout for your muscles so you have a chance of growing more muscle tissues. If you have the benefit of recovering good strength and balance, you may be advised to taper off the use of the e-stim and rely on the strength and endurance training alone. However, I do recommend you continue to train with e-stim to maintain the muscle mass and endurance, in order to maintain your gains. You can reduce the amount of time to 15 minutes per day for the muscle groups involved, or you may discontinue the e-stim and continue daily training without e-stim, but if you do, watch your strength and stamina closely. Are you getting stronger? Are you remaining stable? Or are you slowly losing ground? The challenge is that the loss may be very gradual and you may not be aware that you are losing ground. Certainly, if you perceive that your strength and/or stamina are declining, I urge you to get back to a more vigorous workout schedule, reconnect with physical or occupational therapy, and consider adding back (or starting) e-stim.
- **You should do volitional exercise of the muscles being stimulated during e-stim for best results.** At the very least, do an isometric contraction of the muscles as the current flows into the muscle, causing the contraction. If you are stimulating your gluteal muscles, for example, squeeze your butt cheeks while the current is going. Better yet, do the exercises that your physical therapist or occupational therapist has designed for you while you have the e-stim current going to the muscles you are exercising. Most of us

are sitting for hours each day, making our gluteal (butt) muscles relatively weak. As a result, many people would benefit from doing 45 minutes of e-stim to the gluteal muscles while walking, standing, or sitting and squeezing along with the electrically driven contractions, in addition to the regular exercises they may be doing. Doing volitional exercise, even if it is just an isometric contraction, will help connect your brain and muscles in a way that you cannot achieve if you are passive during the e-stim treatment. Your physical therapist can advise you about the best exercises for you to combine with your e-stim sessions.

- **You need professional input.** Ideally, you will have several training sessions at a clinic with a therapist to learn how to operate the device. There are many different companies and devices available. Your therapist or trainer may use different devices in their clinic. You should be given a specific set of exercises to strengthen your muscles, and you can ask which exercises you should be doing while you are stimulating each particular muscle group. As you get stronger, the therapist will likely advance your exercises and may advance the duration and the intensity of the e-stim. This is all highly personalized to the individual. I urge you to have a therapist evaluate you and design a program specifically for you. Exercise and e-stim are individualized in our clinical trial for each participant. We do not use the same protocol for everyone because each person has a unique set of needs, and a professional can best help you determine what these are for you.

- **You may not tolerate the therapy.** Before you dive into e-stim therapy or spend money on a device or treatment, it's a good idea to do a test session, during which a therapist will determine whether you can tolerate the therapy. Not all people can tolerate the electrical sensations. In our clinical trial, a couple of people found the electrical sensations to be too painful, but 80 percent or more can tolerate sufficient current to generate a strong contraction. Try it first to be sure you are comfortable doing it.

You can do e-stim at home once your therapist is confident you can safely use the electrical therapy device, but stay in touch with your therapist. If e-stim works for you, you may choose to buy your own device. The device

WAHLS TOOLS

E-stim has also been incorporated into exercise equipment. Restorative Therapies (restorative-therapies.com) and Myolyn (myolyn.com) are two companies that make a functional electrical stimulation (FES) cycle. They use electrodes to stimulate the leg and/or arm muscles to push on pedals to maintain muscle strength and endurance. The original work on this was to determine how to use FES cycling to help paralyzed individuals maintain muscle, bone strength, and quality of life. The first patient population that the company targeted was people with spinal cord injuries. In a small pilot study of five patients with primary or secondary progressive MS, researchers found that patients tolerated the FES cycling and experienced faster walking time in the twenty-five-foot walk and higher quality-of-life scores. They report that they have 580 patients using one of their FES cycles. Now some doctors are using the FES cycles to help patients with multiple sclerosis.[32]

More studies have been done showing FES cycling to be helpful for those with MS, even with severe mobility impairment, reducing fatigue, improving quality of life, and improving endurance and strength in the legs, as well as improving overall fitness.[33] FES cycling is likely to be beneficial for improving strength and endurance, but the FES cycles are not FDA-approved as a treatment for MS. You can contact Restorative Therapies and Myolon to see if there is a clinic near you that is using the FES cycle or inquire about having a trial period with a cycle to see if you might benefit.

should be portable and run on batteries. An e-stim device will typically have two to four channels, which translates into two to four muscles that can be stimulated at any given time. Devices that have sufficient power to help grow muscles as opposed to only toning muscles require a prescription to be purchased. Prices vary widely, from OTC devices available for under $100 to high-end devices that can be over $1,000. Also, prescription prices and coverage vary, so the amount you would pay would depend on your insurance plan.

WAHLS WARNING

Use caution if you could become pregnant: Never stimulate the abdomen or gluteal muscles if there is even a remote possibility that you could become pregnant, as the electrical current anywhere near the uterus could affect fetal development and lead to birth defects! Also, no one should use an e-stim machine across the chest, brain, or neck. Do not use an e-stim machine if you have an implantable electronic device, like a pacemaker, or a medication pump such as a baclofen pump for spasticity.

Set goals, start small, and work your way up. If you get the opportunity to try this therapy, the general instruction for athletes is to stimulate the particular muscles that are weak for fifteen minutes a day if you want to prevent muscle atrophy, and forty-five to sixty minutes if you want to strengthen the muscle. If you have a chronic disease, such as multiple sclerosis, the amount of time needed to grow more muscle will likely be different than what healthy athletes need. We do not have precise guidelines for how much time is needed for those with a chronic disease, but the guidelines for athletes are the only guidelines that exist. That was why my personal goal was to add time gradually so I could stimulate each of my weak muscle groups sixty minutes a day. Note that for our extremely disabled study participants, we needed to reduce the e-stim time to five minutes per muscle and slowly advance according to each person's tolerance.

The reason for you to move your body is so you can live your life and not be limited by your disease. It's disappointing and frustrating when you can't do what you used to do, especially when you can't do things with your family that they want to do. However, the people who love you just want to be with you. That's the important thing. Rather than withdrawing into yourself, get up and move as well as you can. Every little bit is good for your body and helps engage you in your life, and with the Wahls Protocol, your progress should be steady.

Chapter 10

WHAT TO KNOW ABOUT DRUGS, SUPPLEMENTS, AND ALTERNATIVE THERAPIES

BEYOND DIET AND EXERCISE, there are many other interesting therapies to consider while on the Wahls Protocol. Many of my patients want to know what supplements they could or should be taking, and I have plenty to say about that. There are other alternative therapies that can also be helpful for some people—should you try them, what will your conventionally trained doctor have to say about it? I have plenty to say about that, too, but before we get into the many fascinating therapies that have the potential to help many people reclaim vibrant health, the very first thing I want to address in this chapter is the medication you are already *taking*.

You may already be thinking about this. If the Wahls Protocol is going to make you better, then you should be able to stop taking all those drugs, right? Not so fast.

Important: About Your Medications

A lot of my patients get very excited about the Wahls Protocol, and that's excellent. Excitement feeds motivation and helps people stick with the diet, even when it feels challenging. Many of these people, however, also get very impatient about the drugs or medications they are currently taking. They want the Wahls Protocol to improve their health (which it will), but they jump the gun and sometimes stop taking their medications in the hope that the Wahls Protocol will "fix everything" in a few weeks. This is not how it works.

You may begin to feel better almost immediately on the Wahls Protocol, but if you are on prescription medications, you must not stop taking your current therapy! This is very important. Do not stop any medication or intervention you are doing right now because you started the Wahls Protocol. Doing so could be disastrous.

It takes several months for the Wahls Protocol to reset your biology and begin the rebuilding process, and then your body must begin healing the damage that has already been done. If you stop your treatment now, you could very likely have another relapse or worsen before you get better. You will be discouraged, disheartened, and more likely to give up. Your friends and family will say, "See? It doesn't work. It's a waste of time and effort and money. Go back to what you were doing before." I can't say this strongly enough:

> **You must stay on your current medications for your medical and psychological conditions!**

In my clinical trials, we do not have the patients stop any treatments, and you must not stop, either. Do the Wahls Protocol *in addition to* whatever you are doing now, then take a deep breath and be patient.

Over the next three years, a new you will be built, molecule by correctly made molecule. Your energy and mood will improve. Likely your blood pressure, weight, cholesterol, and blood sugar (if you are diabetic) will also improve. When you can see and feel the evidence of improved health because you can walk farther, do more, and have more energy, it's time to discuss reducing or tapering off your medication gradually, with your physician's supervision. Some other reasons to discuss tapering off medication after you are solidly on the Wahls Protocol:

- You are on Provigil and you can't sleep at night because the drug is keeping you awake.

- You are on blood pressure medication and now your blood pressure is too low.
- You are on cholesterol-lowering medication and now your cholesterol is too low (less than 200).

If these things happen, don't take matters into your own hands but do work with the doctor who is prescribing the medication. For example, your primary care doctor may be prescribing medication for your cholesterol and blood pressure, and as those numbers improve, those drugs can likely be slowly decreased and potentially eliminated. Talk to your neurologist (or other specialists) for questions about taking Provigil for fatigue.

But what about immunosuppressive drugs? This question is more complex. Your neurologist may agree that your disease has stabilized. Your MRI may show no new lesions. (Likely the lesions already there may remain forever.) However, your doctor may attribute your success to the drugs, not the Wahls Protocol.

Here the question becomes what to do. Do you continue to take the immunosuppressive medication or wean and discontinue?

The research has something to say about this (and I mentioned this early in this book already): It is *very important* to halt disease activity in order to lower the risk of converting to secondary progressive multiple sclerosis. You can disrupt this by discontinuing your medication too soon (or at all). Abruptly stopping disease-modifying drugs is associated with increased risk of acute relapse, rebound, or worsening of disease activity, expansion into other autoimmune diseases, and continued gradual decline—recall the discussion about epitope spreading to review why every flare you have can cause irreparable damage (page 98). While some research does suggest certain situations where discontinuing medication is warranted and does not increase flare risk, it also shows that those who stopped their disease-modifying drugs had a higher risk of progression of their disability than those who did not. This study did *not* examine the effects of diet and lifestyle in this scenario, however, so that is an additional wild card as far as the research goes. I do predict that therapeutic diet and lifestyle reduces the risk of brain atrophy and slow progression, but there is currently no prospective research to prove it. That is why our next clinical trial that will look prospectively at those patients who have declined drug therapy and are using only therapeutic diet and lifestyle. Our results should begin to answer this critical question.

In short, we simply do not know for sure when it is safe to discontinue disease-modifying drug therapy, and therefore I cannot make any general recommendations about when to do this, if ever. Stopping your medication is *not a decision to make on your own or take lightly.* You may very well get to a point where you can stop taking some of your drugs. It could be in six months. It could be in three years. But every person is different, so there is no definitive time frame. I will stress yet again (at the risk of being repetitive) that you must involve your medical team in this decision. The best option is to work closely with a functional medicine provider as well as with your neurology or autoimmune specialist. When everyone agrees you are ready to carefully reduce or discontinue any medication, then and only then should you do so.

In my conversations with conventional neurologists and autoimmune specialists, some have relayed to me that if patients do not have critical lesions in their brains, they could, upon initial diagnosis, quite reasonably give therapeutic diet/lifestyle (such as the Wahls Protocol) three months to see if that will cool off the disease progression, as long as they are seeing the neurologist/autoimmune specialists, every three months. If progression occurs, then they could get a full functional medicine evaluation and get more aggressive with interventions, or add disease-modifying drugs. But the bottom line is that this is a conversation you will have to have with your primary care doctor and your neurologist/autoimmune specialists. I can only share my experience. One of the drugs I was on for MS-related fatigue was Provigil. After just one month into my new way of eating, my fatigue was greatly reduced. At three months, I was sleeping less than four hours a night—Provigil is a stimulant, which is why it is commonly prescribed for fatigue—and my brain had so improved that the stimulant effect was keeping me awake. I wasn't fatigued anymore, and I also wasn't sleeping. It was clearly time to stop this medication, and my neurologist agreed.

When I started biking at six months, I told my neurologist that I no longer wanted to take the disease-modifying medication I was on (CellCept) but would go back on it if the MS symptoms worsened again. He had me take half the dose for a week, then half that smaller dose the following week, and two weeks later I stopped completely. I have continued to do well even though I have not taken a disease-modifying medication in more than twelve years.

What I see in my internal medicine clinical practice is that as patients fully adopt the Wahls Diet, each time we see them back in the clinic, they are looking healthier and younger (I call this "youthening"). Time and time again, I see blood pressures fall, blood sugars fall, moods improve, memory improve, and more. As your cells become healthier, it is likely that your organs will become healthier. As your organs become healthier, it is likely that you, the whole person, will have more energy, more vitality, and more good days and good feelings in your life.

As you become well, it will be apparent to you when you can begin negotiating with your doctor about which medicines to try tapering, and most doctors will see the changes as well and may be more than willing to help you navigate your new, healthier life. I invite you to have an opinion about which medications you want to discontinue first. Consider starting with the drugs with the longest list of side effects and the least immediate benefits to you. The more you can taper off drugs with unpleasant side effects that no longer benefit you, the better your quality of life will be. Just remember, it may take years to repair damage that has taken a lifetime to accrue. Some of it may be permanent, but improvement is possible and always worth pursuing.

WORKING WITH YOUR DOCTOR

Many doctors are happy to work with you as you improve, but unfortunately, not all of them are open to the power of lifestyle modification. If you are not getting the kind of support you really want or feel you need, I would suggest finding a functional medicine, anti-aging regenerative medicine, or integrative medicine health professional to help you decide how to address the immunosuppressive-drug question. They may be more open to attributing your improvements to the changes in your lifestyle. I have successfully been able to get patients in my clinical practice off the immunosuppressive drugs they were on for their autoimmune conditions, but this was under my direct supervision. I have also regressed diabetes, insulin resistance, high blood pressure, mood problems (including PTSD), and continued symptoms after brain injury using diet and lifestyle—but again, I would never want any of my patients to go off their medications prematurely, or without professional supervision. We need to follow people closely as they implement diet and lifestyle changes, to monitor improvements as well as to watch for side effects from medications that are no longer needed because blood pressure or blood sugars are normalizing.

One way to approach the question is to look at the package insert (or find it online) and read all of the side effects of the medication you are interested in tapering off, then talk to your doctors about how many of your current health issues could be the result of the prescription medications rather than the disease. Let that guide your conversations with your doctors about tapering down (very gradually) to see if you can work toward coming off the medication when your improved health justifies it. But again, don't try to quit the drugs yourself without medical approval and supervision. Don't forget that no matter how good you feel right now, abruptly stopping DMTs is associated with higher risk of severe relapse, marked worsening of MS-related (and other autommimune-related) symptoms, and higher risk of developing new and other autoimmune diagnoses.

About Supplements

Now that we have the medication question covered, let's look at some of the many things you can do to support your health as you also practice the Wahls Protocol. Let's begin with dietary supplements.

A huge part of the Wahls Protocol is the infusion of the body, the cells, and the mitochondria with the essential nutrients required for the best possible functioning. This is accomplished primarily through diet, with the 9 cups of fruits and vegetables; the organic, grass-fed, or wild-caught meat and fish; the seaweed and organ meat and fermented food and coconut oil and all the other things I recommend ending up in your blender, in your soup pot, in your salad bowl, and ultimately in *you*.

But wouldn't it be a heck of a lot easier to just take some vitamins? Vitamins and minerals act together to facilitate the chemistry of cells and must be kept in balance, but it is far better (if not easier) to achieve this balance through food, as I discussed in previous chapters. That being said, I do believe that in cases of deficiency, supplementation *in addition to the 9 cups* and the other required foods on whichever level of the Wahls Diet you are practicing may be helpful for some people. If you decide to take supplements, always talk to your personal physician prior to starting them. There are certain conditions for which certain supplements may be contraindicated and certain medications with which some supplements could have an adverse reaction. It won't necessarily state this on the supplement package or the medication.

Also, I strongly urge you to begin one supplement at a time. Keep a log of how you feel in your Wahls Diary, write down any changes in symptoms you observe, and particularly note any head or belly symptoms or skin rashes. If you start several things at once and have problems, you will not know which caused the problem or which was helpful. It is worth being patient and adding things one at a time. If you have no problems after a week, you can add another supplement if you wish. This is the time for you to be a sleuth and pay attention to how you react to the introduction of each supplement.

It is very important that you understand we are all unique, with a unique set of enzymes for running the chemistry of our lives. A supplement that works fine for someone else, even if he or she has the same diagnosis as you have, might not work well for you, and vice versa. Our needs and tolerances are highly individualized. This is why it is impossible for me to give a supplement program (or a diet program or exercise program) that will work for every single person. There will always be those people who have difficulty processing certain foods as well as certain supplements, and others that may need a higher dose than average.

Considering all of this, in addition to your medication, there are some supplements that might be of great benefit to you. These include:

- Vitamin D
- Magnesium
- Essential fatty acids (including gamma-linolenic acid)
- Vitamin E
- B vitamins (methyl B_{12}, methylfolate, and B complex vitamins, including thiamine, riboflavin, niacin, pantetheine, and pyridoxine)
- Coenzyme Q

- Kelp and algae
- Dietary enzymes
- Dietary fiber

Always talk to your doctor about whether you should be taking any or all of these supplements. I suggest beginning with a vitamin D test—most people who do not live in tropical climates are deficient. You can also have tests to determine whether you have other nutritional deficiencies, but the vitamin D test is the one most doctors will not have any problem ordering (they may think other tests are unnecessary, or they might not be covered by insurance, unless you show symptoms of a particular deficiency).

But before you run out and buy a bunch of supplements, let's talk about making sure your supplement use is working rather than causing more problems for you.

THE PROBLEM WITH MULTIVITAMINS/MINERALS

Some people take a multivitamin/multimineral supplement, but they are much more likely to cause problems with nausea and GI upset than some other supplements, so I don't routinely recommend them for my patients.

Vitamin D

A low vitamin D level is associated with higher rates of relapse, more severe disability, more brain atrophy, and higher rates of many chronic health problems. Higher levels are associated with higher levels of function.[1] Furthermore, low vitamin D levels are associated with higher rates of autoimmune disease, mental health problems, cardiovascular disease, and cancer.[2] For that reason I strongly urge you to monitor your vitamin D level and make getting it to an optimal range a priority.

The most natural and effective way to get vitamin D is simply to put your skin in the sun. Vitamin D is an interesting vitamin that is actually also a hormone. We make vitamin D from cholesterol as a result of the ultraviolet radiation in sunlight hitting our skin. When this happens, the liver and kidneys transform the vitamin D into a more active form, and this allows our cells to read DNA instructions more effectively.

Unfortunately, instead of a continuous exposure to the sun the way our ancestors had, with a gradual increase in sunlight exposure over a season and a gradual increase in vitamin D levels and skin pigmentation throughout the summer, we spend hours inside. Think about how our Paleolithic ancestors lived and thrived. They spent most of their time outside. Although they usually slept in sheltered places, during the day they were out and about under the sun millennia before sunblock was ever invented.

We live much differently now. During summer, the heat and humidity in the outdoor world feels uncomfortable to us because we're not used to it and air conditioning feels good to us because we aren't used to extremes of temperature. Even during nice weather, digital entertainment has replaced outdoor play for most people in developed societies. When we do go outdoors, our physicians—especially our dermatologists—warn us to apply sunscreen first. Of course you do not want to burn your skin, but one of the problems with sunscreen coupled with all this indoor time is that many children and most adults are still vitamin D deficient at the end of summer when our levels should be high enough to store vitamin D for the long winter.

Sunscreen blocks the frequency of light that our skin needs to make vitamin D, which is in the ultraviolet B range. The result is chronically low vitamin D levels, which increase the risk of infections, lung cancer, breast cancer, colon cancer, prostate cancer, heart disease, autoimmune problems, preterm labor, toxemia of pregnancy, schizophrenia, learning disabilities, and other mental health problems.

The lab vitamin D target range (meaning your vitamin D level as indicated by a lab test you can get from your doctor) is typically 20 nanograms per milliliter (ng/ml) to 70 ng/ml. Sometimes it is stated as 30 to 70 ng/ml. Because of this target range, many physicians will consider 31 ng/ml to be adequate, but with levels that low, the person is still at four times the risk for autoimmune problems, more relapses, brain atrophy, and cancers as someone with a higher level. The hunter-gatherer societies and those who live in the sun 24/7 have values that range between 80 and 120 ng/ml. It is likely that this is the level most consistent with optimal health.

TEST YOUR OWN VITAMIN D

You can ask your physician to check a total vitamin D level and be sure you get the actual number, not just a note that it is "normal." Alternatively, you can get a home test kit and more information about the health impacts of vitamin D from the Vitamin D Council at vitamindcouncil.org. You can order kit(s) that have what you need to prick your finger, along with a card to collect the blood specimen in six circles. You let it dry and then send the card back to the lab. The lab is fully accredited, and you will receive a letter with the results and general advice about the target level.

In my clinic, we base our target range on what a breastfeeding mother needs in order to have enough vitamin D for her baby in her breast milk: 55 ng/ml or greater. Our target range is 50 ng/ml to 100 ng/ml total 25-hydroxy vitamin D. I tell my patients that 80 ng/ml is an ideal target. In my clinical practice, however, I find that the vast majority (more than 90 percent) are below 30 ng/ml unless they are taking vitamin D supplements, working in an outdoor job with all-day sun exposure with the arms and legs (or torso) exposed, or using a tanning bed regularly. People with pigmented skin living farther from the equator than their ancestors (i.e., African Americans, Pacific Islanders, and Hispanics) are likely to have more severe deficiencies.

So what should you do about this? There are risks and advantages to increasing vitamin D through sun or tanning bed use (your skin) or through supplements (your gut), but my first recommendation is to follow nature's guidance and use your skin to make more vitamin D.

Vitamin D from the Sun

Unlike taking vitamin D supplements, which can cause you to overdose on vitamin D (I'll talk about that next), your skin will not make too much. There are no reports of vitamin intoxication (excessive levels) from sun exposure, and there are studies that show achieving vitamin D levels of greater than 50 ng/ml through the skin leads to a superior immune function than can be achieved using supplements. With the sun, you will make vitamin D in the most appropriate amount and with the most benefit.

This means, however, that you will have to spend some devoted time exposing your skin to the sun and/or a tanning bed. More controversy! Yes, I am an advocate of using light to make vitamin D, even when it comes from a tanning bed. The key point is to gradually increase the time so that you do not get sunburns along the way. When you have enough sun exposure to get a slight pinking without getting a sunburn on your face, arms, and legs, your skin will have made 20,000 international units of vitamin D. There is also evidence that sun on the skin has positive immune effects independent of vitamin D levels.[3]

Hunter-gatherer societies, with their 24/7/365 exposure to sunlight, did not have a particularly high incidence of skin cancers or melanomas. The constant exposure, lack of sunburns, and a nutrient-dense diet may be a factor in why their risk of cancers appears to be much lower than ours.

Of course, you will have to weigh all these factors, and if you have a family history of skin cancer or melanoma, you may be better off taking supplements. But if you like the idea of getting your vitamin D more naturally, I highly recommend more sun exposure, as long as you do not let yourself get a sunburn.

WAHLS WARRIOR Q&A

Q: Are there specific benefits of the Wahls Protocol for osteoporosis, osteopenia, and osteoarthritis?

A: Yes. Osteoporosis and osteopenia are strongly related to a lifetime of vitamin D deficiency and a high-glycemic diet, which tends to draw calcium from the bone. Add to that an increasingly sedentary life and there is very little drive to put calcium back in the bones. Reducing the high-glycemic foods, eating more bone broth, optimizing vitamin D levels to between 50 and 100 ng/ml, and, most important, getting more weight-bearing exercise will all help restore calcium back into your bones.

Another valuable vitamin for mineralization of both bones and teeth is vitamin K2. Eating more greens that are rich in vitamin K1 will provide your gut bacteria with the raw materials for producing an important sub-type of vitamin K2 called vitamin K2mk7, which the liver further metabolizes to another sub-type, vitamin K2mk4. This form is particulary useful for mineralization, helping the body remove ectopic calcium from the blood vessel walls and heart valves and put it into the bones and teeth. Good direct sources of K2mk4 include organic grass-fed ghee, emu oil, and grass-fed liver.

Osteoarthritis (the "wear and tear" arthritis that is not autoimmune-based) can also be helped by consuming a cup or two of bone broth every day so that your cells have the building blocks for maintaining and repairing the cartilage and ligaments around the joints. Eating 3 cups of sulfur-containing vegetables each day will also shore up joints, as will regular exercise. The Wahls Diet will also help to reduce the inflammation that is damaging the joints and provide the nutrients you need to begin repairs.

Vitamin D Supplements

Low vitamin D levels are associated with higher risk of worsening MS symptoms and higher rate of relapse.[4] For that reason I suggest that you get your level checked annually and work with your physician to optimize your level. Taking vitamin D supplements in place of or in addition to sun exposure has its pros and cons as well. If you take supplements, there is a risk that your vitamin D level could become dangerously high (greater than 120 ng/ml), leading to excessively high calcium in your bloodstream, kidney damage, even psychosis. This is because vitamin D is a fat-soluble vitamin. Fat-soluble vitamins have more potential for harm from excessive dosing than water-soluble vitamins. Water-soluble vitamins (B and C vitamins) are excreted by the kidneys, whereas the fat-soluble vitamins are stored in fat, where they can accumulate and reach excessively high levels.

A vitamin D overdose is rare but possible. That is why it is so important to get a vitamin D level test and follow your vitamin D level regularly to know that you are in the ideal range and not becoming excessively high. If you are taking more than 2,000 international units (IU) of vitamin D, I urge you to have a vitamin D level test every three months until you have gotten your vitamin D level to the target level (and are able to maintain it using your current strategy of sun or supplement use), then check it once or twice a year to confirm that you are keeping it in the target range.

Although your supplement needs depend on the latitude where you live, the pigmentation level in your skin, and the amount of time you spend outdoors without sunscreen, many people who live and work indoors need between 4,000 and 8,000 international units (IU) during the winter months when they cannot make vitamin D, and between 2,000 and 4,000 IU per day during the summer when they can get outside and get enough sunshine to have a dark tan, which will make enough vitamin D to maintain healthy levels.

HELPING VITAMIN D WORK BETTER

For vitamin D supplements to work effectively, you also need vitamin K2. Your gut bacteria makes the subtype vitamin K2mk7 from the vitamin K1 in greens, and the liver metabolizes it into the usable K2mk4. The animal version of K2 (K2mk4) is also present in grass-fed/grass-finished organ meat, fermented cod-liver oil, and high-vitamin butter oil from grass-fed cows. (Look for the casein-free version of these oils.) Be sure to eat plenty of these foods if you are taking vitamin D supplements. If you are already following the Wahls Diet, that should be no problem for you.

Note that this is a wide dosing range, so the risk of toxicity from overdosing on vitamin D is real—and I am now finding people with dangerously high vitamin D levels because they are taking supplements but not monitoring their dose. Another problem is that as we increase vitamin D intake through supplement use, we can create a relative insufficiency of vitamins A, K, and E in the cells if those vitamins are not also increased. I recommend eating liver, greens, and nuts. If you don't eat liver, cod-liver oil also contains EPA, DHA, and retinol. If you prefer supplements or feel you aren't getting enough fish oil, you could take molecularly distilled fish oil for the omega-3 EPA and DHA content. (Note that I no longer recommend fermented cod-liver oil.)

WHAT ABOUT CALCIUM?

In the first edition of this book, I recommended taking calcium supplements, but while there may be benefits, calcium supplementation does also have some potential risks. In some people, calcium supplements are associated with ectopic calcifications and cardiovascular disease. To protect against this, calcium supplements should be paired with sufficient vitamin D and vitamin K intake. Vitamin D regulates absorption of calcium from the gut and can increase GI absorption of calcium, and vitamin K regulates mineralization of teeth and bones. Vitamin K can also reabsorb the calcium that gets deposited onto the blood vessel and heart valves and put it back into the bloodstream so it can get to the bones and teeth, where it belongs.

However, our ancestors did not consume dairy products and of course did not take calcium (or any other supplements), yet they had much denser bones than modern humans. My advice is to get your vitamin D and vitamin K2, and also take advantage of gravity (weight-bearing exercise and vibration plate training) to have healthy bones, rather than relying on calcium supplementation.

Also, the amount of vitamin D that you need to take orally will depend in part on the efficiency of the enzymes that handle the production and use of vitamin D in your cells. These are called the single nucleotide polymorphisms, or SNPs ("snips"), that manage vitamin D. If you have several SNPs related to vitamin D, you may not be able to utilize vitamin D as efficiently and you will likely need a higher dose than those who do not have this issue. This is another reason that it is important to monitor your blood level so that you know you have achieved the target vitamin D level. Whatever your individual case, you need to follow blood levels for accurate dosing guidance. Personally, in addition to getting as much sun exposure as I can living in the Midwest, I take additional vitamin D_3 in the form of vitamin D supplements and fish oil or cod liver oil, as well as vitamin K supplements or emu oil. If you are taking 5,000 IU of vitamin D or more, you should also take vitamin K

(I like supplements or emu oil as a source), and check your vitamin D level regularly. See Resources for ways to obtain vitamin D tests to effectively monitor your levels.

However, your nutritionist and primary care medical team may prefer that you do take calcium supplements, and here's why. There is a lower intake of calcium in Wahls Paleo (approximately 950 mg) and Wahls Paleo Plus (750 mg) than in the Wahls Diet (1,450 mg). I suggest that if you are doing either Wahls Paleo or Wahls Paleo Plus (or even if you are on the Wahls Diet), you may consider taking 250 mg of calcium citrate once or twice a day, depending on your gender, age, and which diet you are following. The RDA for calcium for men and for women under the age of 50 is 1,000 mg of elemental calcium. For women over the age of 50, and men over the age of 71, the RDA is 1,200 mg. It is important to intentionally and consistently eat calcium-rich foods—like eating the bones in canned salmon, as well as almonds, bok choy, and collard greens—but supplementation is an insurance policy. The two main forms of calcium in supplements are carbonate and citrate. I prefer calcium citrate because you can take it with or without food and there is less risk of bloating, gas, or constipation than there is when you are using calcium carbonate. Calcium carbonate is less expensive but requires a good amount of stomach acid to be absorbed (and stomach acid declines after age 50). Also, it is important to note again that vitamin D is required to absorb calcium efficiently from the gut, so it is important to monitor your vitamin D level, as discussed previously. Doses of more than 500 mg have been associated with more adverse events, including ectopic calcification of heart valves and blood vessels, as well as increased risk of stroke, heart disease, and kidney stone formation.

Magnesium

Magnesium can be very helpful with reducing spasticity in muscles, improving restless legs syndrome, and improving sleep. (I'll explain more about this in the next chapter, "Managing Stress and Increasing Physical, Metabolic, and Emotional Resilience.") Green leaves are a terrific source of magnesium. If you decide to take additional magnesium, you can take 350 to 400 mg of elemental magnesium by mouth every day as long as you have normal kidney function, but don't take more than that without working with your physician to be sure you are not overdoing the magnesium. Magnesium threonate is the form that crosses the blood brain barrier and is most ideal, but magnesium glycinate is also easily absorbed into your cells. Magnesium oxide is the least expensive form and is less readily absorbed. You could also consider magnesium acetate or citrate if you suffer from constipation, especially if you have concerns about oxalates.

Essential Fatty Acids (Omega-3 Fatty Acids and Gamma-Linolenic Acid)

The next supplement to consider adding to your routine is omega-3 fatty acid. I've already talked about this essential fatty acid when I talked about grass-fed meat and wild-caught fish (and also when I talked about problems with vegetarianism), but although you may be eating these foods, you still may not be getting enough.

There are two omega-3 fatty acids that are very important: DHA and EPA. Your brain needs docosahexaenoic acid (DHA) to make myelin. Eicosapentaenoic acid (EPA) is very helpful in lowering inflammation. You can see why anyone with MS or another autoimmune condition would benefit greatly from these compounds!

In our study, we have subjects take molecularly refined fish oil to increase both the EPA and DHA intake. This is an easy way to standardize intake for a clinical trial. Studies have shown, however, that eating foods high in DHA/EPA is more effective at raising the blood DHA/EPA levels than taking fish oil supplements. Eating wild-caught cold-water fish is best, but if you can't get enough, a supplement may be in order.

There is also an interesting way to get the benefits of both, using a method of supplementation that traditional societies in the far north used for hundreds of generations: cod-liver oil. Cod-liver oil maximizes content of fat-soluble vitamins A, D, and, to a lesser extent, K. If you are not consuming liver, cod-liver oil is an excellent way to get some retinol as well as vitamin D into your diet.

Because of concern for mercury contamination, I suggest you look for highly concentrated, molecularly distilled fish oils with combined DHA and

WAHLS WARNING

Fish oils can prolong bleeding time. As a result, we exclude from our study anyone who takes a medicine to thin the blood, such as Coumadin. If you are on any medication to thin the blood, it is critical that you work with your physician regarding how much and what kind of omega-3 fatty acids you can safely take. If you are taking fish oil, do not take additional flax or hempseed oil without checking with your physician first to be sure you are not increasing the risk of bruising and bleeding. (Note that ground flaxseeds or chia seeds you take for fiber if constipated should not cause a problem.) In my clinic, if a patient is on a blood thinner, I work with the doctor who is prescribing the blood thinner to see if he or she would be willing to replace the blood thinner with high-dose fish oil, since it does the same job. Sometimes that is appropriate and sometimes it is not.

EPA. If you take the molecularly distilled fish oil or cod-liver oil (which is never molecularly distilled), you should also take vitamin E in the form of mixed tocopherols or tocotrienols at 200 to 400 mg per day. (Note that 1 mg equals approximately 1.5 IU; some supplements are labeled with IUs instead of milligrams.) Without the additional vitamin E, you will increase the likelihood that the omega-3 fats will be rapidly oxidized in your bloodstream, which greatly reduces the benefits.

Ideally, ask your doctor to do a lipid panel that includes an essential fatty acid analysis to know what your bloodstream's omega-6 to omega-3 fatty acid ratio is. This looks at the ratio of AA to EPA (arachidonic acid to eicosapentaenoic acid). Your goal is to get that ratio between 1.5 and 3. If you can't get an AA-to-EPA level, don't feel bad. For years, I could not get the AA-to-EPA level at my hospital, either. Instead, I used the standard fasting lipid panel to check on my patients' fish oil dosing. This is an indirect measure of the AA-to-EPA level. The goal is to get the HDL over 60 with a CRP level of less than 1 and a hemoglobin A1C of less than 5.2 percent (your hemoglobin A1C value suggests how highly oxidized your LDL cholesterol is, and a highly sensitive CRP measures your inflammation level—see the "Supplement

Summary" (page 339) and "Annual Tests" (page 345) charts later in this chapter to see which results may warrant additional fish oil supplementation). You may also want to obtain a more detailed lipid profile to understand your cardiac risk factors and to have more precise dietary guidance.

B Vitamins

Many people take vitamin B supplements because the B vitamins—including vitamin B_1 (thiamine), B_2 (riboflavin), B_3 (niacin), B_5 (pantothenic acid), B_6 (pyridoxine), B_7 (biotin), B_9 (folic acid), and B_{12} (cobalamin)—play so many important roles in the proper functioning of the cells. In our clinical trials, we want more specific information. I always check blood levels for folate, vitamin B_{12}, and homocysteine at entry into the study. I also did this routinely in my traumatic brain injury clinic and in my primary care clinics for patients who have a personal or family history of issues that suggest brain dysfunction or inflammation, such as neurological or psychological issues, or cardiac dysfunction, such as coronary heart disease, a valve problem, or a rhythm problem. I want to see the folate, vitamin B_{12}, and homocysteine levels in particular in the top quartile (the top 25 percent) of the suggested reference range.

WAHLS WARRIORS SPEAK

I was diagnosed with MS in 2008, and a hair mineral analysis found that I had high lead levels. Blood tests around that time showed an exposure to tuberculosis, low blood protein levels, and elevated cytokine levels. Between my gluten and dairy intolerances, genetic predispositions, and stress triggers, my body couldn't detoxify and heal itself.

I found Dr. Wahls, started following her diet, and, after ten years of vegetarianism, I am slowly introducing meats and taking a coenzyme Q10 supplement and vitamin D daily. On the days that I don't eat fish or flaxseed oil, I take 15 millliters of high-dose EPA/DHA fish oil. I supplement my banana/kiwifruit/blueberry smoothies with lecithin, acai powder, hemp protein powder, mesquite powder, green tea powder, cacao powder/nibs, spirulina, chlorella, bee pollen, and flaxseed oil. The Wahls Diet satisfies my cravings for good fats and greens in a way that other diets didn't. It gives me direction and incentive because I know I'm eating to improve my myelin sheath, balance my GABA levels, and restore my mitochondria. I've had no relapses for one year and no drug treatment. I've felt improvements in energy levels [and] cognition, lessening brain fog, better balance, reduced weight, clearer vision, fewer migraines, better digestion, clearer skin, and shinier hair and nails. I can run again! My neurologist reported recently that I have no signs of disability. I am ecstatic to be able to keep myself healthy. It is intensive but it is a massive act of self-loving.

—Nissa P., Tasmania, Australia

WAHLS WARNING

Note that any vitamins or supplements that you take should be from a manufacturer that uses good manufacturing processes and has used a third party to test the product and confirm that the product is not contaminated with lead or some other heavy metal and in fact is what it says it is. ConsumerLab.com conducts independent testing of vitamins and supplements and ranks products according to their purity tests. A modest annual membership fee gets you access to their testing information. I think it is money well spent to know which products are the most safe and reliable.

Coenzyme Q10 (or CoQ10)

Coenzyme Q10 is a nutrient that is important for mitochondrial efficiency. It is part of the electron transport chain in the mitochondria that generates the ATP. (See chapter 1, "The Science of Life, Disease, and You.") As we mature, particularly over the age of 50, it becomes more difficult for us to make enough coenzyme Q10, and medications often compromise our ability to manufacture coenzyme Q10. It has been prescribed for heart failure at doses ranging from 100 mg twice a day to 200 mg twice a day[5] and for Parkinson's disease at doses of 300 mg twice a day to 600 mg twice a day.[6] I do have studies using coenzyme Q10 for MS patients showing it is helpful in reducing inflammation markers in animal models of MS. A 12-week study of MS patients showed that 500 mg daily reduced depression and fatigue. Because the heart failure and Parkinson's studies were using only one intervention, it is possible that a smaller dose as part of an entire program of nutritional support (like the Wahls Protocol) would be effective. That is why in our clinical trial we used just 200 mg of coenzyme Q10 total per day. Eating organ meat such as heart (the richest source of coenzyme Q10) and liver (also a good source) will also give you more coenzyme Q10, creatine, lipoic acid, and other critical mitochondrial nutrition. Also, talk to your doctor about the importance of supplementing with coenzyme Q10 if you take statin drugs.

Algae

I already talked about seaweed in chapter 6, "Wahls Paleo," because these are actually functional foods rather than supplements. Technically, seaweed is a type of algae, but there are other types of algae that are not seaweed. The cell walls of algae will bind heavy metals, plastics, solvents, and other toxins, shuttling them out with the stool. While seaweed grows in salt water, other types of beneficial algae grow in freshwater ponds (examples are chlorella and spirulina). Freshwater algae are potent sources of vitamins, minerals, and protein, and all have been used by traditional societies as food sources for thousands of years. However, because of concerns about cyanotoxins in some spirulina and wild blue-green algae supplements, I recommend you stick with chlorella, and pay close attention to how you respond. Algae can generate toxins (as I mentioned previously, red tide blooms that kill fish and close beaches are an example). This has prompted me to be more cautious in my recommendations. Algae is potentially very helpful with detoxification support, but it warrants caution.

You can take algae as capsules—I recommend 500 mg. Take the algae in the morning, as many people experience high energy for several hours after taking algae. If you take it in the afternoon, you are more likely to have problems sleeping. When supplementing your diet with algae, pay attention to how you feel. Some people crave algae and do very well with it, while others find that it causes nausea or loose stools. If it disagrees with you, do not use it.

WAHLS ON THE ROAD

When I travel, it can be difficult to get as many greens and sulfur-rich vegetables as I prefer to have in my diet. I now travel with a head of cabbage. I munch on it in the airport while traveling. Then I have additional raw cabbage each day at the beginning of the day. Cabbage travels well, with or without a refrigerator. Other travel tips:

- I often take liver jerky with me when I am traveling to make sure the nutrient density of my diet does not fall off while traveling.
- I order vegetables, grilled meats, and salads with a wedge of lemon or balsamic vinegar, and berries when they are available.
- I avoid sauces, dressings, and soups, as they often have hidden gluten and dairy.

CALL TO ACTION

Additional travel tips can be found at terrywahls.com/bonus.

While greens are good for us all, remember that all greens have some toxins. If you rotate your greens, including your sea vegetables, you will experience more benefit and less risk. So if you decide to take algae, do so intermittently. I take 500 mg of chlorella every day for a week, then skip the next week. During the summer when I am eating more fresh greens and a wide variety of greens, I stop the algae and resume in the fall when my garden greens are done.

Digestive Enzymes

Our modern bodies carry a heavy load: Not only must we digest cooked food that has had its enzymes destroyed by heat, but most people tend to eat diets high in sugar and carbohydrates that increase the demands on the body's naturally produced digestive enzymes. Years of doing this exhausts the pancreas so that it is no longer able to produce the optimal amount of digestive enzymes for the food we consume.

While I recommend adding fermented foods to your diet in chapter 6, "Wahls Paleo," supplements of digestive enzymes can help your body do an even better job of digesting cooked food.

There are several ways to take digestive enzyme supplements. You can either take one or two capsules with your meals to replace some of the enzymes destroyed by cooking, or you can take one to three capsules on an empty stomach thirty to sixty minutes before you eat. This is the preferable method, because your empty stomach will absorb the enzymes more easily. However, if you take enzymes with your meals, it will make it easier for your body to properly digest food proteins, which will decrease the risk of food sensitivities. So there is merit to taking enzymes with your meals. For those of you with food

WHEN YOU HAVE ACID REFLUX

Another symptom of poor eating habits is heartburn or acid reflux. Ironically, this is often a sign of decreased stomach acid. Digestive enzymes can help to restore the natural balance, but there are some other things you can do to help recalibrate your digestion. Slippery elm powder and licorice teas are both soothing to the stomach. Some find that by adding 1 to 3 teaspoons of apple cider vinegar to a glass of water and drinking it before meals, their heartburn is reduced or eliminated. After the age of 50, everyone's acid production declines (this may be due in part to our bodies making antibodies against our acid-producing cells). Along with digestive enzymes, hydrochloric acid supplements can help restore natural stomach acid balance and may also reduce bloating and improve protein digestion. Finally, prebiotic fiber (you'll get a lot of this from all the vegetables you are eating, but you can also take it in supplement form) helps to feed the gut bacteria that produce butyrate, a short-chain fatty acid that helps with digestion, eases inflammation, and may even help to counter insulin resistance.

sensitivity issues, improving your digestion of proteins is likely to decrease your reactivity to foods.

I take two enzyme capsules first thing in the morning and again at bedtime on an empty stomach, but I worked up to this. I recommend starting with one capsule and gradually working your way up, noting how well you do. When purchasing digestive enzymes, look to see if the product includes at least the enzymes protease, bromelain, amylase, and lipase. Digestive enzymes can increase the effect of blood-thinning medication and need to be used cautiously if you are taking any medication, especially blood thinners of any type, including fish oil. That is another reason for making changes in the dose very slowly.

Additional Dietary Fiber

If you develop problems with constipation, I suggest you take in more fiber. You could use freshly ground flaxseed or chia seed (no need to grind chia) to make more fruit puddings and titrate your dose to the desired effect. That in my opinion is preferable to taking fiber capsules. However, if this isn't doing the trick for you, you might need more fiber. The intent is to take in enough fiber to poop two to three times a day without having an accident in your pants! Look for soluble fiber products made from psyllium husks, inulin, chia seed, or ground flaxseed. Note that insoluble fiber, soluble fiber, microbial-accessible fiber, and resistant starch are all valuable additions to your diet, for your own needs and for the needs of your microbiome. The Wahls Diet and Wahls Paleo are both good sources of all these.

Supplement Summary

This chart shows typical dosages for the supplements I generally recommend, but always check with your physician/health care practitioner prior to starting new vitamins or supplements.

Supplement	Maximum Daily Dose (unless otherwise directed by physician based upon personal evaluation)
Vitamin D	Variable: Follow blood levels and take the amount recommended by your doctor.
Calcium citrate	If recommended by your primary care doctor and you are on Wahls Paleo or Wahls Paleo Plus, 250 mg elemental calcium once or twice a day
Magnesium	350 to 800 mg of elemental magnesium daily, as magnesium threonate or glycinate or other type
Docosahexaenoic acid (DHA)/ eicosapentaenoic acid (EPA), fish oil, or fermented cod-liver oil	2 grams DHA/EPA *or* 2 grams fish oil *or* 2 grams cod-liver oil (if you eat liver regularly, do not use cod-liver oil)
Mixed vitamin E tocotrienols or mixed tocopherols	400 mg, if taking fish oil or DHA/EPA
B complex multivitamin, preferably B-100 (higher potency)	1 caplet
Methyl B_{12} (this form is preferable than a cheaper form of B_{12}, cyanocobalamin)	1,000 mcg (lozenges or drops are preferable—let them dissolve slowly under your tongue for best absorption)
L-methylfolate (levomefolic acid)	1,000 mcg if homocysteine is elevated
Coenzyme Q10	200 to 500 mg
Chlorella	500 mg (intermittently)
Dietary enzymes: protease, bromelain, amylase, and lipase	2 or more capsules on an empty stomach; may interact with blood thinners
Fiber (freshly ground flaxseed or chia seeds soaked for 24 hours, then ground and blended, or inulin, green banana flour, plantain flour, or oligosaccharides)	As needed to have 2 soft bowel movements daily

Optional Supplements

There are some additional supplements that are often promoted for people with brain problems like autism, MS, neuropathy, Parkinson's, memory loss, and mood disorders. You may have heard about them or considered taking them, so I will weigh in. Note that many of these same compounds are promoted for people with heart failure and diabetes. These supplements are not part of the Wahls Protocol but you may consider them, especially if you are not making progress after six months with excellent adherence to the protocol. (Always work with your personal physician if you begin taking any supplement, whether part of the Wahls Protocol or not.)

- **Zinc, iron, and copper.** It is important for your zinc, iron, and copper to stay within optimal range—neither too low nor too high. Excessive copper and iron as well as zinc deficiency either in combination or individually have been associated with increased risk of neurodegenerative disorders such as Parkinson's and Alzheimer's dementia.[7] The increase in copper can occur in part from the copper used in water supply lines or the use of supplements that include copper. The excess iron can occur as a result of supplement use or cooking with cast-iron cookware. Because the uptake of copper is coupled to zinc, avoiding copper supplements (often present in multivitamin-multimineral supplements) and taking zinc (at low levels such as 30 mg daily or three times a week) may reduce the risk of excess copper or zinc deficiency. A baseline zinc level is also a consideration if you plan to take zinc on a regular basis, so make sure you do not overshoot and create a copper deficiency. Because iron is a necessary cofactor for many enzymes in the brain, it is necessary to have an optimal iron level. For that reason, any iron supplementation must be monitored with iron levels to be sure that your iron level does not become too high. Eating organ meats each week (rich in minerals) is better than taking supplements, because you are more likely to avoid creating excess or deficiency problems. This is another reason that I believe eating nutrient-dense food is safer than supplementation done without monitoring the levels of the specific vitamin or minerals levels.
- **Other brain and heart supplements.** Supplements other than the ones I've recommended earlier in the chapter often used in functional medicine practices to help support brain cell process include lipoic acid, carnitine, and creatine. Any or all of these may or may not be helpful to you. At a dosage of 300 to 600 mg/day, lipoic acid has been shown to be helpful in treating painful diabetic nerve damage.[8] Lipoic acid (600 mg) combined with carnitine (1,000 mg) and varying levels of coenzyme Q10 (100 mg to 600 mg twice a day; see previous section) are used for Parkinson's.[9] Lipoic acid

supplements (600 mg twice a day) were associated with less brain volume loss in patients with secondary progressive multiple sclerosis.[10] Lipoic acid may be benficial, but do be sure to follow your kidney function (creatinine blood test and urinalysis) twice a year while taking lipoic acid to be sure you are tolerating it well. The combination of lipoic acid, B vitamins, and coenzyme Q10 has also been shown to be protective in a variety of animal models with brain troubles related to mitochondria that fail[11] and heart failure.[12] Note that two organ meats, liver and heart, are excellent sources of very bioavailable B vitamins, lipoic acid, and carnitine, as well as coenzyme Q10. They are also all found in sardines, oysters, mussels, clams, and kidneys in forms that are more readily absorbed and utilized by the body than the synthetic versions in commercial supplements. You will also have less concern about whether the supplement may be contaminated with heavy metals or solvents from being grown in contaminated soils or during the manufacturing process. I'd rather you spend your money on buying and growing food.

- **Resveratrol** (especially for fasting). When fasting, even for the twelve to sixteen hours suggested in Wahls Paleo Plus, your efforts will be boosted by a resveratrol supplement. This will further stimulate positive changes to your mitochondria.[13] You can get resveratrol naturally from black-colored berries such as aronia and blackberries, purple grape juice, and red wine, or you can take it in supplement form at a dosage of 250 mg once a day.

- **NAC (N-acetylcysteine).** Take 500 mg to 2 grams daily. NAC is approved at much higher dosing for use in acute poisoning and Tylenol overdose and to reduce the risk of damage to kidneys with the use of intravenous contrast for X-ray studies. When I am concerned about detoxification for a particular patient, I may recommend 500 mg to 2 grams of NAC daily for additional detoxification support.

- **Turmeric.** This orange cooking spice helps rebalance the phase 1 and phase 2 detoxification enzymes in your liver and kidneys. I often take turmeric (½ to 1 teaspoon a day, in water like a shot or with coconut milk as a tea), and I have patients who need additional detoxification support take turmeric tea regularly.

- **Organic sulfur compounds.** These are sometimes given as supplements to support detoxification enzymes, reduce cancer risk, and reduce excessive inflammation: sulforaphane, indole-3-carbinol (I3C), and diindolylmethane

(DIM).[14] They are all present in the cabbage family of vegetables, which is why the Wahls Diet includes 3 cups of sulfur-rich vegetables.

- **Antioxidant supplements.** This series of supplements is often used to boost detoxification, reduce inflammation, optimize homocysteine levels, and/or improve the cholesterol profile. Many functional providers will suggest adding some of these when additional interventions are needed, based upon the person's evaluation. I have listed the supplement and put in parentheses the food source for that compound so you can see how the Wahls Diet was designed to maximize these important nutrients: resveratrol (skins of vegetables and dark berries), ellagic acid (berries), quercetin (green tea, onions, and berries), epigallocatechin gallate (EGCG; green tea and yerba maté), aged garlic extract (garlic family vegetables, shown to reduce oxidative stress, improve endothelial function, and improve blood flow[15] through the sulfur components within the garlic family of vegetables—of course you could just eat more garlic), hydroxytyrosol (olive oil that is not heated), and anthocyanins (purple and black vegetables and berries).

- **Probiotics:** The research is rapidly expanding on specific microbes that have health benefits to us. We may soon see mental health, neurologic, and medical conditions treated with specific probiotic species. As data on a variety of species continues to emerge, I recommend rotating varieties for exposure to more species. When I developed antibiotic-associated diarrhea after surgery, I took VSL#3. It has been studied in the setting of inflammatory bowel disease and is associated with fewer relapses in ulcerative colitis patients (but was not shown to be as helpful for Crohn's disease patients). Normally, I rotate through probiotics starting with a lower CFU of 5 billion and working up to 30 billion. If you go very high, to a product with greater than 30 billion CFU, you could increase the risk of developing small intestinal bacterial overgrowth (SIBO), so more is not always better.[16] See the probiotic discussion on page 217.

- **NF-kappaB inhibitors:** Because inflammation is largely driven by NF-kappaB (see page 189), it is a good target for reducing inflammation. Many substances inhibit NF-kappaB and may therefore reduce inflammation. All the substances listed in the previous three bullets are NF-kappaB inhibitors. Some others, which may be in supplement or whole food form, include potassium, potassium bicarbonate, DHA, EPA, crataegus (hawthorn), ginger, licorice, rosemary, extracts of grape seed, garlic, coffee, green tea (especially matcha), fisetin in strawberries, citrus fruits, daidzein, genistein, naringenin, sea buckthorn berry, pomegranate, lycopene, lutein, zeaxanthin, carnitine, alpha-lipoic acid, bee propolis, boswellia, ashwagandha, astragalus, Pycnogenol, ginkgo, milk thistle, white willow bark, glutathione, glucosamine, all the B vitamins as well as vitamins C, D, and E, melatonin, all the essential fatty acids—in short, many different kinds of substances in plants (phytonutrients) and seafood. Rather than looking for all these things in supplement form, however, know that if you are eating your 9 cups and varying your vegetables and fruits to include as many species as you can, and including cold-water fatty fish in your diet, you are likely to get most of these substances.[17]

- **Activated charcoal** and **edible clay are toxin binders.** Some integrative health providers push a number of toxin-binding compounds such as bentonite clay and/or activated charcoal. These compounds act like sticky flypaper to absorb the toxins that the liver transformed from fat-soluble to water-soluble and excreted into the bile. The toxins will stick to the charcoal and/or clay, so you will not be able to reabsorb the toxin back into the bloodstream, and you will excrete the toxin. They also absorb nutrient metals like zinc and magnesium. Therefore, if you are going to take these internally, do so only under the direction of a physician.
- **Joint supplements.** These are often used for joint support for those suffering with degenerative joint disease or rheumatoid arthritis and include

WAHLS WARRIOR Q&A

Q: Why did you simplify the supplement list since your first book, *Minding My Mitochondria: How I Overcame Secondary Progressive Multiple Sclerosis (MS) and Got out of My Wheelchair*?

A: I have learned a lot since I wrote *MMM* and have had a lot of additional research come in. One thing has become very clear: It is best to individualize the protocol. In patients taking a long list of supplements, I have seen more problems with nausea, abdominal pain, and loose stools. For that reason, in my clinic I start with the short list I have provided in this chapter, check labs, take a careful history, do an examination, and then personalize the recommendations. Additions after this point will be more likely to have a positive effect, and the risk of side effects is lower. Requiring fewer supplements is also more cost-effective. I urge all Wahls Warriors to discuss the supplements you want to take with your health care practitioner to decide if they are worth considering for your circumstances, and monitor your reactions to each new supplement carefully. Add them one at a time and make dose changes slowly. Meanwhile, try to get as much of your nutrition from food as humanly possible!

glucosamine, chondroitin, and methylsulfonylmethane (MSM). The best food source for these compounds is bone broth made with knucklebones, chicken feet, and sulfur-rich vegetables.

- **Memory supplements.** These are used to support the clearance of amyloid plaques in patients with Alzheimer's disease (see page 271). Natural substances like turmeric, ashwaghanda, and *Bacopa monnieri* are being studied for their ability to improve clearance of amyloid plaques and tangles and/or improve cognition in those with early dementia.[18]

Finally, remember that targeted use of supplements may be very beneficial, particularly if the homocysteine remains elevated, but keep in mind that the Wahls Diet is designed to increase your intake of these nutrients naturally.

Annual Tests

If you are taking supplements, it's important to have a CBC (or complete blood count—a blood test), a liver function test (alanine aminotransferase or ALT or aspartate aminotransferase or AST), and a kidney function test (creatinine and urinalysis) once or twice a year to be sure you aren't experiencing any toxic reactions. I also recommend several other annual lab tests if you have a personal or family history of brain, heart, or other complex health issues for troubling signs. The following tests are all things your primary care doctor should feel comfortable ordering. I have provided the target ranges that I use and the interventions I typically recommend for my patients in cases of abnormal results, although your personal physician may work with slightly different targets and interventions. You may require refinement of these recommendations based upon your personal health circumstances. To get these tests, just request them from your doctor before your appointment:

Labs	Target Range for the Wahls Protocol	Intervention
Complete blood count (CBC), calcium, creatinine, and alanine aminotransferase (ALT)	Normal values for the target range. (A target range is the value the testing laboratory has defined as normal based on the values that occur in 97 percent of the population.)	These are safety labs to be sure your system is handling the supplements and processing them properly. If the levels become abnormal, you will need to discontinue any noncritical medications and reevaluate promptly to ensure things are normalizing again.
25-hydroxy vitamin D (vitamin D25-OH)	50–100 ng/ml (nanogram/milliliter) or 150–250 nmol/L (nanomoles/liter) (British)	Adjust vitamin D dose up or down according to level. If vitamin D is above target range, then check calcium level to be sure the calcium level has not become elevated, and to best interpret the reason for the elevated vitamin D. If calcium is elevated, you will likely be directed to receive urgent if not immediate attention.
Folate and vitamin B_{12}	In top 25 percent of the reference range for that lab	Interpret with homocysteine (see Homocysteine, below).
Homocysteine	4 to 6.5 micromole/L	If low, eat more protein. If high, switch to the methyl forms of folate (methylfolate) and methyl forms of B_{12} (methyl B_{12}). (Note that less expensive forms of folate and B_{12} do not have the methyl group added.) Also a vitamin B complex like B-100. If still high once folate and B_{12} are optimized, see a functional medicine practitioner for guidance.

Labs	Target Range for the Wahls Protocol	Intervention
Highly sensitive C-reactive protein (hs-CRP)	Less than 1.0 mg/L (milligram/ liter) = low risk (ideal) 1 to 3 mg/L = intermediate risk Greater than 3 mg/L = high risk	If high, eat more vegetables and berries. If still high after consuming 9 to 12 cups/day, see a functional medicine practitioner for further guidance.
Total cholesterol	More than 160 mg/dL (milligram/deciliter) (preferably more than 200 for optimal brain function, although we do not know the optimal upper range for ideal brain function: 250 may or may not be too high). Note: If a person has coronary heart disease or cerebrovascular disease, the treating physicians will usually try to keep cholesterol below 200.	If cholesterol is 200 or less, lower or stop cholesterol-lowering medication. If no cholesterol-lowering medication, increase cholesterol intake—e.g., with ghee. If cholesterol is higher than 250, stop coconut oil and switch to olive oil to reduce saturated fat.
Triglyceride/HDL cholesterol ratio	Less than 3	A ratio greater than 3 indicates probable insulin resistance. Decrease carbohydrate intake and advance to Wahls Paleo or Wahls Paleo Plus Diet. This may indicate need for more fish oil. Note: This ratio is less reliable for people of African descent. In that case, it is better to measure insulin and glucose levels to simultaneously assess insulin sensitivity.
HDL cholesterol (good cholesterol)	HDL cholesterol greater than 60 mg/dL (milligram/ deciliter)	If HDL is less than 60, decrease carbohydrates, increase vegetables and berries, increase fish oil, and increase exercise.

Labs	Target Range for the Wahls Protocol	Intervention
Thyroid-stimulating hormone (TSH) and free thyroxine (free T4)	TSH 0.30–3.00 micro international units per milliliter (IU/ml); free T4 in normal range according to reference lab	TSH is typically checked for those suffering with fatigue. There is some controversy over whether the upper limit of TSH should be 3.0, not 5.0. If the TSH is outside the target range, check free T4; if that is outside the target range, treatment for over- or underactive thyroid is indicated.
Hemoglobin A1C	Less than 5.2 percent	Hemoglobin A1C is typically checked for diabetes. This correlates very well with the level of sugar oxidation of your LDL cholesterol. If hemoglobin A1C is greater than 5.2 percent, lower the carbohydrate content of your diet.
Fasting insulin	Less than 7 microInternal units/mL	Obtain this test to understand how sensitive you are to insulin. Elevated insulin indicates that you are developing insulin resistance and are on your way to pre-diabetes and diabetes, which are serious chronic health problems. If the fasting insulin is greater than 7 I recommend a lower intake of carbohydrates and lower glycemic index foods (less-starchy vegetables, fewer starchy fruits).

Advanced Testing for Personalized Nutrition

With the new advances in data analysis, we are entering a brave new world in which we may soon be able to provide more specific recommendations based on individual genetics and microbiome configurations. It is absolutely true that our genes influence how effectively we can metabolize carbohydrates, protein, and fat and whether we are better suited to a low saturated fat diet, high saturated fat diet, a diet high or low in protein, or a diet high or low in carbohydrates. Genes can also influence how likely we are to develop a food sensitivity to gluten or casein, given the right (or actually wrong) circumstances or triggers. The types of commercial products currently available analyze your genes and the known research about the various single nucleotide polymorphisms (SNPs) you have, to give you recommendations about your ideal macro (protein, carbohydrate, and fat) ratios and whether particular supplements are more likely to be helpful or harmful in improving your health. These products will continue to evolve in sophistication and usefulness. GenoPalate is one good company making these tests right now. You can use the results to guide you in your quest to determine whether to use coconut oil or olive oil as your source of fat, if you want to try Wahls Paleo Plus and get into ketosis (see page 235). For DNA-based tests available right now, see the Resources. You can also visit my website to order your own basic and advanced health tests, at http://yourlabwork.com /wahlsprotocol/. See the Resources for more information.

Microbiome Testing

Microbiome tests are even more sophisticated than DNA tests because they analyze much more data. The best tests examine the microbes living in your bowels (not just the bacteria), their metabolites, and the microbial genes. Since we have about 25,000 genes and our microbes have 5 to 9 million genes, this is incredibly useful information. All of the data from your health history and the microbiome analysis are used to develop recommendations. One company called Viome uses artificial intelligence to continue to learn and refine its advice to consumers. Also included with Viome is a second follow-up assessment so you know the impact of your new dietary intervention. This is the most optimal way to personalize the dietary recommendations. There are other similar companies doing this high-quality level of testing and service, such as BIOHM Health. If you have the funds, it is a worthwhile test. For more information on currently available microbiome tests, see the Resources.

Self-Monitoring Technologies to Improve Health

As technology allows us to measure and monitor more of our biological functions—nutrition, movement, heart rate, blood pressure, brain waves— we are becoming increasingly able to use big data computing and artificial intelligence to provide much more specific recommendations about how to optimize our health. We can obtain feedback to more quickly achieve meditative states, more muscle growth, less (or more) body fat, superior fitness, cognitive training, better blood pressure, improved heart rate variability, and more.

Devices such as the Apple watch and the Fitbit tracker (there are many others) can monitor many physiologic parameters to provide real-time guidance on how we can enhance our health and performance. Many of these devices can monitor activity levels, step counts, calories burned, heart rate, and more. HeartMath monitors heart rate variability (and therefore the output of the sympathetic and parasympathetic nerves). There are a variety of devices that monitor brain waves, too, and can detect meditation states. Examples are Muse and Melomind. The Quantified Self movement uses technology to optimize health and human performance—and you can learn more about how to use self-monitoring technologies at. It's an exciting new world with an even more exciting future! For information about these companies and more, see the Resources.

Complementary and Alternative Therapies

I am a conventionally trained internal medicine physician practicing at an academic center, so it's probably not surprising that, prior to my diagnosis, I was skeptical of alternative and complementary medicine. I believed people were wasting a great deal of money on these alternative, unproven therapies—that is, until I became a patient with a progressive disease for which there is no cure.

In my research, I found numerous studies showing that MS and other autoimmune patients use complementary and alternative medicine therapies, usually as adjuncts to their conventional medicine treatments. How could I not consider this option when I had so few choices left?

That is when I began looking at alternative medicine. Yet I did this with the eye of a conventionally trained doctor: In everything I read, I looked for some common sense, and sometimes I found it. Not always, but sometimes. When I found evidence, I kept an open mind. There are many alternative medicine modalities that are not science-based, or that have a seed of science at their core but that take that and speculate or extrapolate. This is where you have to be careful. When I looked at alternative therapies, I asked myself whether the treatment balances potential benefit with potential harm in a responsible way, even if the treatment isn't FDA-approved. Is there any research backing it? Does it make scientific sense? I urge you to ask yourself these questions before trying something new:

WAHLS DIARY ALERT

If you decide to try any new therapy, keep detailed notes in your Wahls Diary about how you feel before the treatment begins, what you hope will improve, and how long you are going to try the new treatment before deciding if it is helpful or not—say, three months. Put a note in your Wahls Diary on the day you are going to reevaluate how you are doing, and put a note on your calendar, too. Then make notes once a week about how you are feeling. When the date comes for you to evaluate whether you have made any progress, you will have a little more information to help you decide if the new treatment is worth continuing. It can be hard to look back and remember how you felt before. Also, sometimes you may think the treatment isn't helping, but when you stop taking it, you realize how much it really has been benefiting you.

---

1. What are the risks? They should be minimal. For example, going gluten-free for 100 days to see how your body reacts has very little, if any, risk.
2. How much will it benefit the specific disease I am suffering from? Is there any proof that it will, or that it has done so in others with my specific disease? Are there published studies in peer-reviewed scientific journals? Pubmed.gov is where I search.
3. How much will it benefit (or potentially worsen) my overall health? Is there proof that it has done so in others? Are there documented side effects that could be troublesome or intolerable for me?
4. How much will it cost to do this, how often will I need to do it, and what kind of monitoring, if any, is needed if I try this? Is there a way to test whether it is working?

5. Does it make sense in terms of potential mechanism of action? Would a doctor or scientist say it is impossible, just improbable, or actually quite possible?
6. Can I do it easily on my own or with my family's support?
7. How will I decide if it is improving the quality of my life or my family members' lives enough to continue?

Even if the therapy you want to try doesn't pass every test, you may still want to try it. We all have our own level of risk tolerance. Some people prefer to wait for clinical trials that garner FDA approval for a drug or surgical treatment. If that is what makes you comfortable, then that is the appropriate choice for you. (You may, however, want to read the package insert of potential side effects for those prescription drugs!) Others do not want to wait and are more comfortable seeking new things to try to improve the quality of their lives, even if they aren't proven just yet. However, I do recommend that you evaluate new treatments with this rubric and create a plan that will help you decide if the intervention is helping you. I suggest doing this for every new treatment (FDA-approved or not) that you begin. Keep a record of your progress and don't hide what you are doing from your personal physician.

The list of potential alternative therapies is a long one, but there are some that I find particularly low-risk and potentially useful for MS, autoimmune problems, and other chronic diseases, as well as for other brain issues. There are other alternative therapies that I did not include on the list because of space limitations.

Low-Risk Alternative Therapies

- **Oil pulling.** To avoid an unfavorable bacterial balance in the mouth (dysbiosis), it's important to brush your teeth (I use coconut oil and a drop of essential oil, such as oregano oil or tea tree oil) and floss. Oil pulling takes this process a step further. It involves swishing oil around in your mouth for about a minute—coconut oil, olive oil, or emu oil are the most typical—and it could help to reduce the occurrence of a pathogenic bacteria called *Porphyromonas gingivalis* that has been linked not just to periodontal disease but also to atherosclerosis, rheumatoid arthritis, and the autoimmune process.[19]

- **Reiki /Healing Touch/Therapeutic Touch.** This is a form of therapy that supposedly manipulates energy so it moves better through the body, promoting balance and healing. The use of Reiki, Healing Touch, or Therapeutic Touch therapy uses light or proximity-only touch to interact with the biofield energy of the body. *Biofield* is the term used to describe the field of weak electromagnetic energy surrounding the human body. With the development of quantum mechanics, the tools to build monitors that can measure these fields now exists, and it is the same quantum mechanics that allow for magnetic resonance imaging (MRI) scanners that have become critical to imaging the brain. Reiki and Healing Touch/Therapeutic Touch techniques interact with the person's biologic energy, using the energy of the person who is giving the therapy to provide support to the person receiving the treatment. Biofield therapies are being added to cancer treatment centers and have been shown to be clinically helpful in reducing pain and improving quality of life, and are now being shown to improve immune cell function.[20]

- **Movement therapies.** This group includes practices like yoga, Pilates, and tai chi. These three styles of movement all include stretching, balance, strength training, and awareness of your position in space. As such, they are all excellent for improving the connections between your brain and your body. I do both yoga and Pilates as part of my morning workout. I have also attended tai chi classes. If you can find a good, experienced instructor, I recommend any of these therapies highly. Another option is to obtain a DVD and begin doing them at home. The advantage of an instructor is that she or he can be very helpful in learning how to do the moves correctly, adapting them to where your body is presently, and helping you advance what you are doing as your strength and balance improve. (For more on these and all types of exercise, review chapter 9, "Moving for Healing.")

- **Bodywork.** This includes body manipulation by someone else, as you would experience in massage, trigger point therapy, and reflexology. Our skin is filled with skin receptors that send information back to our brains. The touch that we feel can help downregulate the number of inflammation molecules and restore a more optimal balance to the hypothalamic-pituitary-adrenal function.[21] In other words, massage can reset your stress hormone levels back to idle. For years I could not tolerate massage therapy, as even the lightest massage felt painful to me. Now, however, I find that massage, even the most vigorous deep-tissue massage, is very helpful. It is relaxing and provides a deep sense of calm and contentment following the massage. If you can have massage therapy on a regular basis, by all means, do so. If all you can do is simply massage and stroke your own skin—or have a family member or friend do this for you—you will still enjoy plenty of benefits. Even if you do get massages, I also recommend that you spend some time stroking your face, ears, hands, and feet daily.

- **Reflexology.** This is the art of applying pressure to specific locations in the feet to reduce symptoms and improve function. Studies of reflexology and multiple sclerosis have shown benefits in reducing pain and fatigue.[22]

This next list of therapies come with a slightly higher risk, but you might want to consider them.

Moderate to High Risk but Potentially Beneficial Alternative Therapies for Some

- **Chiropractic care.** Many people with multiple sclerosis have lesions in the cervical (neck) spinal cord. If the cervical bones are not in proper alignment, they can put pressure on the spinal cord. Chiropractic manipulation, if done properly, can lessen malalignments and decrease the pressure. In a study of chiropractic care to the neck using forty-four multiple sclerosis patients and thirty-seven Parkinson's disease patients published in the *Journal of Vertebral Subluxation Research* (a chiropractic journal), 91 percent of the MS and 92 percent of the Parkinson's patients improved.[23] If you have cervical lesions, an evaluation by a chiropractor may be beneficial to you, but choose someone with a good reputation who has experience treating patients with your disease.
- **Acupuncture.** Acupuncture is a therapy involving the insertion of tiny needles into predetermined points on the body. Practitioners study where these energy centers are and which ones can be stimulated to resolve particular issues. Acupuncture can be done using needles or electrical stimulation of particular points in the body to improve the flow of energy, or

chi, through the body to reduce symptoms and improve function. Two studies showed the benefits of the use of acupuncture to treat fatigue in multiple sclerosis patients. In one study, twenty subjects who had fatigue that was not helped by drug therapy underwent twelve sessions of acupuncture. Fifteen of the twenty had clinically significant reductions in fatigue.[24] In another study of thirty-one patients with relapsing-remitting MS who were given immune modulator drugs and acupuncture therapy or sham therapy (a placebo), the active acupuncture group had greater reductions in pain and depression than the placebo group.[25]

- **Pulsed electromagnetic therapy.** Magnetic forces may have biologic effects on our cells, in part due to the documented improvement of the flow of electrons through the electron transport chain in mitochondria in an electromagnetic field. There have been several uncontrolled small studies that have shown the benefits of using pulsed electromagnetic fields (PEMF) in the setting of MS. There has now been a randomized, double-blind (meaning neither the patient nor the investigator knew who had active treatment), placebo-controlled study that used two study sites to examine the effect of PEMF in multiple sclerosis. In this study, subjects received four weeks of therapy, then a two-week washout period, and then two weeks of the other therapy. One hundred seventeen subjects completed the study. There was significant improvement found for fatigue and overall quality of life for the active device (the device that actually delivered PEMF, as opposed to the sham device or "placebo device" used in the study). (No benefit was seen for bladder control.[26]) In another study using PEMF, using Bio-Electromagnetic-Energy-Regulation (BEMER) therapy, thirty-seven subjects were randomized for a double-blind twelve-week treatment of active therapy versus placebo and were then followed three years after the initial randomized crossover controlled trial. Again the PEMF was associated with reduction in fatigue and improved quality of life in the short term and also in longer follow-up studies.[27]

- **Light therapy:** Light therapy using low-level lasers or near-infrared light has a long history of use for pain management and dermatological issues. It has been used for everything from hair regrowth to Achilles tendinitis, and many things in between, such as tinnitus, TMJ and dental pain, arthritis, skin rejuvenation, neck pain, wound healing, muscle fatigue, carpal tunnel syndrome, even reduction of heart attack. Low-level laser therapy is proven to be useful for pain control and may even help with memory loss and neurodegeneration, as well as "electrical acupuncture."[28] While there are a few risks—you need to wear eye protection and should never use it if you are pregnant or have a cancerous lesion, and you should probably not use light therapy over your thyroid[29]—the dangers are easy to manage and the pain relief and other benefits may make it worth trying.

- **Detoxification/colonics/cleanses/chelation.** There are many practitioners whose goal is improving detoxification pathways of the kidneys, liver, and sweat glands. Some of the practitioners use intravenous drugs to pull out the toxins. The potential harm of intravenous detoxification is that more toxins will be pulled from the body than the liver, kidneys, and sweat glands can process, which will lead to the transfer of the toxins back to the storage sites in the lipids (fats) in the body, including the brain. For that reason I would be very cautious about any intravenous detoxification strategies. Other detoxification strategies (beyond those I talked about in chapter 8, "Reducing Toxic Load") include colonics or colon hydrotherapy, which is the use of water or other fluids to wash out the colon. Although the FDA regulates the devices used to introduce the fluid into the colon, it does not regulate the practice. Conventional medicine does not consider colonics to have any scientific merit. I cannot find any studies of colon irrigations in PubMed.gov, nor do I have any experience with colonic lavage, personally or in my patients. Therefore I cannot give you an opinion on its benefits and/or potential harm. Intravenous chelation therapy is costly and potentially hazardous if not done correctly. Work with a physician who has been trained and certified so that you are not harmed by removing the toxins more quickly than your liver and kidneys can metabolize the toxins. When that happens the toxins are transferred from your belly fat to the fat in your brain—not a good thing to do!

- **Fecal transplants.** This is a new therapy a lot of people are talking about because it has shown some real benefit and promise for those who suffer from chronic *Clostridium difficile* (C. diff—a serious, potentially life-threatening bacterial infection) and inflammatory bowel diseases, specifically Crohn's disease (CD) and ulcerative colitis (UC). The technique involves implanting the feces of a healthy donor into the colon of an afflicted patient. The patient must undergo multiple transplants. The issue to consider is the risk of health consequences. Although we know how to analyze stool samples, we cannot detect everything they contain— any given sample may be harmless to the person it came from, but could affect someone else in a harmful way. The microbiome is powerful and influential, and there is some evidence that health issues in the donor, such as obesity or mental health problems, could be transferred to the recipient along with the beneficial bacteria in the stool sample. So far this treatment is only approved for chronic C. diff, but there is a lot of research into this area and attempts to approve it for other conditions. I do not contest that fecal transplants have been transformative, even lifesaving, for some people, but right now, we still have no data on adverse event rates, and changing one's microbiome so quickly and drastically could have both unforeseen positive and negative effects. There has been a death reported with fecal transplant, so this does have some risk associated with it. Also, trying this yourself at home could have dangerous and toxic effects, so please don't attempt fecal transplants on your own! However, if your doctor recommends this procedure for you, it might be worth a try.

- **Worm therapy.** Ever since we've had gastrointestinal systems, we have had many things living in them, and one of those things is worms. While many people consider worms to be parasitic, I question that conclusion— over the course of human history, the presence of worms has become an advantage to some degree, helping to regulate our immune systems and reduce the risk of autoimmunity. The absence of worms is actually associated with higher rates of autoimmune disease and also of Alzheimer's disease. A major program in India that dewormed 1 million children resulted in the wormed kids being no better off than those who did not receive the treatment.[30] A more recent study in China also showed no benefit to worming children.[31] I ask you this: If 80 percent of us have worms and they are not noticeably harmful, are they really parasites, or are they actually symbionts, living in cooperation with us for mutual benefit? Specifically, the helminths known as pig whipworms and rat tapeworms are being purposefully introduced into the systems of people with autoimmune conditions, in an attempt at treatment. This is certainly an alternative treatment, but these two worms are the safest for us. Any adverse responses are most likely easily resolved, and these worms cannot migrate to other parts of the body. I have mixed feelings about this potentially beneficial treatment—Americans want a "magic pill," and helminths are no magic pill. They will not cure autoimmunity, but they could nudge it toward a calmer, less reactive immune state. They certainly do not release you from your other obligations to your own health, and should be used *in addition to* dietary and lifestyle changes. I definitely do not recommend trying a DIY approach and giving yourself worms—there are many dangers that could result, including the introduction of parasitic worms that could cause serious harm. Only try this under the direct supervision of an experienced practitioner.

- **DMT.** Not to be confused with "disease modifying therapy," DMT is dimethyltryptamine, a psychedelic drug that has been shown to have an immune modulatory effect on NF-kappaB and may prove to be beneficial for autommune, neurologic, and mental health conditions in the future.[32]

- **Cannabis.** I avoided talking about cannabis in the first edition of this book. Recreational cannabis is not legal in the state where I live, but now that it is legal—especially for medical purposes—in so many states, I have decided to weigh in at last. The research on cannabis is decidedly *mixed*. There is some evidence that it helps with spasticity, pain, and incontinence.[33] Other research is less promising. There is also some evidence that cannabis, or the cannabidiol (CBD) it contains, may be useful for inhibiting NF-kappaB and reducing inflammation. If it is legal where you live, you can get a prescription, and if you want to try it to see if it works for you, that is probably fine. Some people say they experience pain relief through the use of cannabis, while others say they don't notice any effect, or even say they have negative responses to THC. If you know you react poorly to THC, definitely avoid cannabis. There has been more research into CBD oil, which can contain no THC (the compound that gets people "high"), but we still don't know what dose is therapeutic and whether there are actual benefits beyond those people report. We do know that adverse events are unlikely. Hemp oil may be useful because it has a favorable omega 6:3 ratio, but hemp oil is purely nutritional, not therapeutic.

- **Low-dose naltrexone.** This drug is not really "alternative medicine," although I list it here because it is a narcotic agonist used for the treatment of opioid addiction and alcoholism. It also happens to be a potent anti-inflammatory that calms inappropriate activation of microglia in the brain, lowering the cytokine response. Many patients with MS as well as inflammatory bowel disease, fibromyalgia, cancer, and chronic pain take very small doses of this drug to good effect. Its main side effect is vivid dreams, and not everyone responds to it—the standard advice is to stop taking it if you don't notice any difference after three months. Research has shown that low-dose naltrexone improves the quality of life in patients with multiple sclerosis[34] and a variety of other autoimmune and other conditions (such as mast cell activation syndrome, postural hypotension syndrome, fibromyalgia, inflammatory bowel disease, chronic pain, cancer, and skin conditions). If you are interested in this therapy, talk to your doctor about whether it would be appropriate for your individual situation.

- **Cryotherapy.** This treatment involves therapy in a cryotherapy chamber, which is kept at very cold temperatures. It is used for many different things, including pain management, inflammation reduction, reduction in muscle spasms and spasticity, and swelling management. Risks are related to staying in the cold too long, which can cause irritation or damage to the skin. Do not use cryotherapy if you have any history of heart attack, high blood pressure, cardiovascular disease, stroke, seizures, bleeding disorders, kidney disease, respiratory illness, or a pacemaker, or if you are under 18 years of age. I will talk more about cryotherapy in the next chapter, when I talk about physical and metabolic resilience.

- **Stem cell therapy.** This is a medical treatment with significant risk and costs involved. However, keeping in mind the high risk, I do occasionally recommend it to patients who have fully implemented functional medicine 100 percent and are still declining. It can also be a good therapy for those who had stroke or concussion/head trauma, and it may become a more common strategy in the future as the research continues and technology improves. Right now, there are limited published papers supporting its benefits. Stem cells come from the patient (their own bone marrow or fat cells) or from someone else. The hazard of using stem cells from someone else is that it can cause a graft-versus-host disease in which the new stem cells set up an immune system that thinks its new host body is foreign, resulting in an all-out autoimmune attack. The consequence is a need for long-term immune suppression. Harvesting a patient's own stem cells is also complicated. The bone marrow stem cell harvests usually involve a fairly intensive immune suppression via drugs as part of the procedure, with all the involved risks, and a small risk of graft-versus-host disease. The fat stem cell transplant requires harvesting your fat cells, releasing the stem cells, purifying them, and then reinfusing them into your bloodstream.

A review of stem cell transplants that come from fat included cases in which this therapy was apparently beneficial for a wide variety of symptoms and clinical outcomes. However, I have not been able to find a prospective randomized clinical trial of fat-derived stem cell transplants, so while fat stem cells have become widely available, the lack of research and regulation surrounding them warrants caution.

Several medical centers have patient registry or case series of patients using hematopoietic stem cells (from bone marrow or blood). There is some evidence that this kind of stem cell transplant could result in fewer relapses and less progression,[35] and the evidence continues to grow supporting the use of stem cell therapy in the setting of aggressive multiple sclerosis that has not responded to the most potent conventional disease-modifying therapies. Stem cells may have an immune cell resetting effect, but I still suggest caution. If I were to investigate stem cell transplants, I would look for someone with A4M or IFM expertise to ensure that the practitioners fully investigate and address all of the patient's underlying environmental factors (diet, toxins, food sensitivity, hormonal imbalance, etc.), to ensure maximum safety and permanent results. If you don't get to the root cause of the dysfunction, the effects of stem cell therapy likely would not last.

The bottom line is that this therapy is out there, available, expensive, risky, but potentially beneficial. There is much to consider, and you should do thorough research before committing to something this extreme, but it is possible that it could help you. If you want to pursue this therapy, look for practitioners who have completed an A4M stem cell fellowship, ideally with a patient registry or in a country that regulates stem cell therapy.

Finally, there are a few approaches I do not recommend.

Alternative Therapies I Do Not Recommend

- **Color therapy, crystal therapy, and aromatherapy.** There isn't really anything wrong with these harmless therapies. If you are using these as part of your meditative practices to lower your stress level or improve your sleep, please continue to use them. They are certainly not dangerous. However, I cannot find any published peer-reviewed literature offering proof of their effectiveness or supporting their use specifically for autoimmune conditions (though I admit those studies may exist and I simply have not found them).

- **Bee venom, scorpion venom, and other biologic toxin therapies.** These have been reported to be remarkably useful for some individuals in uncontrolled studies of MS and other autoimmune conditions, but randomized controlled studies have been mixed at best.[36] I chose not to pursue those therapies because the risk for adverse reaction is significant.

- **Liberation therapy (angioplasty for blocked vessels) for chronic cerebrospinal venous insufficiency (CCSVI).** I discussed this earlier when I reviewed Dr. Paolo Zamboni's work studying patients who have clogs in the veins that drain the brain.[37] Liberation therapy is a costly surgical procedure with significant risks, and I expect that if the underlying environmental factors (diet, toxins, food sensitivity, hormonal imbalance, etc.) are not addressed, any benefits achieved will likely not be permanent. Dr. Zamboni himself no longer recommends it.

Navigating a disease can be difficult and frustrating, especially when you don't feel like you are making progress. However, unproven, risky treatments are not the answer. Stick with sound, sensible approaches that feed your cells and promote repair and healing. Stay on your drugs and work with your personal physician to individualize these concepts for you. As you provide your cells the building blocks they need to do the chemistry of life properly and remove the toxins that interfere with doing the chemistry of life properly, your cells will begin repairing themselves.

Chapter 11

MANAGING STRESS AND INCREASING PHYSICAL, METABOLIC, MENTAL, AND EMOTIONAL RESILIENCE

S TRESS, INCLUDING PHYSICAL, metabolic, and emotional, is necessary for life. Growing up on a farm gave me excellent bone density because of all the stress on my bones from manual labor. When humans enter a weightless environment, with no gravity pulling on bones and muscles, their bodies begin to lose strength and their muscles shrink. Likewise, brains need the stress of learning and adapting to change in order to produce the hormones (nerve growth factors) that nurture brain cells and direct them to make new connections. Without the stress of learning, our brains make less nerve growth factor and begin the process of atrophying (shrinking).

This is an adaption from our Paleolithic days. We needed that spurt of adrenaline from our adrenal glands to get away from predators or catch prey for dinner. That adrenaline as well as the surge of cortisol that comes from physical or emotional stress sharpen our vision and hearing and improve muscle strength and endurance. We are more likely to get away and survive with this boost of energy and keener senses.

This applies to our lives now, too. It is beneficial to experience a challenge, release the hormones that result in energy, take physical or mental action (or both), learn something from the experience, then relax afterward as the stress hormones subside and the challenge is over. This is the process that allows you to quickly jump out of the way of a speeding car, have a good workout, learn a new language or musical instrument, give a speech or a presentation, jump off a diving board, take a test, or even get the courage to tell someone something difficult. Afterward, you can relax with a "Whew! I'm glad that's over!"

Stress, however, is meant to be acute, not chronic. Chronic high stress without that important recovery period is maladaptive, damaging the body and the brain. After stress, our bodies are supposed to rapidly metabolize (process and eliminate) the stress hormones circulating through the system so we are back to a safe state of "idle." When our adrenals are constantly putting out stress hormones—when we are never able to feel that "Whew, I'm glad that's over" moment because it never seems to be over—then we can't get back to that important safe state. Our biochemistry becomes deranged as a result, leading to excess inflammation in the body and in the brain. We are more likely to become obese and/or diabetic, have clogged arteries (atherosclerosis), have mental health problems, develop autoimmune problems, and even create ideal conditions for the proliferation of cancer cells. Chronic stress wears down the body and uses more than its fair share of your internal resources, so you are less effective at building, rejuvenating, and healing. Chronic stress can trigger chronic disease, but chronic disease also increases chronic stress—it's a vicious circle that is hard to escape.

Your Autonomic Nervous System

The stress response is complex, but one way to look at it is through the lens of the autonomic nervous system. This is the set of nerves that connect brain to body and govern all the things that happen in your body automatically, like digestion, breathing, and the beating of your heart. This is also the system that determines whether you are currently in a dangerous situation or all is well and you can relax.

The part of the autonomic system that reports when you are safe and all is well is called the parasympathetic system. When that system is in charge, your cells know they are safe and can focus on doing the work of living. That means digesting food, making hormones, removing toxins, and building proteins to create new cells, support your immune cells, repair damage, and grow.

There is another part of the autonomic nervous system that kicks in when your brain signals that you are not safe and are indeed acutely threatened. This is called the sympathetic nervous system. When the sympathetic nervous system takes over, everything changes. The work of living, including digestion, normal hormone production, detoxing, and protein building, comes to a screeching halt. Your cells switch gears, priming the body for only one of two things: either to run away or to fight an attacker (the fight-or-flight response).

In order to do this, two glands—the adrenals and the thyroid—change tactics. You can think of them as the tortoise and the hare. The adrenal glands are the hare. They respond rapidly to a threat, immediately revving up the metabolism and secreting stress hormones like adrenaline, noradrenaline, and cortisol. These make your heart speed up, enable your eyes to see more acutely, and divert blood from your bowels to your muscles so you can run faster and longer. They also make your blood sugar and insulin levels increase so you have more energy to use for fighting or fleeing. This is all very effective—for a short time. Once the threat has passed, we go back to a safe state, digesting our food again and conducting the chemistry of life normally. If this happens too often, over time it exhausts the adrenal glands and they lose their reserve. At that point the person begins to develop adrenal fatigue, which just feels like plain old bone-tired chronic fatigue. The adrenals may look "normal" from a conventional medicine perspective, but the adrenal reserve is compromised.

Meanwhile, the thyroid has a longer view. It adjusts the metabolism according to what the adrenals are doing. If there are a lot of threats, the metabolism may stay idling at a higher speed, just to make sure the engine is ready to go whenever necessary. However, if the adrenals are always pouring out stress hormones and don't get to calm down because the brain never signals that the threat has passed, the thyroid thinks the motor has to be racing all the time, Your thyroid will pick up the baton the exhausted adrenals have dropped in order to keep your energy and metabolism up; but when your thyroid can't keep up with your continual stress, it, too, will begin to fail. Your body will do the best it can to keep your metabolism running. By that time, you are likely experiencing deep, near-constant fatigue.

WAHLS WARRIORS SPEAK

I have a traumatic brain injury that occurred during a bicycle accident in 2008. Secondary to that, I've dealt with epilepsy, aphasia, cognitive problems, memory loss, major depression, vertigo, and the inability to go back to my previous position as a pediatric nurse practitioner. A few years after my accident, I was craving a diet high in dark green vegetables, fruits, and salmon, and my doctor recommended that I meet Dr. Wahls. Among the many improvements I've noticed since starting the diet three years ago, I've been able to cut my antidepressant medication in half because my depression has improved a great deal, as has my mental clarity. I truly love and need exercise, so I do cardio or strength-training exercises nearly every day. I meditate and nap daily, get a massage once a month, and use deep breathing whenever I'm stressed out. Being out in nature and having some quiet time alone are so necessary for me. I also utilize my medical knowledge to share my story of survival with others. I believe all of these have helped me, and giving talks about my experience when I'm able has been a wonderful therapy as well.

—Bridgid R., Coralville, Iowa

Now that these two systems are out of whack, this can cause a ripple effect throughout the entire endocrine system, disrupting the entire hormonal system and causing widespread trouble in your body and brain. In addition, chronic stress can also damage the lining of the blood vessels throughout the body, including the ones in your brain and in your heart, so that they become too porous and leak proteins, allowing more endotoxins to enter into the bloodstream and other parts of the body where they don't belong. These leaky vessels, leaky brain, and leaky gut put you at greater risk for developing or worsening your autoimmune problems. Our cells simply aren't built to work that way over the long term, continually bathed in high levels of stress hormones.

The Stress/Insulin Resistance Connection

In addition to the damage to your blood vessels and hormone levels, stress can also lead to system-wide inflammation by causing an increasingly common and dangerous condition called insulin resistance. Here's how it works: Stress hormones acutely increase blood pressure, heart rate, blood sugar, and insulin levels. When there is a constant elevation of stress hormones in the body, that leads to a chronic elevation of blood sugar, which then produces chronic high levels of insulin in an effort to keep the blood sugar at a safe level.

One of insulin's main jobs is to shuttle sugar out of the bloodstream and into the cells of muscles, fat, and the liver, where it can be stored or used for energy. Insulin especially prefers the fat cells around your middle, also known as visceral fat. Not only does this lead to weight problems, but it also leads to inflammation, because visceral fat is hormonally very active. It produces hormones and inflammatory cytokines (little protein molecules that act like hormones) that markedly increase inflammation in the bloodstream and in the brain. If this goes on for too long—especially if the person is also eating a high-sugar, high-carb diet—the insulin response can become blunted. If the "doors" in the muscle and organ cells become resistant to letting the glucose in, so that it remains in the bloodstream, despite insulin's efforts to push it out, the doors will get more and more "stuck" over time. The high sugars are dangerous, so the body goes into alert mode and the pancreas pumps out even more insulin. An insulin-resistant person needs much more circulating insulin than a healthy person to keep the blood sugar in the normal range. If this is happening to you, you may be diagnosed with metabolic syndrome, which is considered a precursor or warning sign that diabetes is in your future. If you continue the way you are going, your pancreas will eventually lose the ability to keep your blood sugar in the safe range. Diabetes is the result. You will begin spilling sugar into your urine, and the damage to your blood vessels and brain cells dramatically increases. People often have diabetes for many years before it is diagnosed, inflicting damage on the nerves and brain cells all the while. The high levels of insulin in the brain compete with the enzymes that help clear the amyloid out of the brain. This can worsen the accumulation of amyloid plaques and tangles, which are part of the toxic load that increases the risk of developing cognitive decline and dementia. This is one of the reasons why changing the diet to reduce carbohydrates (and protein) can be beneficial—this can reduce the risk of elevated insulin, which can help reduce amyloid buildup and the risk of worsening cognition.

This is another vicious circle: Stress keeps blood sugar higher, and the pancreas responds by making more and more insulin, which also leads to more and more visceral fat, which will make more inflammation cytokines and hormones responsible for revving up the inflammation in your bloodstream. To make matters even worse, these changes also increase a person's appetite for carbohydrates, further driving this entire cycle. As you can probably see, continuing to eat a high-carbohydrate diet when you are fighting inflammation is the worst thing you can do—it's like dripping gasoline on a fire while the firefighter (your doctor) is trying to put out the fire with water from the hydrant (conventional medicine). You also need to know that high protein intake increases insulin as well, which is why I prefer a moderate

TEST YOUR INSULIN SENSITIVITY

A simple and inexpensive test for insulin sensitivity is the fasting triglyceride/HDL cholesterol (good cholesterol) level in the bloodstream. A ratio of greater than 3 suggests insulin resistance and that the insulin level is way too high. Keep in mind that this ratio is less predictive in people of African descent. If that group includes you, ask your physician to check your blood glucose along with an insulin level to check insulin resistance or sensitivity. The best way to improve insulin levels is to reduce the demand for insulin production by eating a moderate-protein, high-healthy-fat, very-low-carbohydrate diet. Wahls Paleo and Wahls Paleo Plus fit the bill perfectly. They are both intentionally lower in carbohydrates, greatly reducing or eliminating not just sugar and grain but starchy vegetables and starchier, sweeter fruits. You can obtain a fasting insulin level with the goal of having that number be less than 7 µIU/mL. If you are eating a low-carb diet and your insulin level is still 7 or higher, you probably also need to reduce your protein intake. Many people don't realize that protein also stimulates insulin release (although it is to a lesser degree than carbohydrates do).

protein intake, as opposed to a high-meat or meat-only (carnivore) diet. You are making it much harder to put out the inflammation fires as long as you keep your insulin levels high. Go to the root cause and lower the stress hormones through the stress management techniques we will talk about in this chapter *and* a lower carbohydrate, moderate protein intake. (Wahls Paleo is ideal for this, although you can do a low-glycemic version of the Wahls Diet by eliminating starchy vegetables.)

In addition to the very real risk of diabetes, insulin resistance is also associated with higher rates of brain problems like apoptosis (early or accelerated brain atrophy), more damage to nerves (like painful diabetic neuropathy), and more amyloid protein tangles typical of Alzheimer's dementia. That is because insulin interferes with the enzyme that normally clears these harmful protein tangles.[1] The visceral fat produces cytokines, which drive up the inflammation in the bloodstream and brain, making autoimmune problems worse. Insulin resistance is also a major contributing factor in the development of atherosclerosis, polycystic ovary syndrome (a leading cause of infertility), hirsutism (facial hair on women), and erectile dysfunction and low testosterone in men. Insulin resistance wrecks your hormones and metabolism in many profound ways.[2] You don't want to go there!

The Bright Side of Stress: Physical, Metabolic, Mental, and Emotional Resilience

All this may be making you fear stress; maybe at this point you are contemplating how to avoid it completely. But as I said at the beginning of this chapter, stress can be a good thing. In fact, when you purposefully use stress to increase your resilience, it can actually improve your health and increase your vitality.

Imagine someone who has never encountered any stress—whose life has been easy. Imagine this person has never encountered any difficulty, any danger; she has never been questioned and nothing has ever been demanded of her. Imagine this person has never been in an argument, never experienced self-doubt or guilt, never been told she cannot do something she wants to do. She has never experienced any temperature extremes, never been sick or injured, never eaten a large amount of sugar, never gone hungry. She has never broken a sweat—never even had a raised heart rate or a spike in blood pressure.

Then imagine what would happen to this person in a stressful situation—whether something dramatic like war or extreme injury, or even something minor like getting yelled at. Even a small disruption might feel extreme. A large disruption might be catastrophic and not survivable.

People who undergo mild to moderate stress intermittently become increasingly resilient. In this circumstance, every stressor we encounter makes it easier to encounter the next time we face it. We learn that we manage that problem and move on. If you have an autoimmune disease or other chronic disease, *you* have become resilient. You have encountered problems and have learned how to manage a variety of challenges to get where you are today. And while chronic stress can weaken us, periodic stress can strengthen us and improve how our cells and bodies function. Let me explain how stress can become a tool for improving your health.

There are four different different kinds of stress you can employ in the service of your wellness.

Physical Stress

Physical stress is anything that stresses your physical body—your muscles, skeleton, heart, lungs, etc. Examples of physical stress include things that you would not want to do, like getting injured, but it also includes beneficial things, like exercise. Exercise is a prime example of physical stress. When you do cardiovascular exercise to the point of sweating and being out of breath, that is physical stress on your cardiovascular system. Weight-lifting workouts are physical stress on your muscles. Walking and jogging are physical stress on your skeleton, muscles, and cardiovascular system (if you push yourself to the point of being short of breath). Dry brushing makes your skin more resilient.

Anything that is uncomfortable, tiring, or difficult increases your physical resilience. This is why exercise trainers often encourage people to work just outside what they call the comfort zone. Of course, that doesn't mean going *way* outside your comfort zone. Extreme discomfort can be traumatic and injurious, but mild discomfort increases resilience.

BALANCE TRAINING

Balance declines with age because our proprioception declines with age. We can slow that loss with intentional balance training, which is another type of stressor. Balance practice can easily be incorporated into daily activities. Put one foot in front of the other, at first wide apart, then closer together, as if you were on a balance beam. Eventually stand with one foot on top of the other foot. Then practice turning your head side to side while you stand on one foot. Gradually make your balance training more challenging, but always stay safe!

For example, you might decide to lift weights, doing enough reps that you can't do any more, working your muscles to fatigue (muscle failure, so that you are unable to complete the third round of a weight-lifting exercise in your circuit of exercises—after which you should take a day off before you lift weights again). The goal is to damage the muscle *slightly* so the immune cells come in and repair and rebuild a stronger muscle. Note the emphasis on *slightly*. I am not talking about extreme damage.

You can do the same thing with walking or jogging. Walk just a little farther than feels comfortable (but just a little, then take a nice rest). Depending on your mobility, physical stress could be something as simple as walking across the room before sitting to recover. It could mean stretching your muscles so they begin to feel just a little uncomfortable. Many people with chronic disease become afraid of exertion, but this is a mistake. When you stop moving, stop challenging your muscles, stop flexing your joints, and stop putting pressure on your skeleton, your muscles will atrophy, you will begin to accumulate more body fat, and your body will begin to remove minerals from your skeleton. You will lose strength, mobility, and function. As you can see, you can purposefully stress yourself physically (just enough to send the signals to your immune cells to keep repairing and rebuilding a stronger you), and then you can purposefully end the stress appropriately so your body can recover and grow stronger.

Physical stressors for building resilience:

- Begin an exercise program or class.
- Begin a strength-training program, such as body weight yoga, lifting free weights, or using weight machines.
- Begin walking, jogging, or biking (as you are able) on a regular basis.
- Buy a mini trampoline with a handrail and jump on it for a short while each day.
- Rotate your exercises so you never do the same thing two days in a row.
- Lift heavy things whenever you get the chance.
- Rub and/or brush your skin every day.

Metabolic Stress

Metabolic stress is anything that stresses your metabolism, or the mechanisms that control the chemistry of life. This can include the complex processes that turn food into energy, regulate your internal temperature, control your breathing and heartbeat, manage your blood pressure and blood sugar, and much more. Stressing these processes teaches your metabolism that environments change and it must adapt. This makes your metabolism more resilient so it can more easily fluctuate to keep your systems regulated under many different kinds of conditions. Living in a temperature-controlled environment so that we are always between 68 and 72 degrees markedly decreases our metabolic resilience. Our ancestors learned how to live in winters and summers without central heating and air conditioning. Their bodies could tolerate living and working in cold and hot weather. Spending time out in the weather is one great way to improve your metabolic resilience.

So examples of metabolic stress would be going outside and spending time outside where you live. Do go outside in cold weather and in hot weather. Be sensible, of course—wear appropriate clothing and take precautions to avoid dangerous hypo- or hyperthermia. But do try to go outside every day. I walk every day, in cold and hot weather, but I did forgo my walks when the weather recently became extreme, with a −60 wind chill. Don't mess with polar vortex wind chills! (But I still went out and got the mail and stood outside for just one minute.)

As you improve, likely your tolerance for cold and heat will improve. Take your time and gradually increase your exposure to cold and heat.

Fasting (including intermittent fasting) is another useful metabolic stressor. Eating afterward relieves that stress. Even feasting on occasion is a metabolic stressor—your metabolism gets used to adapting to no food or a lot of food, even though most of the time, it is sustained by a moderate amount of food. The composition of your diet can also be a metabolic stressor. Changing the macronutrient ratios of your diet so your body sometimes must rely on carbohydrates or protein or fat (or fasting) also improves metabolic resilience. I intentionally go through periodic fasts (or do a fasting-mimicking diet) followed by a three-day re-feed with a higher protein intake than usual. During the fast, my stem cells are getting boosted, and during the re-feed, the stem cells are rebuilding a younger, more vigorous body. Note that I do *not* recommend eating foods that are harmful, such as gluten, dairy, trans fats, high-fructose corn syrup, highly processed foods, foods with added sugar or food-like chemicals added to them, or anything that you are allergic or intolerant to—this is an extreme stressor that can harm rather than strengthen your metabolism.

Metabolic stressors for building resilience:

- Don't be afraid of the cold or heat. Try to get outside every day, even when it is very cold or very hot. When it is chilly outside, bundle up, but go out there, even if just for a few minutes (as long as it is safe—and don't slip on the ice!). And do heed warnings about extreme weather, frostbite risk, and heat index.
- Try a cryotherapy session. Cryotherapy exposes your body to extremely cold temperatures for very short periods of time (just a few minutes). Cryotherapy may help with pain, improve mood, resolve skin conditions, reduce restless legs symptoms, improve sleep quality, and more. It also improves metabolic resilience. There may be a cryotherapy chamber near you, or look for one when you are in a big city. Or, you could simply take cold showers or cold baths, a less expensive way to get your cryotherapy sessions. This is what I routinely do!
- Use an infrared sauna, if you have access. I put one in my house because I use it so frequently, although I admit this is expensive. Some of my patients do "car saunas"—they sit in their cars for a few minutes on a hot day until they begin to sweat—no cost! Near-infrared and red light therapy may also improve metabolic resilience.

- Swim in a cold pool or take a cold bath. At first this feels very uncomfortable, but I have learned to love doing this. I feel that it is very good for me. This is especially helpful for metabolic resilience if you combine a sauna and then a cold pool or bath because of the extreme temperature difference.
- Eat until you are 80 percent full. This is the practice of the Okinawan centenarians. Modest calorie restriction improves metabolic resilience and is excellent for anti-aging. But every so often, have a feast meal. Stick to your food list, but let yourself enjoy more calories than you normally do. This is natural for the human body because sometimes food was available in abundance, and other times, it was scarce. I use holidays and special occasions as an opportunity to practice feasting.
- Try intermittent fasting. Going for periods of time without eating (even if it's just twelve hours per day—fourteen is even better) is a great practice for increasing metabolic resilience. The shorter your "feeding window," the better for your resilience. I recommend aiming for eating within a six- to eight-hour period and fasting for the remaining sixteen to eighteen hours. (See page 262 for more information about how to do this smartly and safely.) You can even extend this to periodic fasting (fasting for two to five days). Our ancestors have all had to endure periods with little or no food. Periods of fasting stimulate brain nerve growth factors, stem cells, and mitochondrial efficiency.
- Go to high elevations. Not only can this improve heart health but it also improves metabolic resistance because your body has to adapt to less oxygen.
- Practice holding your breath. This helps your body adapt to the temporary reduction in oxygen. (Be sensible and don't do it for too long!) An easy way to do this is while you are walking. Hold your breath for a certain number of steps, then breathe normally again. Do this whenever you think of it (but not to the point of dizziness).

Mental Stress

The more cognitive work you do, especially when it feels difficult, the more mentally resilient you will become. Examples of mental stressors that increase resilience are playing brain games (see page 91), doing math, or reading difficult books, learning a new language, learning a musical instrument, or doing anything mentally challenging that you don't normally do, like having to give a speech to a group or having to figure out a problem in your personal accounting.

Many people try to build resilience by doing a puzzle every day, but if you do a crossword puzzle every day and doing crossword puzzles has become easy for you, then you are not getting the benefits of mental training. It's better to mix it up with number puzzles or different kinds of word games that will be more of a surprise to your brain, so that it will learn to adapt. This is what builds resilience. Even addressing a new kind of problem at work, having to figure out the logistics of vacation travel, or teaching your children new skills, such as how to balance their checkbooks, can build mental resilience. But remember to pace yourself. The tasks should be challenging, but not exhausting, and what is challenging but not exhausting for you depends on many factors. Remember, helpful stress is meant to be temporary. Don't push your brain activities so far that you are exhausted or develop a migraine in response!

Mental stressors for building resilence:

- Do a different kind of brain challenge every day—crossword puzzles, sudoku, word jumbles, or find a puzzle book with many different kinds of puzzles in it. Even a jigsaw puzzle works.
- Do different brain games on your computer or smartphone.
- Play card games, board games that require some strategy, like chess or Risk, or even strategy video games. I'm afraid I don't know of any strategy video games, but I am told there are many.
- Designate tasks during which you will do everything with your nondominant hand, such as brushing your teeth or eating your salad.
- Learn a new musical instrument, or get reacquainted with an instrument that you used to play but never fully pursued, such as the piano or the guitar.
- Learn a foreign language, or continue learning one you learned in school but did not pursue beyond your classes. There are many audio lessons and local community college classes that offer language lessons.
- Practice driving places without relying so heavily on your GPS or smartphone. Notice landmarks as you pass and really tune in to your

surroundings. You can also memorize turns, such as right, left, left, right, left, then reverse them on your return trip. Keep your GPS or phone with you, though, just in case you get lost!

Emotional Stress

Emotional stress is the kind of stress that many of us think of when we hear the word *stress*. Unproductive emotional stress includes anxiety, panic attacks, depression, and other extremes of emotion (or lack of emotion). However, you can build emotional resilience by purposefully acknowledging uncomfortable emotions rather than avoiding them. For instance, have a difficult conversation with a colleague at work, a friend, or family member. Feel the uncomfortable feelings and wait 90 seconds, then continue with the difficult conversation. You may find that acknowledging the discomfort and then facing the uncomfortable situation becomes easier with practice. Also practice going to social events, especially new ones, even those where you may not know many or any people. These all build emotional resilience.

Emotional stressors for building resilience:

- If you feel sad, angry, or lonely, consider writing about those emotions. Write about what you feel, and what you would like to see change.
- If you have a situation you have been avoiding, such as a problem relationship, write about the circumstances and what you would like to communicate to that person. What would you like to have happen? When you are ready, schedule a time to communicate with that individual.
- Spend more time with your friends—especially the ones that you can laugh with or cry with. If you don't have many, get out there and find like-minded people. Social groups for people with common interests, church groups, or classes can all be good ways to find your tribe.
- Do something you normally avoid because of anxiety or fear. Don't put yourself in danger, but do expose yourself to something that makes you uncomfortable, such as talking with people you do not know, joining a social event that is larger or smaller than you normally would do, or volunteering to do a presentation to the public, working your way gradually toward greater courage. The more you do it, the less scary it will seem.

- Become more social. Engaging in social events requires a lot of emotional skill. Find ways to expand your social circle. Participate in events with your colleagues at work or at your religious community or your school. Invite neighbors, friends, or family to tea. This is a great way to deepen any relationship.
- Learn to say no to things you really don't want to do. It's not up to other people to dictate what you do with your time. If you don't have time for it or you just don't want to do it, you can politely decline. There are many ways to say no, but usually it's sufficient to say, "I'm so sorry, but I just can't fit that in right now."
- If you feel like crying, don't choke it back. Find a private space and let it out.

THE PRICE OF LONELINESS

I often mention the importance of a supportive family, friends, and community. The presence of these support systems is crucial to success in the Wahls Protocol and in keeping a positive attitude and a can-do spirit in the face of adversity. But even when you have support with things like cooking and driving, if you do not have emotional support, you may become lonely. Loneliness and social isolation are literally bad for your health, both mental and physical, and are also associated with poor health habits.[3] A UCLA loneliness scale assesses loneliness based on (among other measures) whether people feel like they have no one to turn to or talk to, lack companionship, do not feel close to anyone, do not feel known or understood by others, and/or feel unhappy about being withdrawn.[4] One study showed that loneliness increases as disability worsens and is associated with an increased risk of heart disease, stroke, and all-cause mortality.[5] This is why it is so important to maintain social connections, even if it is through social media, phone calls, or letters. There are many groups of people on social media with common interests, and this can become a fulfilling solution to loneliness for those who are housebound.

- Figure out what you really love to do, what gives you joy and a sense of purpose, and prioritize it in your life. Whether it's painting or woodworking or volunteering at the animal shelter, doing something truly meaningful to you builds emotional resilience.

Stress Management the Wahls Way

Now you know that there is good stress and bad stress, and you may already be practicing ways to build your own resilience. But it is just as important to manage the bad stress as well as to make sure that even the good stresses are only temporary. That means knowing how to relieve stress so your body can benefit from it. You don't build physical, metabolic, mental, or emotional resilience while you are stressed. You build it after the stress is gone.

But how do you get your stress hormones back to the resting state or idling so your body can recover and your chemistry can normalize again between bouts of stress?

Fortunately, stress management is an important part of the Wahls Protocol, and it's not difficult. In fact, it feels fantastic. All you have to do is switch the autonomic nervous system control from the sympathetic back to the parasympathetic to signal that you are safe. This reduces the demand for stress hormones and gives your poor adrenal glands a break.

There are many ways to flip this switch, so choose the activities you enjoy the most. I recommend doing something stress-relieving several times each day, such as one thing in the morning, one thing in the middle of the day, and one thing in the evening before you go to sleep. You need only spend a minute or two doing some of these activities. Every single one of the activities in the following list is something you could not and would not do if you were in an emergency situation. If you were in danger, would you be meditating with your eyes closed? Would you be strolling through a park or working in the garden or writing in your journal? Of course not. Activities like these will trigger the brain to signal the adrenals that they can relax again. You are meditating, so all must be well. You are gardening or napping, so obviously you are safe. This helps the whole cascade of stress response actions in the body go in reverse. Thus you eventually, with some practice, get back to your normal state.

Here are some ideas, and remember my prescription: three per day!

- **Spend time in nature.** Walking or jogging outside in the fresh air and sunlight is incredibly rejuvenating and a good way to de-stress, especially if you typically spend a lot of time indoors feeling tense.

- **Garden.** Gardening has multiple benefits. It is incredibly calming, as well as light exercise. You are outside in the sunlight, producing more vitamin D. Your eyes *see* sunlight, which helps to align your internal clock with the external clock, improving your circadian rhythm and hormone balance. You are communing with nature and doing something productive, like beautifying your yard or growing your own food. You are also learning about how to nurture and care for something.

- **Exercise.** Any kind of exercise (aerobic, strength training, stretching) can work for stress relief. See chapter 9, "Moving for Healing."

- **Meditation and/or prayer.** When I traveled to and lived in Nepal for six months, I became close with my Hindu and Buddhist clinic staff. I traveled with them to their holy places and had the opportunity to do prayers with them, using prayer beads, prayer wheels, prayer flags, and doing walking meditations. This instilled in me a much deeper appreciation for the power of prayer, religious chants, and rituals. If you do have a religious practice, it can be deeply comforting and healing, but even simple meditation can be done just a few minutes several times a day without any religious affiliation. There are many different forms of meditation, from simply sitting and breathing to chanting a mantra to visualization of peaceful situations. You could have a meditation teacher show you how to do it, or you could learn from books or videos. There is no right or wrong way to meditate, as long as it relaxes you. Whatever type you enjoy is the type for you.

- **Journaling.** Write in your Wahls Diary about the problems you are facing or have faced in the past. Spend at least forty-five minutes over the week writing about your deepest concerns or struggles. No one else has to see the journal. You don't have to read the journal entries again, and you should write in pen and not correct yourself. This is called free writing, and it helps you develop new insights into your experiences. This actually helps the brain send less energy down the sympathetic nervous system to the adrenals. That translates into less adrenaline and cortisol in your system, resulting in better immune cell function and better health. Continue to journal a few minutes each day or fifteen minutes three times a week.

- **Regular contact with a supportive group of people.** When people have a supportive group of peers, they are more successful at adopting behaviors that promote health. Dr. Mark Hyman completed a project with the Saddleback Church in Lake Forest, California, where he coached the church through the adoption of health behaviors to combat obesity and diabetes, with tremendous success.[6] Dr. Hyman taught the church community about functional medicine and diet, but the small support groups the church formed to help their members along seemed to have the greatest impact. I suggest you do something similar for yourself. Find a support group of like-minded people and you will feel your stress drop.

- **Contemplate your higher purpose.** Finding that higher purpose beyond the self can provide inner calm, direction, and guidance that is reassuring and healing. (See chapter 3, "Getting Focused.")

- **Forgive.** Carrying a grudge for prior injustices and wrongs burdens the person who continues to hold the grudge.

- **Yoga, tai chi, qigong.** With their focus on breathing and postures, yoga, tai chi, and qigong also reduce stress hormones. There are many different types, from strenuous to meditative. Almost anyone can find a variety that they enjoy.

- **Massage.** Our skin expects to be touched and massaged. While receiving a deep-tissue massage has many measurable health benefits,[7] getting a daily professional massage is impractical. In our clinical trial we teach people to give themselves a simple self-massage as part of their daily routine. They can use a couple drops of an essential oil (such as grapefruit, lavender, or sandalwood), or an omega-3-rich oil (like walnut oil), or no oil at all. I ask them to begin by massaging the sole of the right foot and all of the toes. The fingers should press as firmly as desired into the ball of the foot and the arch, then massage the toes. Repeat with the left foot. Then, using both hands, gently massage the calf and leg muscles, pulling toward the heart. This will improve the return of lymph fluid to the heart. Move to the right hand and massage the palm of the hand and the fingers. Massage the left hand. Next massage the arm, stroking toward the heart. Massage both earlobes between the fingers, then move around the entire earlobe and ear. Then massage the forehead, cheekbones, and chin. Massage the scalp. Do the massage yourself as part of your evening routine, just

WAHLS WARRIORS SPEAK

In addition to daily exercise and deep breathing, I spend time in nature every day, and occasionally I meditate for about ten minutes. Learning many new cooking techniques has also been good for my brain. One improvement since starting the Wahls Diet and retiring is that I have resumed piano lessons. Playing piano is therapeutic for my weak left hand, which has begun to function better, a wonderful development because I am left-handed. Playing piano is also good for my cognition, and I have developed a deeper appreciation of music. That's good for my brain, too!

Like Dr. Wahls, I am a Unitarian Universalist. I am surrounded by a terrific community of friends! They are quite a reassuring comfort and source of strength, security, and love. I'm not just feeling sorry for myself and thinking about my health concerns. While my activism is limited now due to my low energy levels, I remain connected to the larger issues in our world and maintain a global perspective. I just make sure to bring my own meals to the frequent potlucks endemic to my UU social life.

—Toni C., Cave Creek, Arizona

before bed or upon arising. Of course, if you have someone in your family who will give you a good back rub, that's just icing on the cake.

- **Take an Epsom or Dead Sea salt bath.** Chronic elevations of stress hormones lead to depletion of minerals, especially magnesium. That is why Epsom salt (magnesium sulfate) and Dead Sea salt baths can be so soothing. They help reduce the stress hormones and begin to replenish the magnesium.
- **Take a nap.** Sometimes, a 20-minute catnap is all it takes to restore your energy and calm your mind.

The Importance of Sleep for Stress Management

Sleep is an important part of maintaining the health of all mammals. We need to sleep. It's a requirement for life. Without sleep, our brains will become disorganized. We will hallucinate and become psychotic and nonfunctional. For our bodies, sleep is equally critical. During the eight or nine hours of sleep that our biology requires, the body doesn't consume as much energy because it doesn't have to move, digest, or engage in rational thought. That leaves more available energy for toxin removal, hormone manufacture, and infection fighting. When we fail to get enough, our bodies may not complete those important tasks, increasing the chance of developing problems due to excess toxins, inflammation, and hormone imbalances.

Sleep is also incredibly important for stress management, especially for people with autoimmune conditions. Many people who are stressed have trouble sleeping even as they suffer from fatigue. The relationship between sleep quality and duration and health has been well established across multiple studies,[8] and because sleep problems are more frequent in those with MS than the general population, and restless legs are a common problem for MS patients,[9] this is worth dealing with right now.

Even with my MS fatigue, I never slept a lot. I liked thinking I needed only four to six hours of sleep to function normally. This was back in the days when I was reading scientific literature at night after my family was in bed. Once a week, I'd crash and sleep a lot—sometimes ten hours—then I'd be back to not needing much sleep.

When I learned how critical sleep is to normal biology, I began to rethink my strategy and address my sleep behaviors so that I could get a regular seven to nine hours of sleep. Even if you think you thrive on less than seven hours of sleep a night, your body and your brain are paying a heavy price. You will be at a much higher risk of heart attack, obesity, diabetes, early memory decline, and autoimmune problems. Your cells need you to sleep if you want to have optimal health. That is why I pay attention to sleep now.

Sleep is such a natural activity that it's a wonder so many people have trouble with it. However, if you look at how we live, it isn't such a surprise. We do many things that interfere with getting a good night's sleep. Here are some of the most common and what you can do about them to improve your sleep:

- **Caffeine.** People often drink caffeinated beverages throughout the day to compensate for not having enough energy (often because their diets are so poor), and that caffeine can stay in the system for hours, increasing wakefulness even when it's time to sleep. Some people are much more sensitive to the effects of caffeine than others. For best sleep, stop drinking caffeinated beverages after eleven A.M. and switch to drinking a chamomile tea or an herbal blend with chamomile in it in the evening.

- **Alcohol.** People often drink alcohol in the evenings "to relax." However, alcohol can interfere with sleep quality throughout the night. On the Wahls Protocol, I prefer to limit alcohol use to "occasionally" (three or fewer drinks per week). Consuming it more often may compromise the health of brain cells. Also, consuming alcohol increases the probability of awakening in the middle of the night with difficulty resuming sleep. For this reason, do not consume alcohol for two to three hours prior to going to bed.

- **Sleeping pills.** People often use a variety of medications to induce sleep (sleeping pills like Ambien or other preparations intended for a different use, like Benadryl or NyQuil). These also interfere with the normal sleep cycle and should not be used for more than three days in a row. In numerous studies, individuals who used benzodiazepines or antihistamines—the classes of medicines most often used as sleeping pills—had a higher risk of falls and hip fractures.[10] Definitely not worth the risk.

- **Irregular sleep hours.** Many people stay up too late or go to bed at different times every night. People also use electronic devices late into the night, sitting at the computer or watching television. Because we want to finish what we're doing or watching, we tend to prioritize that over sleep.

EPSOM SALTS AND DEAD SEA SALTS

Epsom salts are an excellent remedy for relaxation. Make an Epsom/Dead Sea salt bath (with warm or cool water) part of your regular evening routine. Taking a bath for twenty to thirty minutes just before bed will relax you, and Epsom salts can also help support your body's detoxification processes, as well as providing supplemental magnesium and sulfur. Dead Sea salts contain more than twenty-six different minerals that are nutrients our cells need to conduct the biology of life, including magnesium, calcium, zinc, potassium, lithium, sulfur, boron, phosphorus, manganese, and more.

This confuses our bodies. If you set up and strictly follow a bedtime routine—such as always having a cup of chamomile tea, listening to relaxing music, having a warm bath, and then meditating, praying, reading, or journaling before bed—your body will get in the habit of relaxing and will naturally induce sleepiness.

- **Exercising at night.** Aerobic exercise early in the day can actually improve sleep later, but exercise right before bed can make sleep more difficult for some because it is stimulating.
- **Stress.** Most of us have chronic elevations of stress hormones that keep us alert, making it more difficult to initiate and maintain sleep. Manage your stress!

A few more sleep-inducing tips:

- **Taurine** is a sulfur-containing amino acid found in fish that boosts the production of gamma-aminobutyric acid (GABA). Taurine supplements (500 mg) and a few cups of chamomile tea may also help to induce natural sleep.
- **Write** a note to yourself about the issues that you want to address in the coming days, or make a to-do list for the next day. This can prevent your waking up to fret about what you have to do or what you don't want to forget during the night. Once it's down on paper, you can release it from your mind.
- Give your face, ears, hands, and feet a **massage** with lavender oil as soon as you get into bed. Other calming oils include frankincense, chamomile, sandalwood, patchouli, and ylang-ylang. I place a small amount (½ teaspoon) of another oil such as emu oil, coconut oil, or almond oil on my hand and 2 to 3 drops of the lavender or other calming essential oil and massage into my skin.

Try to sleep between eight and nine hours every night. You won't believe how much better you'll feel if you can get in this habit!

About Melatonin

Much of our ability to get a good night's sleep has to do with the brain's ability to manufacture melatonin, the hormone made by the pineal gland that is key to the wake-sleep cycle. Your brain secretes melatonin (making it out of serotonin) in response to the world becoming dark, and increases in melatonin are associated with shorter times falling asleep. You get to sleep a lot faster if you have a melatonin spike in your brain in the evening with the onset of darkness.

The problem is that our current lifestyles conflict with the melatonin cycle. For instance, we use artificial lights, which confuse the brain. Is it the sun? Is it daytime? Your brain doesn't know. Also, melatonin is a potent antioxidant and anti-inflammation molecule. You want to have your brain making plenty of it! Here are some things you can do to help regulate your melatonin cycle:

- Have some daylight exposure in the morning or noon hour and spend at least thirty minutes looking into the blue sky or clouds to get your dose of natural blue light to your retina, which will help your brain to trigger your melatonin cycle.
- Go to bed just after sunset, ideally between eight and ten P.M.
- At dusk, put on yellow, orange, or red glasses to block the blue light spectrum. I tell my patients with sleep problems to do this. You can wear these "blue blockers" for several hours before going to bed. This corrects the natural light exposure to your eyes and therefore your brain, increasing the production of melatonin, because the blue portion of the light is what suppresses the melatonin surge. I often use low-blue-light glasses when I am awake past sundown, working in my home. Depending on the time of year, that could mean I wear the glasses for just a few minutes or for several hours before going to bed.
- Wear a sleep mask at night so your eyes see only darkness when you are in bed. Because many with MS have balance issues, you will want to leave some kind of yellow light on to avoid nighttime falling in case you do have to get up. We use a sea salt night-light in the bathroom, which gives off negative ions and a soft golden glow. If you don't have a yellow night-light, don those yellow glasses so that you don't stimulate your retina with the blue light spectrum.

- Although fixing light exposure is the most effective way to boost your melatonin, you can also take melatonin by mouth. Start with 1 mg of melatonin one to three hours before you wish to sleep. Check with your physician regarding the top dose for you. Fixing your light exposure is the real solution for correcting your melatonin levels. (If you use melatonin, be aware that some people have reported increased dreaming or even nightmares.)

IF YOU HAVE RESTLESS LEGS SYNDROME

Restless legs syndrome (RLS) is a disorder in which people have an uncontrollable urge to move their legs, usually in the evening when relaxing or at night when trying to sleep. RLS can involve feelings of pain, cramping, spasms, electrical sensations, tickling, itching, or a "crawling" feeling in the legs. It can also be characterized by an intense need to move the legs without any particular feeling in the legs. It can occasionally affect other limbs, but the legs are most common.

Although primary RLS is idiopathic, meaning there is no known cause, it has been observed at higher rates than in the normal population in people with autoimmune diseases including multiple sclerosis, as well as with neurological disorders like Parkinson's disease and peripheral neuropathy, and with other conditions like diabetes, thyroid disease, fibromyalgia, and attention deficit hyperactivity disorder (ADHD). The underlying mechanism for restless legs has to do with a drop in the levels of the neurotransmitter dopamine in the brain. Dopamine levels fall in the evening, allowing us to sleep, but that drop in dopamine may also trigger RLS symptoms.

The biggest problem with RLS, other than being an annoyance and sometimes painful, is that it can severely interfere with sleep. The frequency of restless legs increases with age, but even young people in their teens can develop restless legs. The treatment from conventional medicine is to prescribe medications that boost available dopamine to counteract the effect and/or to prescribe benzodiazepines at night to make the person sleep more deeply. (This will increase the risk of falling and also the risk of dependence on and addiction to benzodiazepines.) I prefer to use alternative approaches, including getting sufficient iron, B vitamins, omega-3 fatty acids, magnesium, calcium, and trace minerals. You should get all these things in sufficient amounts on the Wahls Diet, Wahls Paleo, Wahls Paleo Plus, or Wahls Elimination. Higher doses of magnesium, B vitamins, and omega-3 fatty acids are sometimes needed to calm restless legs.

You might also try using essential oils at bedtime. Massage 1 teaspoon of liquid emu oil or A&D ointment onto your legs. Then add 2 to 4 drops each of cypress, frankincense, and lavender oils onto your hands and massage into your legs. You can do this as many times as you like during the evening and night. Another helpful topical is menthol or camphor ointment applied to the legs at bedtime. Ointments like Vicks VapoRub, Tiger Balm, and Biofreeze provide a mild topical anesthesia to the leg and help calm the restlessness. Essential oils such as lavender or cypress oil (diluted with a carrier oil such as emu oil) may also be helpful. Reapply as needed.

A cold bath (or cryotherapy) reduces inflammation and symptoms of restless legs syndrome at night. You could also massage your legs with ice to drop the skin temperature. This can help as well.

Additional magnesium can be very helpful to soothe the spasm and reduce the restless legs. Taking additional elemental magnesium at bedtime may be helpful. Magnesium threonate will be the most effective. Speak with your personal physician about whether a higher dose of magnesium may be helpful for you.

Finally, boosting your brain's ability to make gamma-aminobutyric acid (GABA) may be helpful, both for restless legs syndrome and for helping the brain calm down, making it easier to fall asleep. In addition to taurine supplements (mentioned earlier in this chapter), compounds that boost your brain's ability to make GABA include N-acetylcysteine (NAC, 500 mg to 2 grams) and lipoic acid (600 mg once or twice a day). Prescription medications that boost GABA, including baclofen and gabapentin, can also be helpful in extreme cases. Many people with MS are on one or both of these compounds anyway because of muscle stiffness or spasticity (baclofen) or pain (gabapentin). Somewhat higher doses may resolve the restless legs for you. Talk to your doctor about seeing if a higher dose is an option for you.

It's rather amazing that stress and sleep deprivation can have such a profound effect on the body, but they do. Manage that stress proactively and take these important steps to getting a full, sound eight to nine hours of sleep per night, and you will be taking a huge leap forward in your healing because your body will have the biochemical environment and the time it needs to perform the many subtle and pervasive cellular repairs, corrections, and manufacturing you require.

Chapter 12

RECOVERY

Y ou've come a long way. You've worked through the Wahls Diet, perhaps staying there, or you've progressed to Wahls Paleo or Wahls Elimination, or perhaps you've even tried out Wahls Paleo Plus. You've instituted changes in your routine. You may be exercising more, practicing stress management, and sleeping better. Now it's time to step back and take a look at how far you've come. This is your chance to assess your progress. Are your improvements greater than you expected? Are you right on track? Or are you not seeing the results you hoped to see?

If you are seeing dramatic results, I am overjoyed for you! If you are seeing mildly positive results, know that you are headed in the right direction. If you are not seeing results yet, I will help you determine what to do next in this chapter. People are impatient. People with chronic illness are even more impatient—they want to be well! At least, they want to be well right up until they give up on ever feeling better.

Do not give up! Recovery is a highly individual process, but I've watched it happen time and time again in my traumatic brain injury clinics, in my primary care clinics, even in my own family. People are standing up to witness about their own recoveries in my public lectures. And me? I'm walking.

Riding my bicycle. Working. Enjoying my family. Writing another book. I can't believe how far I've come.

Great Expectations

Many of my patients have very high hopes for the Wahls Protocol, and many of them see their hopes fulfilled. For others, however, when progress is slow, it can be incredibly frustrating. They see what happened to me and they want those same results, but my road was an incredibly long one. Do not give up hope.

There is always hope. We constantly replace our cells and the molecules within cells. The lining of your gut is replaced every week to two weeks. It takes about a year to replace your skin. It takes approximately one to three years to replace the cells in your liver and kidney. Blood vessel cells (endothelial cells) are continually repairing themselves. It takes seven to ten years to replace the myelin insulation around the nerves in your brain, in your spinal cord, and out to your body. It takes fifteen years to replace the muscle cells in your heart. It takes twenty years to replace the minerals in your bones and teeth.[1] It is happening right now inside you. Every day your cells are replacing molecules, replacing mitochondria, growing more mitochondria, and rebuilding themselves. It may happen quickly or slowly, but it is happening.

However, we all have a unique combination of genetic vulnerability because of the mix of efficient and inefficient enzymes that we have, courtesy of our DNA from our parents. If you have more inefficient enzymes, it will take fewer insults to make disease happen to you, and it will take more work to reverse the process. Depending on who you are and how you are made, there will be variations in the rate of healing.

How are you doing with your motor skills? Are you feeling accomplished? Are you excited about the changes? Are you disappointed in your progress when you read about the speed and depth of my recovery? Keep in mind that I worked very closely with a physical therapist who had years of experience treating athletes with electrical stimulation. I trained with him three times a week in a clinic, and spent hours each day doing the rehabilitation exercises and e-stim that he prescribed (I still do it!). The remarkable speed of my recovery is likely the result of the intensive nature of all the interventions plus the intense commitment that I made to doing the hours of physical work. I started small, saw my therapist frequently (who used the rehabilitation principles that he used on his athletes), and kept advancing what I was doing. Plus, I worked incredibly hard—in fact, much harder than I had ever worked as an athlete!

Rehabilitation is like that. Before I was diagnosed with MS, I trained as an athlete in tae kwon do, competing nationally in full-contact sparring. In my rehab, I put in more hours than I did training for my competitions. It was my therapist who told me it was possible, who pushed me to keep advancing my exercise and e-stim programs, who kept increasing the weight I was lifting, who saw that I could get stronger. Having someone like that monitoring your rehabilitation can make a profound difference. If you can, find someone who will work to rehabilitate your function, with experience working with athletes and electrical stimulation of your muscles if you have strength, balance, or coordination issues.

Most important, do not give up. Keep looking to find someone who can assist with your physical training. Keep moving and following all the tenets of the Wahls Protocol as you are able, and you will become increasingly able.

This may be a good time to repeat the Medical Symptoms Questionnaire you filled out in your Wahls Diary when you began the protocol. You may have progressed more than you realize. When you begin to feel better, it's easy to forget how bad you used to feel. You are unique, so I can't give you an exact timeline of what your progression should look like, but I can give you some averages based upon what I have seen in my clinics, in my followers, and in the practices of other functional medicine health care practitioner colleagues.

CALL TO ACTION

To help people learn more about e-stim and rehabilitation, we have created an e-course, which you can purchase here: terrywahls.com /estimcourse/.

WAHLS WARRIORS SPEAK

I was diagnosed with RRMS in 1985 and SPMS in 2004, and I started the Wahls Diet in June 2012 after hearing about it from my mother. I feel as if the disease has halted as opposed to progressed. I used to walk with two sticks, but now I just use one. In addition to improved balance, I've noticed much more strength and energy and an increase in my walking speed. I practice water exercise and stretching daily, and I use e-stim and Reiki as well. With the diet, I love eating organic fruits and vegetables, and I have fun looking up new recipes that fit in the Wahls Protocol. These are early days in my recovery, but I know there will be great things in the future.

—Debra F., Napa, California

- **More energy.** Fatigue is usually the first thing to improve. Many will see energy begin to improve within a few weeks, but nearly always within the first three months. This is often accompanied by improved mood and motivation.
- **Better mobility.** Mobility usually takes longer and is less predictable. Many will see mobility improvement, however slight, within six months, but it could take a year or more to begin seeing improvements in your ability to walk. For others, the most that may happen is halting the steady decline—which is its own victory. Have you started working with your physical therapist or occupational therapist so they can guide your exercises and rehabilitation? Did you add e-stim sessions, or if your gait is severely impaired, have you added an FES bike (see page 308)? The evidence continues to grow that e-stim and FES improve function and physiology.
- The reasons for poor walking ability are varied. It could be a problem with the balance-sensing part of the brain, problems with the muscles of the legs or torso, poor coordination, generalized and diffuse weakness, or problems with pain. In addition, much depends on how severe the damage is, how severely disabled you are now, how much of the Wahls Protocol you adopt, and what your burden is of broken biochemistry, toxins, hormone imbalance, and genetic vulnerability. I had one patient take up

jogging and another began lifting weights at the gym after just six months on the Wahls Protocol. Others have had their energy, memory, and mood improve, but their walking hasn't changed much, even after a year. One patient told me that even though she is still not walking, and in fact has lost some functions in the last year, the losses are occurring at a much slower rate and she is much better than she was in many other ways, including energy, thinking, and mood. For her, this is a huge success.

- **Weight loss.** I have consistently observed that people who are overweight steadily lose weight with minimal hunger when they adopt any of the Wahls diets. The weight loss begins with the first week of full implementation of any of the three diet plans and is usually sustained until the person is back to a normal body mass index (healthy weight), often the weight they had in their early 20s.

- **Improvements in diabetes.** People with diabetes—especially those who are overweight—who start with Wahls Paleo come back reporting that they are losing weight without being hungry and have more energy than they have enjoyed in years. In many cases, we see blood sugar going down into the normal ranges within two weeks, leading to steady reductions in the medications needed to control blood sugar. Because your blood sugar rapidly improves as you adopt the Wahls Protocol—sometimes within days, certainly within two or three weeks of strict adherence to the protocol—it is critical to work with your diabetes doctors and monitor your sugars closely to adjust your medications as you improve. The more completely the patients adopt the diet and the protocol, the more rapidly the sugars normalize.

- **Improvement in blood pressure.** High blood pressure develops because the proteins designed to provide elastic support to blood vessels become oxidized and stiff from the high levels of inflammation, blood sugar, and insulin in the bloodstream. As you adopt the diet and protocol, those incorrectly made, oxidized, and stiff protein molecules are replaced with correctly made, flexible molecules. We see blood pressure steadily improve over the next three years, with the medications needed steadily declining, often down to none. Occasionally, blood pressure dramatically improves within weeks, sometimes within days. It is very important to work closely with your prescribing physician/medical team to adust your blood pressure medications as the blood pressure normalizes. You do not want to be fainting!

- **Improvements in heart disease symptoms.** Patients with heart disease— who are usually overweight, and many of whom are diabetic—report weight loss, more energy, and better lipid levels. Again, the root cause of clogged arteries is the high level of inflammation in the bloodstream, the cholesterol that has been oxidized by the high sugar in the diet, and the high levels of inflammation and stress from poorly working mitochondria. Or, the problem is closely linked to higher levels of lead, cadmium, or other heavy metals, leading to more inflammation in the blood vessel walls. The Wahls Protocol improves all of those things. People who have heart failure are often on medications that interfere with the body's ability to manufacture ubiquinone (coenzyme Q10), a crucial element for the heart muscle. Helping the person improve his coenzyme Q10, B vitamin, and mineral status is key. The improved blood pressure, better blood sugar, lower insulin levels, lower inflammation, and more effective mitochondria do wonderful things for people suffering with heart disease. People typically feel noticeably more energetic within three to six months, sometimes within weeks.

- **Fewer abdominal complaints.** Those with autoimmune problems that target the gastrointestinal tract (like inflammatory bowel disease) report fewer abdominal complaints and more energy, again typically within three months. It is common for those with chronic abdominal complaints ranging from irritable bowel to severe Crohn's disease or ulcerative colitis to find that once they go on the Wahls Elimination Diet, their abdominal discomfort dramatically improves. Some can tell things are improving within two weeks when experiencing dramatic improvement, but some improve slowly over three to six months. The vast majority report that the diarrhea and belly pain are markedly lessened and usually completely gone within two weeks.

- **Less pain.** Pain was the most common reason people came to see me. The pain was from autoimmune issues, polyneuropathies, diabetic neuropathy, phantom pain after amputation, war wounds, fibromyalgia, and chronic back pain. We treated all of those individuals with diet and lifestyle interventions only. Typically, the pain began to reduce within six weeks. The pain wasn't resolved, but it was often reducing for the first time. People needed steadily fewer narcotics and were often able to discontinue narcotics entirely. They also had improved function.

- **Improved sexual function (resolution of erectile dysfunction), improved fertility, and less pelvic pain.** Many young men and women (in their 20s) that we saw in the therapeutic lifestyle clinic had marked decline in libido. Men in their 20s had erectile dysfunction. Women had severe pelvic pain, painful periods, and lack of desire. Within three to six moths, these young men consistently reported improved libido and resolution of erectile dysfunction. The young women also reported resolution of pelvic pain and painful periods, often within six months. Several young women who had gone through IVF trying to get pregnant found that within six months of starting the protocol, their pelvic pain resolved and they were able to conceive and carry pregnancies to term. We have many hormone-disrupting compounds in our food, water, and environment that confuse the sex hormone signaling in our bodies. In addition, unrecognized autoimmune conditions create inflammation in the fallopian tubes and uterine lining, making it difficult for embryos to implant. Improving our detox pathways, reducing stress, and sleeping at night improve hormone balance, and taking out the foods to which we may be sensitive reduces the autoantibodies interfering with fertility.

- **Fewer skin problems.** We have had many people report their psoriasis and blistering skin problems and acne steadily improve over the first 100 days, and often entirely resolved as long as they followed the protocol. Recurrent hives take longer to resolve, and are more likely to require the Wahls Elimination diet.

- **Improvement in headache severity and frequency.** Chronic, often daily headaches are a common disabling problem in our society, even for those without any diagnosed chronic disease. Again, many of my patients and followers with chronic headaches discover that unrecognized gluten and/or casein sensitivity is at the root of their daily headaches. In my clinic, I suggest a two-week or month-long experiment on a gluten- and dairy-free diet to see if the headache frequency reduces. At the end of the trial period I have them try a test meal with gluten. The following week I have them do a test meal with dairy. In nearly every case, headache frequency and severity steadily diminish and often disappear on Wahls Paleo, and the gluten meal triggers a recurrence. The dairy meal will trigger a recurrence in about 80 percent. This convinces patients to eliminate gluten and usually dairy permanently. It's also an opportunity to test other foods they have given up, to see if they also cause reactions. I also have patients keep a food symptom diary in which they write down the ingredients of what they are eating each day and whether they develop a headache in the next seventy-two hours, then look for patterns. Many find multiple sources of sensitivity or allergy. (To do all this in a more structured manner, see the section on the Wahls Elimination Diet, beginning on page 122.)

- **Less irritability.** Irritability is another common problem with anyone who has had any kind of psychological or neurological problem, including concussions, post-traumatic stress disorder, depression, and autoimmune disorders involving the brain. We each have 10 billion brain cells with 10 trillion connections between those cells. If we have had a concussion, severe psychological stress, or chronic inflammation in the brain due to MS or some other autoimmune problem, some of the connections between brain cells are strained and/or broken. As a result, brain cells have less cross talk between them. People can have brain cells ready to engage in mortal combat over nothing at all, just to protect the person, and without that cross talk, those brain cells aren't "supervised" and don't have much feedback about whether a situation is a big deal or whether they are prompting an overreaction. (Frankly, the reason we aren't all in jail for fighting everyone we meet is that our brains have cross talk going on that restrain us.) When people who are suffering from irritability start the Wahls Protocol, typically within ninety days of adopting the lifestyle changes, they tell me that things are beginning to improve: The kids are not as annoying, it is often easier to get along at work, and they are not fighting as much with their partners. These are huge improvements in quality of life. In children, this improvement shows up as better behavior and less opposition and defiance. You greatly help your children by adopting the Wahls Protocol as a family. You are helping them now, with likely improved brain function, less inflammation, and less risk of future autoimmune and chronic health problems.

- **Better mental focus.** We have many patients report less brain fog and better memory that is often noticeable within 100 days. In children, this shows up as fewer problems with attention deficit, better grades, and more confidence at school.

Troubleshooting the Wahls Protocol

If you haven't improved as much as you would like, it's time to assess what you are doing. One potential reason for a lack of progress is new exposure to potential food allergens, molds, stress, toxins, or infection. If your Medical Symptoms Questionnaire (MSQ) score is greater than 40, toxin overload is likely a factor contributing to your health challenges. Go back to the detox chapter and think about what you might have been exposed to. People with high MSQ scores often have problems with toxin elimination; this is unfortunately quite common in people with any type of brain disorder, obesity, and/or diabetes. Another potential cause is excessive stress hormones due to unresolved conflicts and other stressors. Remember, those high cortisol levels derail the healing environment.

The most common problem I see in my patients when they aren't improving or are improving too slowly, however, is certainly compliance. What sometimes happens is that patients are excited and perfectly compliant at first. Over time, however, following the diet strictly may become difficult, especially if you are doing well and think that this gives you license to take it easier. You will be tempted to eat the foods you know are problems for you (cheat) as you feel better. You might also be tempted to eat those excluded (but oh so tasty) foods if you aren't feeling better and it seems like too much work or restraint for no payoff. In either case, the old familiar comfort foods that you eliminated when you started the diet may creep back in because you don't realize that the very reason you are doing so well is because you have been following the rules so carefully—or that the very reason you aren't doing well is because you have never really strictly followed the rules!

Sometimes people slide back into bad habits so gradually that they don't realize it. A little exception here, a little splurge there, and suddenly you're having so much fatigue that you can't get through the day. In the clinic, if the MSQ is slowly improving or under 20, we consider that a satisfactory score.

WAHLS DIARY ALERT

Keeping motivated is tough when temptation is all around you. To help you keep track of what you are actually doing, especially if you are not progressing as quickly as you would like, it is critical to record what you do every day, including what you are eating and whether you are meeting the goals for the Wahls Diet, Wahls Paleo, or Wahls Paleo Plus.

Writing down your dietary plan as well as your symptoms in your Wahls Diary will also help you keep it all organized as you keep track of the guidelines for the level of the diet you are currently on and your success in meeting those requirements. It can also be a great source of inspiration. See how far you've come when you're having a bad day by looking back at your initial Medical Symptoms Questionnaire or reading what you wrote about what you were eating, how you felt, and how much you were moving and doing on a day in the past. Your Wahls Diary is your support system here, so make the most out of it. If you aren't writing it all down, you are missing a tremendous opportunity.

But I should also tell you that the longer the person is on my program, the more likely he or she is to get the score all the way down to near zero! If the MSQ begins to rise or gets stuck and stops falling, we explore with the patient or study subject how well they are complying with the study diet and all of the "beyond food" parts of the protocol: stress reduction, sleep quality, toxic load, exercise, and the recommended supplements. Nearly always, our people with rising scores admit that they have been slacking off and allowing prohibited foods back into their diet. One woman thought that by eating twelve servings of vegetables each day, she could have pizza and ice cream with her friends on the weekly girls' night out. It would be wonderful if this trade-off worked, of course, but in her case, these little indulgences were sabotaging her progress. When she stopped the pizza and ice cream and went back to 100 percent compliance—gluten-free and dairy-free in this case—her energy markedly improved.

Others like me have experienced an immediate (within twenty-four hours) severe adverse symptom such as a sharp increase in pain, worsening vision, or motor weakness, if they slack on the protocol. Actually, I talk a lot about the gift of my face pain. When it turns on, it is still the most severe pain I have ever experienced—much worse than childbirth, broken bones, or the emergency C-section I had without anesthesia when my daughter was born. Still, I am grateful for its intensity. If I have gluten, dairy, or eggs, in six to twenty-four hours, the electrical zingers in my face begin. I cannot ignore them, so I am meticulous with the protocol, even while traveling on the plane with my cabbages in my suitcase.

If you have negative symptoms that come back in close proximity to deviations from the protocol, it is a huge gift because you are getting feedback. Your body is telling you that your cellular environment is no longer optimal. It is deranged, and it is calling to you for help. For this reason, I hope you have symptoms that call out to you if you stray from the protocol. Listen deeply to your body. Find the symptoms (feeling well and energetic) that tell you when your cells are working optimally, and the symptoms (pain, fatigue, sensory problems, cognitive problems) that tell you your cells are not working properly.

It is incredibly hard to stop eating the standard American diet for some future benefit. The food we eat has been designed (by the commercial food industry) to be addicting. But we can do it for acute symptom reduction. To sustain change, we will be much more successful if symptoms come back when we fall off the protocol to remind us that our cellular biochemistry is going berserk, that our bodies are becoming inflamed, that destructive inner processes are damaging you.

But in the absence of direct and immediate feedback? No, it is not easy to sustain change in our diet and lifestyle choices.

Our brains are wired to reinforce behaviors and food that stimulate dopamine. The more we engage in an activity, the more hardwired that activity becomes in our brain. Stopping those ingrained behaviors is quite challenging. Think of the individuals who are addicted to drugs of abuse, such as methamphetamine, cocaine, or nicotine. Or those who have become addicted to video games or gambling. It is a long process from the time people recognize they have a problem to the time when they decide they want help to the time when they learn how to re-create their lives without that addictive behavior or substance. It means removing that item and associated paraphernalia from their home, their work life, and their social life. They can't continue friendships that involved their addictive activities.

It is much the same when someone decides they need to stop eating sugar, gluten, and casein. These foods are highly pleasurable and addictive, and the cravings for them can be extremely challenging. Finding ways to socialize with friends and families while still keeping your environment free from the addictive compounds is important but difficult, especially at first. Making changes as a family is the best strategy for maximizing success. The more your extended family and friends also make the changes and/or fully support yours without leading you into temptation's way, the more likely you are to succeed.

Missteps are part of life. We learn from our errors and make adjustments. Each time you fail in your resolve, pick yourself back up and start again. Pay close attention to your environment. What do you need to do to make your environment more supportive for success? Do you need less exposure to certain things? Do you need more exposure to certain things? Keep tinkering to make your success easier to achieve—your new path is a great experiment, and experiments don't always go exactly right. They need recalibration; sometimes they require starting over. Keep tinkering to make failure more difficult and success more attainable. I am still learning, still tinkering, still adjusting my routine and my environment. I plan to be learning forever. Why would I ever want to stop when there is so much to learn? That means I will be adjusting my daily routine and my environment as I learn—for life. I hope you will commit to doing the same.

I spend a lot of time working with our patients to grow their internal motivation to take on the challenges of adopting and sustaining change. We ask the person to reflect on what exactly they are seeking better health in order to do. Next, we talk about Dr. Martin Seligman's work on positive psychology and the elements of the pleasant life, the good life, and the meaningful life. Which of these do you want? It's nice when things are pleasant, but it is better when they are good, and it is even better, with a ripple effect far into the future, when life is meaningful. We have people reflect on strategies they could use to achieve these various levels—the pleasant, good, and meaningful— that are consistent with their values and their family structure.

Then we discuss Joseph Campbell's work on myth and the hero's journey.

We discuss how the hero's journey relates to their struggle and their life experiences, and how they are the hero in their own journey. I ask them to tell me what they need to learn while on this healing journey. As they progress, we begin to talk about when they will feel ready to re-engage in their community and share their hard-earned insights.

I have come to learn that these exercises are very powerful for most individuals. Completing these steps gives people the insights that allow them to grow their internal motivation to take on doing the hard work of adopting and sustaining new health behaviors. It also gives them the grit to restart the work each time they falter, until the new behavior is a well-ingrained habit.

Sustaining change becomes much easier the more we understand why we pursue it and why these behaviors are so powerful. This is why I have given you so much information in this book—I want you to understand why these things work, to the extent that we all understand it (some of it is still a mystery). It is also easier the more effectively we have removed the harmful elements from our environment and the more available and convenient the helpful elements are in our environment. Sometimes it's just a matter of looking more closely at what you are (and are not) doing and how closely it aligns with your goals.

If you find it hard to stay 100 percent on your food plan or to keep moving every day or to fit in the self-care or stress-reducing activities, just remember, it's not about getting away with something. The Wahls Protocol exists to help you, not to restrict you. It is your ticket to a better life. Keeping that in mind, think about the last two weeks, and check any boxes that apply:

☐ Have any gluten grains crept back into your diet? Have you had gluten even once in the last two weeks? This can cause a major reaction in gluten-sensitive people.

☐ Do you read all the labels carefully to know the food items that are truly gluten-, casein-, and egg-free?

☐ Have you been eating sugar? Even natural sugars like raw sugar, honey, and real maple syrup will feed the bad bacteria and yeasts in your gut.

☐ Are you eating dairy? A little cheese here and there?

☐ Have you been eating eggs, since they are on "regular Paleo" and you thought they would be okay even though you might be sensitive to them?

☐ Are you really eating your 9 full cups of vegetables and fruits? If you are on Wahls Paleo Plus, are you getting at least 6 full cups of vegetables and fruits?

☐ Do you have inflammatory bowel disease or autoimmune issues involving joints such as rheumatoid arthritis? You will probably continue to be symptomatic until you adopt the Wahls Elimination Diet. It is harder, but probably necessary.

☐ Are your vegetables and fruits evenly distributed between leafy greens, sulfur-rich vegetables, and deeply colored vegetables and fruits, or are you eating a lot more colorful fruit than anything else?

☐ Are you getting enough animal protein? Remember, you need at least 6 ounces per day, and preferably closer to 12 ounces. On Wahls Paleo, you need 9 to 21 ounces.

☐ Are you eating mostly organic produce and organic wild-caught fish and/ or grass-fed meat? Are you using organic cleaning and personal care products? (Chemicals and other impurities in your food and other household products could be interfering with your recovery, even though you are getting sufficient nutrients.)

☐ Are you following all the rules for the dietary level you've chosen?

☐ Are you limiting cooking fats to only coconut oil and animal fat as prescribed?

☐ Are you eating enough fat? If you are on Wahls Paleo Plus, are you eating enough coconut oil and/or coconut milk or olive oil every day?

☐ Did you go off your medication prematurely? (You may be able to do this eventually, but you must not stop before you and your doctor determine you are ready. Review pages 317–322.)

☐ Have you been sedentary? Are you neglecting daily movement, exercising your heart, lungs, muscles, and joints?

☐ Did you have some success with e-stim but have stopped doing these sessions?

☐ Did you find a physical or occupational therapist or personal trainer to work with?

☐ Are you working to fully rehabilitate your motor strength, or at least to reduce the metabolic damage of inactivity? If you want to improve your motor function, you will be more successful working with a therapist who will incorporate e-stim or FES cycling into your physical training.

☐ Are you getting enough sleep? Can you take steps to get more?

☐ Are you beset with stress and not taking steps to manage it?

☐ Did you have an emotional setback and lapse into other bad habits because you were upset?

☐ Do you have unresolved issues with family, friends, or coworkers?

Nobody is perfect. We make mistakes and bad decisions. Sometimes we go off our diets or stop taking our medicines because we are hopeful that we are better and don't need to try so hard anymore. This kind of regular evaluation is incredibly useful and informative as you track your own progress and continue to take charge of your own health because you will have a record of when things aren't working. I encourage you to complete the MSQ once a month for a year and use the scores to monitor your progress. Whenever you see an upward tick in the score, you will know it's time to reexamine how well you are implementing the whole protocol.

If you began to see progress but then your progress stalled, it may be time to move up to the next dietary level. If you are on the Wahls Diet, consider advancing to Wahls Paleo. If that's not quite giving you the rapid results you want, it may be time to move up to Wahls Elimination. If you are still not where you want to be, it is time to consider Wahls Paleo Plus.

There are many aspects to pursuing health, many opportunities to succeed, and many risks for failure, but persistence is necessary. Even a little grit. You have suffered, and you have that grit somewhere inside you. Find your supportive people and press on. The changes are coming.

What a Functional Medicine Doctor Can Do for You

If you are following the Wahls Protocol carefully and you still aren't seeing the results you want to see, it may be time to consult a functional medicine doctor who can evaluate you in a highly individual way that a book could never do. A functional medicine doctor will approach your health from the broadest possible standpoint. As part of the initial evaluation, a functional medicine health care provider will likely have you complete several detailed questionnaires about your life's story, from the time you were in your mother's

THE BENEFITS OF A HEALTH COACH

Health coaching is a new burgeoning profession. For people who are interested in health and helping others but do not have the time, resources, or inclination to become a doctor or pursue an advanced degree, health coaching is a great option. Many of my Wahls Warriors have become health coaches after learning about the Wahls Protocol and advancing their knowledge through specialized training. But what I really want to say about health coaches is how beneficial it can be to hire one, especially when it comes to staying compliant with your Wahls Protocol. Health coaches have been trained in many aspects of health, including nutrition, and many are already aware of the Wahls Protocol. Some of them have even become certified in coaching the Wahls Protocol. These experienced professionals can help you stay on track, with weekly or even daily calls to help you stay focused and stay true to your goals. You can ask them questions when you aren't sure about something, and they can help you make a workable plan for your life. Best of all, they help you follow up and stay motivated. They check in with you to be sure you are keeping at it. They can be an excellent investment, especially if you find someone who clicks with you and understands your unique situation and goals for your health and life.

CALL TO ACTION

For a current list of health professionals who attended the Wahls Protocol Health Professional certification course, go to terrywahls.com /find-a-wahls-protocol-health-professional/. These professionals have many different types of qualifications—doctors, chiropractors, nurses, and more. Many of these professionals are health coaches who can work with you remotely.

uterus. (They may look similar to the MSQ in this book.) You will answer questions about the various infections, vaccinations, toxin exposures, and health issues that led to this point in your life.

After reviewing those forms, your doctor will ask more questions and then do a physical examination. The next step is to look at the various health problems that you have experienced and how those problems fit into the big picture of how your body works. There are seven big-picture physiologies a functional medicine doctor will consider:

1. Energy production (how well your mitochondria work)
2. Assimilation (how well you digest and absorb nutrients)
3. Defense and repair (how well and appropriately your immune cells are working and the health of your "old friends" living in your bowels, your nose, and your skin)
4. Biotransformation and elimination (how well you process and eliminate the harmful compounds that your cells encounter, including both the trash the cells make as they do the work of living and the toxic stuff we absorb through our skin, our lungs, and our gut)
5. Communication (how effectively your cells can communicate with one another through hormones, neurotransmitters, and other signaling molecules)
6. Structural integrity (the structural integrity of the tiny things like cell membranes as well as big things like muscles, ligaments, and bones)
7. Transport of fluids through the body (blood and lymph)

Your functional medicine doctor will also want to understand your personal health behaviors, which are the bedrock of health (or disease). These are the very things that you have been tuning up and optimizing as you implement the Wahls Protocol: (1) sleep and relaxation, (2) exercise and movement, (3) nutrition, (4) stress and resilience, and (5) relationships. Then the doctor will ask about your spiritual practices and your mental and emotional beliefs. They will also ask about the potential triggering events and health events that may be a factor in your health status. This could include things like major life events, antibiotic history, infections, water-damaged buildings, childhood trauma, or other traumas. These may be triggering events. When all of that is complete, the functional medicine health care provider will tell the story back to you of how your problems fit into the matrix, what the antecedent risk factors are (your genetic vulnerabilities), what your triggers are, and what is likely keeping your disease active. This will help your doctor explain where your various health problems fit in the seven physiologies and how your health behaviors are likely contributing positively or negatively to your current health. They will also talk about your resilience factors—your spiritual, mental, and emotional life—and how these are supporting or inhibiting your progress on your healing journey.

Once the matrix has been completed, then you and your functional medicine doctor will develop a plan to move forward together. If you are following the Wahls Protocol, you will already be doing many of the things functional medicine recommends, but this careful individual assessment can tell you much more about how you as a unique being can benefit from additional targeted guidance. Your doctor may order specialized testing and prescribe customized natural therapies for you that would not necessarily be appropriate for everyone. As you progress, your functional medicine doctor will also be there for you, helping you to adjust your plan based on your individual reactions to the lifestyle, vitamin and supplement usage, and other changes and prescriptions. For those tough cases that don't respond sufficiently to the Wahls Diet, this is your best plan for making faster progress.

Functional Medicine Tests to Consider

One of the benefits of visiting a functional medicine provider is that you will have access to certain kinds of tests that conventional medicine doesn't normally use. The types of testing that a functional medicine health care professional[2] can request and evaluate include the following:

Genetic Tests

Genetic testing is usually an ethical quagmire when it is used to predict if you might have a specific disease such as Huntington's disease or cystic fibrosis or the gene increasing the risk of developing breast cancer. That is not the type of testing I am discussing. There are also tests that can elucidate the efficiency of some of your enzymes that run your cell chemistry, particularly the ones involved in how you are able to utilize certain nutrients, eliminate toxins, and manufacture brain neurotransmitters. Once you understand which

enzymes are not optimal, you can use dietary choices, vitamins, and/or supplements to bypass the less effective enzymes and lower the risk for a variety
of health problems such as brain disorders, heart disorders, toxic overload,
and even cancer.

We are getting ever more sophisticated in our understanding of the
interplay between our genes and the genes of the "old friends" in our microbiomes. People can use genetic testing, such as 23andMe, to get their DNA
sequenced, and then run it through various other programs to receive guidance on how to optimize their cellular physiology through supplement and
food choices. Other labs can assess your microbiome and figure out how it
relates to your medical history and current symptoms. See the Resources section for more details on companies that provide this service, and page 349,
where I discuss these tests in more detail.

I have used genetic testing and microbiome testing to understand my risks
and condition more thoroughly. They do provide useful insights, especially if
you still do not feel as well tuned as you would like to be.

Keep in mind that genetic testing doesn't tell you everything. For example, it can tell you which enzymes are mutated, but it won't necessarily tell you
about function. You can, however, assume that mutated genes are probably
less effective (often but not always the case), and this may be helpful in understanding which vitamins and supplements can make up for this.

Toxin Load Assessment

For someone with an autoimmune problem who continues to struggle, understanding the body burden of toxins may be very useful. Often this is done
with a twenty-four-hour urine collection and a provocation agent to draw
toxins out of fat storage. Depending on the clinical circumstances, the test
may be for heavy metals, solvents, or pesticides. Often the person also has a
genetic vulnerability in his or her detoxification enzymes that exacerbates the
toxic effect. If the person is toxic, the next decision is whether to do a long,
slow detoxification based on food or to utilize a more rapid removal via chelation under the direct supervision of a physician trained and certified for managing chelation therapies.

WAHLS WARRIORS SPEAK

We have been following the Wahls Protocol for six weeks. My husband (57 years old) has been exhibiting Parkinson's symptoms and has been seeing a neurologist since July 2011. In just six weeks, his PD symptoms showed significant reversal, the most dramatic being the restoration of his balance and the return of his normal walking gait. His asthma was gone in one week, and we noticed improvements in his blood pressure, speech, sleep patterns, energy levels, and mood. We started to reintroduce foods at five weeks on the four-day rotation and found that sweet potatoes work fine, but dairy showed up within hours—general digestive upset, headache, slurred speech, and nasal/throat congestion/drip. Amazing! We will continue being grain-free, legume-free, and dairy-free and following the rest of the Wahls Diet until all symptoms are gone. Thank you, Dr. Wahls. This is very exciting!

—*Dorothy W., Philadelphia, Pennsylvania*

Nutritional Testing

It is possible to have a comprehensive assessment of your nutritional status in terms of your levels of vitamins, minerals, essential fats, and antioxidants, and to look at how efficiently your mitochondria can generate energy, how well your brain cells can make neurotransmitter molecules, how well you produce myelin, and more nutritional details. These types of tests are helpful in showing how well your own personal chemical factories are functioning and where the blocks (inefficient enzymes) are located. A functional medicine physician can then guide you to the foods, vitamins, and nutraceuticals (herbs) that can help unblock the ineffective biochemistry. This may be a good alternative to using genetic testing to identify which enzymes are not working as effectively. There are a variety of companies that provide these types of assessments.

As science continues to learn about how to evaluate big data and the shifts in our metabolites in the bloodstream, this type of nutritional testing will become increasingly affordable and likely increasingly helpful. I can envision a day when we are able to obtain a genetic analysis of our genes and our microbes' genes and a measurement of the precise chemicals in our bodily fluids and tissues. There are tens of thousands of different chemicals (metabolites) currently being assessed in scientific studies. Tests of these metabolites allow us to assess the metabolism of the mammal (that is us) and the metabolisms of our old friends (the microbes living in our body). These tools, which will become increasingly available, will allow for a very precise personalization of the diet, and will also include supplement and lifestyle recommendations to achieve optimal biochemistry for our cells, with the goal of maximizing the health of each individual. I am very excited about the future of this science—this is how we will really be able to drill down to the question of how effectively we are able to conduct the chemistry of life in our cells! See the Resources for a list of labs that currently offer nutritional testing.

Gut Health

You may need to have a comprehensive assessment of your gut function. The first level might be a DNA analysis of your stool, which would specify which bacteria, yeasts, and parasites are living in your gastrointestinal tract. Many

---

AUTOANTIBODY LEVELS TO DETECT THE PRODROMAL STATE

Are you in the prodromal state I talked about back on page 45—that state prior to diagnosis where your body is already making autoantibodies but you are not yet sick enough for a doctor to diagnose you? There are labs that can perform comprehensive autoantibody testing to see if you are. This is a terrific evaluation to obtain if you are having symptoms that no one can diagnose. If those autoantibodies are present, you now have biological markers and you can use your therapeutic diet and lifestyle interventions. You can then monitor your results and watch those autoantibody levels fall!

---

labs also do analyses for sensitivity to the common nutraceuticals and pharmaceutical agents in order to treat the troublemakers that may be contributing to your problems.

Other labs do cultures and microscopic examination to look for the yeasts, bacteria, and parasites. The key point is to find a lab with extensive experience, as most conventional physicians do not routinely have access to labs that are experienced with the evaluation of dysbiosis (microbial imbalance). This comprehensive gut health assessment will also look at digestion enzymes and acid production in the stomach. See the Resources section for labs that test your gut health and function.

Food Allergies and Sensitivities

If you need a lab test to convince yourself or your family member to give up gluten, dairy, or other potential foods that are creating trouble, then food allergy/sensitivity testing is money well spent. Since I could not get these tests in the VA, I needed to convince people to go gluten-/dairy-/egg-/soy-free for a month and assess how they did; but if you have access to food allergy tests and you want to go that route, ask your functional medicine doctor about the best ones for you.

However, you should know that these tests are controversial. Many conventional physicians do not agree that they are accurate or that they relate to any clinical signs of allergy, and it is true that there is limited scientific proof that they do.[3] Some papers do however report that food sensitivity testing may be helpful in identifying food triggers for symptoms,[4] and a good reason to do the tests is that it can be difficult to determine every sensitivity through an elimination diet. Many people have delayed reactions to foods. Although most reactions to food occur within seventy-two hours, occasionally the delayed reaction can be as long as seven to fourteen days. If you are still having trouble after adopting the Wahls Elimination or Wahls Paleo Plus Diet, it can be helpful for you to get a food allergy assessment of some type and eliminate the foods to which you are sensitive. They may be foods you never suspected. The best way to use this information is in conjunction with an elimination diet, such as the Wahls Elimination Diet in this book, so you can confirm whether eliminating the foods your test results suggest makes an actual difference in how you feel.

If you want to be evaluated for food allergies, sensitivies, or intolerances, your doctor may go about this in any of several ways. Each has its benefits and drawbacks:

- **Elimination diet.** The gold standard for understanding whether you have a food sensitivity or allergy is completing an elimination diet, in which you essentially go on a supervised fast and then, starting with the food least likely to be troublesome, reintroduce foods one at a time every other day (or sometimes every third day). During this time, you keep a detailed food symptom diary and monitor your pulse rate before and after eating each new food.⁵ Any food that evokes a jump in heart rate or a problem symptom such as pain or fatigue is put on the suspect list and removed from the diet for six months and then retested. This is difficult to do on your own and is most effective under the supervision of a nutritionist or functional medicine doctor because you will be less likely to cheat, which would completely skew the results. Also, fasting is not safe or recommended for everyone, which is another reason why medical supervision is important.
- **Modified elimination diet.** Another approach is to go on a diet that eliminates the most common allergenic or sensitizing foods: gluten, dairy, eggs, soy, corn, potatoes, tomatoes, eggplant, peppers, citrus, peanuts, shellfish, and fish. This is similar to the Wahls Elimination Diet I talk about starting on page 122. Ideally, you will also eat strictly organic foods to avoid genetically modified foods and toxins. After a specified period of time (eight weeks, a hundred days, or six months, for example), you test the eliminated foods one by one to look for reactions. The reactions can be headache, fatigue, abdominal complaints, rash, allergy symptoms, asthma, or acne. As you heal your gut and stop having a leaky gut, some sensitivities may diminish to the point where you could have the offending food once a week without a problem (but if you return to daily consumption, you are likely to develop problems with that food again). (For more specifics about how to do this yourself, go to page 123.)
- **Blood test.** One blood test option is the ALCAT (Antigen Leukocyte Cellular Antibody Test), marketed by Cell Science Systems. It is capable

of assessing delayed responses to 350 different foods. Another lab, NowLeap, does cellular immune response (innate immune response) testing. Yet another option is to measure blood levels of immunoglobulin IgG and/or IgA in response to various foods (adaptive immune response). Because 2 percent of the population does not make a normal amount of IgA, if you have a negative test, you should also check your IgA levels to be certain that you can make a normal amount of IgA before trusting that negative test. See the Resources section.

- There are more commercial labs that offer IgG testing to foods. Because each lab generates its own antigens for the test, there is variability between labs and variability with how reliable the tests are. Ideally, you can find a functional medicine doctor who can assist with finding a reliable lab for food sensitivity testing and guide you in interpreting your results.

- **Stool test.** You could get what I unceremoniously call the "poop test" for the most common food groups. This is more sensitive than the blood test because abnormal antibodies to foods are secreted in the stool sooner— sometimes years sooner—than they are detectable in the bloodstream. However, this test detects fewer food items. You can get your own stool test from EnteroLab without a doctor's order, but insurance won't cover it. Another advantage of stool testing is that EnteroLab will do genetic testing to see if you have the genes that put you at risk for developing gluten sensitivity, and they can also test for sensitivity to dairy, *Saccharomyces cerevisiae* (baker's yeast), eggs, soy, and nightshade vegetables (potatoes, tomatoes, eggplant, and peppers). The stool test is also less likely to give a false negative. (Note that *Saccharomyces cerevisiae*, such as the kind in kombucha, and *Saccharomyces boulardii*, the kind in probiotics, compete with *Candida albicans* and can be very helpful at reducing and controlling symptoms related to *Candida* overgrowth. However, although it's rare, some individuals, most often those with Crohn's disease or SLE, will react to *Saccharomyces cerevisiae*.)

WAHLS WARNING

Many people ask me about gluten sensitivity testing and are surprised to learn that I do not recommend getting a blood test for gluten sensitivity through your primary care doctor's office. A negative test does not rule out gluten sensitivity, and even though your doctor will likely tell you that you can eat gluten, you actually should not. The test is not worth the money spent and could even slow down your healing. I have had many people with a negative blood test for gluten sensitivity experience remarkable improvements to their health after going gluten-free.

Infections

We are used to thinking of an infection as an acute illness caused by a virus, bacteria, fungus, or parasite. Our immune cells begin attacking the infecting agent and a war ensues. If we win, our immune cells clear out the infection and we return to good health. If we lose the war completely, we die.

There is also, however, a middle ground. When our immune cells are unable to clear the infection completely, it may continue to smolder. For example, people who have irritated gums (when they brush their teeth vigorously, their gums bleed) have a low-level infection of their gum tissue that can increase inflammation and the probability of developing an autoimmune disease, heart disease, stroke, diabetes, and other chronic diseases.[6] As vitality declines, we are more likely to be infected with something else. If we don't have the proper nutrition for our immune cells or we have too many toxins impairing the immune cells, we have troublemakers living in our bowels, our hormone signals are confused, and our white blood cells are less capable. As a result of any of those factors, our immune cells are less effective at clearing the infection. Furthermore, once a person's immune system is weakened by having one of these chronic infections (or overgrowths in the bowels), he or she is more susceptible to having a coinfection with a second organism or more.[7]

If you are still struggling with fatigue and brain symptoms, it may be very helpful to have a comprehensive assessment to test for these types of chronic infections or coinfections, especially if the Wahls Protocol is not resolving issues like chronic fatigue or symptoms of MS, ALS, Alzheimer's disease, or Lyme disease. These could be due to a viral infection (such as Epstein-Barr, herpes 6 virus, or herpes simplex) or a bacterial infection (such as *Borrelia burgdorferi*—Lyme disease—chlamydia, and *Bartonella*).[8] A functional medicine doctor can evaluate you for the possibility of these indolent (painless, asymptomatic) chronic infections. If you do have an infection or coinfection with several organisms, a functional medicine doctor may treat you with nutraceuticals, pharmaceuticals, or a combination of both, depending on the type of infection and your individual health situation. Some protocols require years of treatments and ongoing support to clear and stay clear of chronic infections, particularly if there are multiple infecting agents, so finding someone who has considerable experience evaluating and treating chronic infections will be essential. Your healthy immune cells are the most potent antibiotic. Thus I strongly favor intensive support of your cellular health and a long-term look at how to nurture a healthier microbiome. I prefer to minimize pharmaceutical long-term use of antimicrobials, although there are times when antimicrobials do become necessary.

Hormonal Balance

Hormones are the molecules that our cells use to communicate and regulate how the other cells in the body will function. They instruct other cells to work harder and faster or when it's time to relax and slow down. When the hormones are finely tuned, your body works like a beautiful symphony; but when the hormones get out of balance, health declines.

Classic signs of hormonal imbalance include fatigue, foggy thinking, and irritability. Immune cells become less effective when hormones are imbalanced, and you may become more vulnerable to both infection and cancer. People with hormonal imbalance may also be much more likely to develop an autoimmune problem.

Scientists continue to discover that our bodies have multiple layers of hormone communication that provides many layers of feedback to help keep the potassium, sodium, calcium, magnesium, and other minerals in the correct concentration in our bloodstreams and in our cells. Hormones also regulate your hunger, thirst, and sleep. Maintaining an optimal hormone balance means providing your hormone-secreting glands (pituitary, adrenal, thyroid, ovaries, and testes in particular) with support so that each gland has a healthy reserve.

The Wahls Protocol should accomplish this for most people, but if you are still having trouble, you may need a more comprehensive assessment of the interplay between your adrenals, thyroid, pituitary, and sex hormones to understand and correct persisting hormone imbalances. Consult a functional medicine or an American Academy of Anti-Aging Medicine (A4M) doctor who has experience in hormonal balance for more advanced hormonal testing and a more natural but specifically targeted program of nutrients, supplements, and medications, if necessary, to address your issue. A functional medicine doctor will view your hormonal imbalance based on the big picture of your physiologies and personal health behaviors, so your treatment will be more comprehensive and individualized.

These are the primary tests that could be done in a functional medicine clinic. They are generally not covered by health care insurance, often because they are not yet FDA-approved. The tests can cost many hundreds to many thousands of dollars if you investigate every potential imbalance, so your functional medicine doctor will likely recommend only the tests that are indicated based on your functional medicine matrix and then help you prioritize which ones to obtain first.

These tests can be useful and meaningful, but in many cases, they are not essential. In my clinical practice at the VA, I relied on careful history and laboratory evaluations that I could obtain through my conventional pathology departments. We then focused on maximizing all the health-promoting behaviors of the Wahls Protocol. I referred those who want to pursue the comprehensive testing I discuss here to another functional medicine provider in the community to complete the testing. I saw terrific results without advanced testing, but at times it may be very helpful when the person is not responding despite full implementation of the Wahls Protocol.

Now that I have a private practice, I am able to offer more detailed comprehensive assessments that allow me to provide more specific guidance. However, obtaining the most basic tests from primary care providers, implementing the Wahls Protocol, and working closely with your personal physician/medical team will improve the environment for your cells. As your cellular environment improves, your health will improve. I saw terrific results in my patients at the VA without doing comprehensive advanced testing. Thousands of our patients and followers report similar success working with their primary care team, using basic primary care labs outlined in this book. Work with your doctor to implement and follow the Wahls Protocol using the primary care labs I discussed earlier. If you do not achieve the level of recovery you hoped for, then do seek out someone who can do these more advanced investigations and provide you with more personalized recommendations.

Finding a Functional Medicine Practitioner

Many functional medicine and anti-aging restorative medicine practitioners come from the ranks of conventionally trained medical professionals: medical doctors (MDs), osteopathic doctors (DOs), advanced registered nurse practitioners (ARNPs), physician assistants (PAs) and nutritionists and registered dietitians (RDs), and more. To find a functional medicine practitioner near you, go to the Institute for Functional Medicine website at functionalmedicine.org and click on "Functional Medicine Resources." Then click on "Find a Functional Medicine Practitioner." You will then be able to enter your address and how far you are willing to travel. You will be presented a list of individuals who have completed the training course called "Applying Functional Medicine in Clinical Practice." The Institute for Functional Medicine has a certification program for those individuals who have completed additional training and have successfully passed an examination. The individuals who pass the certification process will be Institute for Functional Medicine Certified Practitioners, with the designation of IFMCP.

Or, go to the American Academy of Anti-Aging Medicine website to look for their pratitioners (a4m.com). They have a directory and membership information where you can seek practitioners in your area. A4M has fellowship programs for additional training in metabolic and functional medicine, integrative cancer therapy, and stem cell therapy. I am on the faculty for both IFM and A4M, and am impressed with the training provided by both organizations. Ideally, you can find a practitioner who has gone through and received certification by IFM or fellowship training for A4M, so that you can be confident that your health care provider is familiar with the latest research on how to create the most healing environment for your cells.

Once you have some names, visit a few (if you have more than one option). Ask some questions so you can get to know the practitioner and whether you will feel comfortable working with her or him. Some questions to ask:

1. Where and when did you get your training in functional medicine or anti-aging and restorative medicine?
2. What percentage of your practice is functional medicine or anti-aging medicine?
3. Do you assess and treat problems related to high body burden of toxins, food allergies, gut microbiome problems, and parasites?
4. Do you take medical insurance? (Note: Most of the providers do not take medical insurance because it would not cover all of the time involved. The assessments and evaluations are expensive and time-consuming, and some providers may choose not to do much testing, preferring to focus on a careful history, physical examination, and lifestyle intervention.)

If you cannot find someone close to you who is in the Institute for Functional Medicine or anti-aging and restorative medicine databases, you can still look for health care providers with an integrative medicine background or interest. Talk to the provider about the issues of toxic load, food allergy and sensitivity, the microbiome (who is living in your bowels), digestion and assimilation issues, and hormone issues to see if the practitioner is trained and has a good knowledge base in those areas. Naturopathic doctors (NDs) and doctors of chiropractic (DCs) are often more focused on using nutrition than MDs or DOs. In fact, they receive more training in nutrition than most medical doctors and can do these types of comprehensive evaluations and know how to treat with food and nutraceuticals. They are definitely health care providers to consider.

If you still can't find anyone, work with your primary care physician/medical team as you adopt the Wahls Protocol. Many primary care physicians are more open-minded to the power of diet and lifestyle interventions than the subspecialists and are willing to learn about different approaches to healing, especially for chronic issues like autoimmune disease that aren't responding to conventional treatment. The best doctors rely on a good history, a thorough physical exam, and basic lab tests. Some are more than willing to learn something new. Others are not. If you can, help lead your primary care doctor to do just that. If you can't, perhaps there is a better doctor for you out there. Only you can make that call, of course.

This is the Wahls Protocol, in all its simplicity and complexity. Now it's your turn to make it what you want it to be. You can simply adopt the Wahls Diet. You can go all the way to Wahls Elimination or Wahls Paleo Plus. You can integrate an exercise program, cleansing techniques, supplements, alternative medicine, stress management, and of course the Wahls Diary. You may or may not take on the services of an official functional medicine practitioner, but the bottom line is this: *You* are now in charge of your own health. Your future, your progress—even your happiness—is up to you. Your destiny is in your hands, and that is a wonderful and powerful thing to know. I hope you will make the most of it. Your future can be filled with health, hope, vitality, and connection. I've given you the tools. Now it's up to you to use them.

EPILOGUE
The End of My Story,
The Beginning of Yours

Y OU KNOW MY story of decline. You know I got out of my wheelchair. Now I'd like to finish that story.

When my body began to heal, I didn't fully understand what was happening at first. In spite of the changes occurring with amazing speed, I still did not consider that I might recover. I had accepted for years that people with secondary progressive MS did not improve. It did not occur to me that the improvements I was experiencing could continue. It was not until nearly six months after my symptoms began to reverse that I first dared to wonder if recovery might be possible.

I began to dream of biking again. On Mother's Day weekend in 2008, I was feeling so much better and my mobility had improved to such a great degree that I decided to try riding a bike. I went to the garage, picked up a helmet, and walked to my bike. Five years earlier, when I got the wheelchair, I'd given my bike to my son, Zach. Now I wondered if I was ready to take it back. I adjusted the seat downward, clicked on my helmet, and began rolling the bike out.

My kids heard me in the garage and came to investigate. Zach grabbed the bike from me and called out for Jackie to stop me. We all looked at one another. I told Jackie that if she thought I wasn't ready, I wouldn't attempt it. She responded by getting out her bike helmet and bike and told Zach and Zebby to jog alongside me.

We all got into position. Jackie gave the all clear that there was no traffic. I pushed off. The bike wobbled, but I did not fall. My kids cheered as they ran behind me. Tears streamed down my cheeks as Jackie and I pedaled around the block. When I stopped, Zach, Zebby, Jackie, and I all stood together, holding one another and crying. I had a new future ahead. I had proof: I had ridden my bicycle. My steady decline was not the rule, not anymore. I was rewriting my future and who knew what it might become! I still have tears in my eyes when I tell that story. I am still crying as I read this again while I proofread this revised edition. I will every time. This story is and always will be miraculous to me.

Doctors and scientists don't often believe in miracles. My getting up from that chair wasn't really a miracle from a scientific perspective, even though it felt like one to me at the time. My getting out of the chair and onto a bicycle was just the facts related to my body's ability to regain strength and health. We may not fully understand all the facts, but it's science that my team is working hard to reveal. This is the basis of the clinical trials we've undertaken in order to understand the mechanisms of why the Wahls Protocol is effective and who can best be helped by it.

As the basic science has advanced, we now have a deeper understanding of how our food choices influence our health. The evidence continues to grow that the composition of our microbiome influences the risk of MS and severity of disease.[1] The microbiome influences the level of inflammation in the body and in the brain, and the production of neurotransmitters in the brain and its periphery. The food choices we make each day are the strongest drivers of what microbes live in our guts. The exercise choices, stress reduction choices, toxin exposures—in short, all of our environmental exposures—also speak to our genes, influencing which genes are turned on and which are turned off. This information is becoming mainstream—the world is catching up to the idea that diet and lifestyle matter a great deal to our health, and the proof is rolling in.

New ideas always meet with both skepticism and enthusiasm from scientific colleagues. Our work is no different. We have our champions and our detractors. But we will keep doing our work, submitting our papers, applying for grants, and raising money through the Wahls Research Fund, which is managed by the University of Iowa. Philanthropic support that allows us to collect pilot data for these studies is crucial, allowing us to make grant proposals much stronger. We have already received generous support and hope to secure more so that we can build on these proposals, generate pilot data, and submit more competitive grants to the National MS Society and the National Institutes of Health. Please contact my team (giving@foriowa.org) at the University of Iowa Center for Advancement to learn more about the research proposals we are doing to continue and expand our work. If you'd like to become a member of the team and donate to the Wahls Research Fund, please see the Appendix for more details on how to support our research team.

Money is incredibly hard to get for research, with less than 2 percent of applications being funded now. Researchers must show preliminary data with grant applications to have any hope of getting their grants funded. Having philanthropic support has allowed us to collect additional data that we use for grant proposals. The generous support has allowed us to collect additional biospecimens (blood, stool, diet quality data).

I am very optimistic about the future. I see the public more and more interested in using diet and lifestyle choices to create more health for themselves and their families. I see more funding for dietary and lifestyle research, and more papers about diet and lifestyle interventions for wellness.

In the summer of 2007, I thought I knew what my future held: worsening disability, and a life in which I would eventually become bedridden, demented, and riddled with intractable pain. But I kept going on, doing the best I could because my children were watching. My Jackie was by my side, whispering that we would get through this together. And on that journey, I discovered ancestral health principles, paleo principles, functional medicine, and now anti-aging medicine. I have found my way back to biking, hiking, and a full and vital life. And I have found a new purpose: creating an epidemic of health.

It is an exciting time. I have to meditate each night, to quiet the mind so I can sleep. I am just so thrilled by how far we have come, and how rapidly the scientific community is validating the power of diet and lifestyle to favorably influence disease risk and disease activity. The public is more and more interested in therapeutic diet and lifestyle for their wellness programs. My scientific and clinical peers are inviting me to teach them about our clinical experience and our research all around the world.

I cannot wait for all my conventional medicine colleagues to catch up, and neither should you. Yes, I will continue to do the research to deepen my understanding and to publish those findings in peer-reviewed scientific journals. I will continue to lecture around the world to integrative, functional, and anti-aging clinicians and research scientists. I will also continue to teach people directly, because nobody should have to wait for information like this. You can join our membership site to get access to my recent lectures, ask questions, and use the tools we provide to make adopting and sustaining the Wahls Protocol easier. The premium membership includes menus with recipes and shopping lists for a year. The membership site also has current lectures and methods for submitting topics you are concerned about and for asking questions. We also have live events—the Wahls Protocol Seminars— and you can attend to experience a community of hundreds of other Wahls Warriors on a similar journey. You can learn the latest research, participate in our group functional medicine assessment, and identify your key health events and the most useful interventions. You can practice skills, make new friendships, and discover your why, as well as a community that will support you in your healing journey. Just go to terrywahls.com and look under the Resources link.

Scientific inquiry is a long and complex process, often taking twenty to thirty years for proven successful treatments to become accepted clinical practice or the standard of care. I could have waited for randomized double-blind studies before talking to the public. But that seemed immoral to me. I needed to tell the public and let the public decide for themselves what to do.

What will you do? Will you wait for more clinical trials? Or do you want to begin turning your health around *today* using the commonsense things under your control, like the food you eat and what you choose to do every day? I choose to let the public decide. The public can choose whether to take back their own health by learning how to adopt the many wonderful health behaviors embedded within the Wahls Protocol. Let the public decide whether the

Wahls Protocol works for them and their loved ones. I don't want you to have to wait for FDA approval to try the low-risk but powerful interventions described in the Wahls Protocol.

I acknowledge that not everyone is helped in my clinics or in my trials. Not everybody will be able to adopt all of the Wahls Protocol, and not everyone will be able to get up from the chair. But what if you could? What if you will? The Wahls Protocol has already worked to reverse debilitating health symptoms in thousands of people—millions, if you count the lives touched by the TEDx talk. Why shouldn't you be one of them?

Everybody can maximize their own functioning. One person's best may be quite different from another person's best, but you can be *your* best. It may be that you have a condition that is associated with steady progressive decline such as Alzheimer's disease and Parkinson's disease; I recommend you look for someone who can assist with a functional medicine approach to your health. We have had people with cognitive decline and Parkinson's disease improve their memory and function using the Wahls Protocol. We have observed improvements in memory and in motor function as people have implemented the protocol. We have even had some individuals with ALS use the protocol and report back that their function has stabilized and they are still able to play golf three years into their illness.

Whatever your chronic disease, I recommend you consider the concepts in this book. The Wahls Protocol may not be able to make you fully well, but by following it, you can have the best function that is possible for you. We're learning new things every day about the body and disease, but what I do know is this. When you align yourself with what nature intends for you, remove impediments to your biochemical functioning, and restore what your mitochondria and cells are missing, you can maximize your biochemical health at the cellular level to optimize your life, whatever your health challenge. The Wahls Protocol gave me my life back. Give it the chance to restore yours.

WAHLS RECIPES

Adopting any of the Wahls Diet plans is a challenge. Reducing and/or eliminating grain and dairy means we have to reimagine our breakfasts without the cereals, pancakes, breads, and eggs typical of the standard American breakfast. I recommend that you start the day with a smoothie that provides some of the 9 cups of vegetables and fruit and high-quality protein. The following section provides guidance on creating smoothies for your household. Experiment with flavors.

Basic Smoothie

You can use anything that qualifies for your 9 cups in a smoothie, especially greens. To begin with, most of us need the sweetness of fruit to mask the bitterness of greens. Soy, almond, or coconut milk will also mellow the flavor nicely. Boxed milks often have extra calcium added, which is helpful, since by decreasing dairy you are lowering your intake of that essential nutrient. Always check the nutrition label to verify.

The ratio I recommend starting with is:

- 1 part greens
- 2 parts fruit or 2 cups organic soy milk (Wahls Diet only), coconut milk, or other nut milk, preferably unsweetened

❖ Add water and ice and combine in a high-speed blender until desired consistency.

There are endless smoothie combinations: combine kale, collard greens, romaine lettuce, beet greens, or cilantro with blueberries, strawberries, grapes, peeled orange segments, pineapple, and mango as well as other vegetables like broccoli or cucumber. Beets yield a brilliant magenta smoothie. As you get more used to the taste of green smoothies, you can gradually shift your ratio until you get greens and fruits in an approximately 1:1 ratio or switch to greens only and an approved nondairy milk. You can also add greater proportions of coconut milk. Having fat with your greens reduces bitterness and also lowers the glycemic index of the fruit in your smoothie. I personally always use full-fat coconut milk in a can to make smoothies and soups and to add to my teas.

You can also add a few unexpected nutrient boosts to your smoothies. Spices such as cinnamon, cardamom, ginger, or nutmeg can also cut the bitterness and add more nutritional benefits. I like to add 1 to 2 tablespoons of nutritional yeast, because it is a powerhouse of B vitamins, minerals, and RNA. Great stuff! Use nutritional yeast whenever you can in your smoothies or sprinkled on top of your vegetables. You'll get a lot of wonderful nutrition. The yeast in nutritional yeast is *Saccharomyces cerevisiae* that has been killed. Still, the inactive *Saccharomyces cerevisiae* is believed to suppress the harmful *Candida albicans* that can overgrow with a high-carb diet. Occasionally, some people have headaches with the nutritional yeast. If it bothers you in any way, omit it.

My breakfast protein sources are usually leftover meat from the previous night's dinner, liver pâté, or pickled herring. That way my breakfasts are fast and easy. When I was still eating three meals a day, my lunch was essentially a repeat of breakfast. I took a thermos with some of my morning smoothie in it and leftovers from the night before. Again, quick and simple.

Parsley (or Lovage) Green Grape Smoothie

SERVES 1

THIS IS A terrific way to get children excited about green smoothies. Parsley and green grapes pair particularly well. Lovage, which is a perennial parsley-like green that we grow in our garden, is easy to grow, and will grow to about 5 feet tall, unless you are picking the greens (which we do!). It is a very inexpensive way to have plenty of greens for your smoothies. The carotenoids (antioxidants) in the greens are more readily absorbed with oil. If you do not have parsley or lovage on hand, you can experiment with other greens. I use a mixture of green herbs that are growing in my garden such as lemon balm, oregano, basil, rosemary, or savory. If I use a more bitter green such as dandelion greens, I double the green grapes. The level of bitterness is a reflection of an elevated pH or alkalinity. Adding lemon juice lowers the pH and can reduce this bitterness. Freeze any extra green grapes you have on hand for future smoothies.

> *1 bunch parsley or lovage (leaves and stems), or approximately*
> *2 cups*
> *1 cup green grapes (fresh or frozen)*
> *1 cup ice*
> *1 cup water*
> *1 tablespoon olive, hemp, or flax oil*
> *Lemon juice (optional)*

FRESH HERBS

I grow fresh herbs in my garden, so during the spring, summer, and fall, I can harvest fresh herbs almost daily. I mince them either by hand or in my food processor. I place the fresh herbs on the table and we add them liberally to our meals. The addition of fresh herbs adds a wonderful zest to salads. You can stir the fresh herbs into an olive oil/flax oil combination to make a delicious sauce to drizzle over your cooked vegetables and meats. Store-bought salad dressings are usually made with lower-quality oils and a wide variety of food additives that are harmful to your microbiome, and they often include excitotoxins. Instead, use fresh garden herbs, your own high-quality olive, flax, or hemp oil, and lemon juice, lime juice, or vinegar to make your own fresh salad dressing. Herbs that I grow in my garden include parsley, cilantro, thyme, oregano, basil, rosemary, sage, lemon balm, dill, and tarragon. Herbs are also easy to grow in a pot on your deck and are an excellent way to begin growing just a bit of your own food.

❖ Chop the parsley or lovage leaves and stems coarsely and place into the blender. Add the green grapes, ice, water, and oil, and pulse. Add more water or ice to achieve the desired texture.

Mitochondria Support Smoothie

SERVES 1

REMEMBER FRESHMAN BIOLOGY class where you learned about mitochondria? You may recall they look like small ovals with a lot of squiggly lines inside. All those lines are the membranes inside and outside the mitochondrion, which hold the proteins that do the work of making the ATP (energy). All those membranes are composed of fat. To keep your mitochondrial membranes healthy and young, you need a lot of phosphatidylcholine (PC), along with omega-6 and omega-3 fats. This smoothie is PC-rich, so it is great for increasing the vitality of your mitochondria. PC isn't the best-tasting substance in the world, but the cocoa masks the taste, and the cinnamon and ginger cut the bitterness of the cocoa. If you have never taken PC before, start with 1 teaspoon to 1 tablespoon of PC and gradually work your way up to the desired amount. In my clinics, I occasionally have people take up to 4 tablespoons per day. Another bonus: The inulin feeds the butyrate-producing bacteria in your microbiome that promote a healthier mix of microbes. This is also the base recipe for the Mitochondria Support Pudding in the dessert section of this chapter (page 462).

SEE THE RESOURCES for the best sources of PC. The PC supplement is expensive, but it is an excellent anti-aging, mitochondria boosting, and brain repair ingredient.

2 cups water
1 teaspoon to 1 tablespoon PC (or up to 2 tablespoons as you adjust to it)
1 tablespoon organic hemp oil
¼ to ½ teaspoon organic extra virgin cod-liver oil
½ to 1 cup fresh or frozen berries (optional)

1 to 3 tablespoons inulin powder

1 to 2 tablespoons organic cocoa powder

1 tablespoon ground cinnamon

¼ to ½ inch coarsely chopped or sliced gingerroot (optional)

1 teaspoon powdered lion's mane mushroom (optional)

1 teaspoon powdered medicinal mushroom (e.g., turkey tail, reishi, chaga, or other medicinal mushroom blend)

1 teaspoon matcha green tea powder (organic)

❖ Blend the water, PC, hemp oil, and cod-liver oil in a high-speed blender for 1 to 3 minutes (it should look like cream). Add the remaining ingredients and blend on high until everything looks thoroughly combined.

Note:

Don't skip the long blending time for the water and oils. This is required to make liposomes, which are a form of fat more easily absorbed into the bloodstream and brain. You can have this twice a day, for up to 4 tablespoons of PC per day.

SNACKS/APPETIZERS

Bacon-Wrapped Dates

THIS HAS BECOME a family favorite treat for special occasions, and you can use pork, lamb, or turkey bacon. If I have liver pâté and/or almonds on hand, I stuff those into the dates (a teaspoon of pâté and/or a single whole raw almond) to make an even more spectacular treat.

12 thick slices of bacon (gluten-free, nitrate-free)

24 pitted dates

Almonds (optional)

Liver pâté (optional)

❖ Preheat oven to 400°F. Cut the bacon slices into half. Wrap half a bacon slice around one date. Hold in place with a toothpick. Place on a brownie sheet or broiler pan. Continue until all of the dates are wrapped in bacon. Bake for 4 to 5 minutes. Then flip the dates and bake another 4 to 5 minutes. Serve at room temperature. (You can also add almonds and a small amount of liver pâté inside the pitted date before baking.)

Bacon-Wrapped Lamb Liver

MY DAUGHTER, ZEBBY, makes this as appetizer for a fancy meal. She'll add avocado slices or guacamole and hot sauce as a dipping sauce. It has been a hit with all of our friends.

> *1 pound lamb liver*
> *12 thick slices of bacon (gluten-free, nitrate-free)*
> *Guacamole (optional, homemade or store-bought without*
> *   additives—if on Wahls Elimination. watch for the addition of*
> *   tomatoes to the guacamole)*
> *Hot sauce (optional)*
> *Horseradish sauce (optional)*

❖ Cut the lamb liver into 1-by-2-inch rectangular blocks. Cut the bacon slices in half. Wrap a bacon slice around each lamb liver chunk. Hold in place with a toothpick. Place on a brownie sheet or broiler pan. Continue until all of the liver chunks are wrapped in bacon. Bake at 400°F for 4 to 5 minutes and then flip. Alternatively, we have also used a broiler. Watch closely so you don't overcook the liver.

❖ Serve with guacamole as a dipping sauce or an avocado slice. This also pairs nicely with a hot pepper sauce as a dipping sauce. If you are following an elimination diet, you could use a horseradish sauce as a dipping sauce instead of hot pepper dipping sauce.

Cauliflower Dip

IF YOU HAVE decided to do an elimination diet that includes no legumes, this is a delicious alternative to hummus.

2 heads garlic
1 head cauliflower
½ cup olive oil
¼ cup nutritional yeast
2 tablespoons lemon juice
½ teaspoon sea salt

❖ Preheat the oven to 350°F. Cut off the head of the garlic to expose the top of all the garlic cloves. Cut up the cauliflower into 2-inch pieces (include the core and outer leaves). Place the garlic and cauliflower pieces on a baking sheet and roast them in the oven until slightly browned, approximately 30 minutes. Place the cauliflower, garlic, olive oil, nutritional yeast, lemon juice, and sea salt in a food processor and pulse until a thick puree forms. Add additional olive oil if needed to achieve the desired texture.

NUTRITIONAL YEAST

I like to keep a jar of nutritional yeast handy. I have a bowl of it on the table, too, as a condiment for meals (so much better than a sugar bowl!). Nutritional yeast is a powerful source of B vitamins and minerals. In addition to nutritional yeast, brewer's yeast (they are both strains of *Saccharomyces cerevisiae*) can reduce symptoms related to *Candida* overgrowth. I use them both liberally—they provide a delicious cheesy flavor without the negative effects of dairy cheese, and excellent nutrition. My goal is to have one to two tablespoons per day.

SKILLET MEALS

In the evening, after both Jackie and I have worked all day, we usually have a skillet meal for dinner. I'm typically the chef in our house, and when I get home, I prefer to be able to eat within twenty minutes of starting to cook. If it takes more than twenty minutes to make something, it is much less likely that I'll have that dish often. Skillet meals fit the bill: simple dishes with animal protein, lots of vegetables, and savory spices. These meals are prepared in a skillet on the stove and are generally ready in less time than it takes to cook a frozen pizza. Using my family's big skillet, I add coconut oil and some wine or vinegar. Then I sauté onions or mushrooms and add meat. Since I tend to like my meat rarer than the rest of my family, I put my piece in three to four minutes after the others. Two minutes before all the meat is finished cooking, I add other vegetables, and that's it. I can usually have the meal done within fifteen minutes from the time I start, and I serve the meal from the skillet. Because the meals are prepared and served in a single skillet, there are fewer dishes in the cleanup.

Before I give you the basic directions, here are a few general things to keep in mind:

- Grass-raised and grass-finished means an animal was fed grass until slaughter. This should be your first choice. Grass-raised, grain-finished means the animal was fed grain during the last six weeks of its life, which skews the ratio of omega-6s to omega-3s unfavorably but is still preferable to conventionally raised meat.
- Farm-raised fish means grain-fed fish, which leads to a much higher omega-6 fatty acid level than found in wild fish. Look for wild-caught fish.
- Garlic and other members of the onion and cabbage families all contain sulfur. This sulfur stabilizes in the crushing and cutting of the vegetable. Therefore, if you are cooking with these vegetables, crush, mince, and/or chop them and then allow them to sit for five to fifteen minutes prior to cooking. You'll lose less of the sulfur-rich antioxidants as you cook the food.
- Seaweed: Remember that ¼ teaspoon powdered kelp equals 1 teaspoon dulse flakes. You can use them interchangeably in the recipes, and I

encourage using a variety of seaweeds for maximal health benefits. Alternating between kelp and dulse is superior to using the same seaweed each day. *Remember that it is important to introduce seaweed and algae into your diet gradually.* If you eat too much of these too suddenly, it can cause problems with your thyroid. Follow your tastes and gradually increase the amount. When you are accustomed to it, have up to 1 serving per day. The amounts listed are optional and you can always leave seaweed out of any recipe if you choose, but do try to have it at least a few times per week, as recommended at the Wahls Paleo level. I recommend adding seaweed because collards—and all cabbage family vegetables—compete slightly with the iodine uptake in your immune cells and all of your endocrine glands, including the thyroid.

- Vinegars: I like balsamic vinegar. It does have more sugar, but it also has more antioxidants and flavonoids than other vinegars. Other vinegars I particularly like are unpasteurized, unfiltered apple cider vinegar with the "mother" or SCOBY. (SCOBY stands for symbiotic colony of bacteria and yeast—these are terms referring to the bacterial colony that transforms fermented alcohol into acetic acid to make vinegar.) Also try wine vinegar, rice vinegar, and coconut vinegar. Feel free to experiment with other vinegars. You can also substitute citrus juice for vinegar in any recipe.
- Sea salt has trace minerals but does not contain iodine. Be sure you are cooking with plenty of seaweed if you use sea salt. I use iodized sea salt for the iodine boost.
- Black pepper and other spices support cellular health; use spices and experiment with new ones.
- Cook at lower temperature for more nutrition. Mix water, vinegar, or wine with cooking fat to keep the temperature lower as you cook on the stove.

Do feel comfortable modifying these recipes by adjusting seasonings to taste and using the meats and vegetables that are available in your community and beloved in your culture. It is far better to use your local greens than kale or mustard greens that have been shipped in. Rotate through the varieties available to you and try new combinations. The magic is in eating fresh, in season, and local. As my mother said, recipes are only suggestions. These are my suggestions for easy meals.

Basic Meat and Greens
Skillet Recipe

SERVES 4

THE BASIC PRINCIPLE of this versatile recipe is to cook meat in a skillet with coconut oil, vinegar, and spices, then to add greens in the last 2 minutes of cooking. I chop chard, mustard greens, spinach, and most other varieties of greens but usually add kale whole because kale leaves are delightful to slice with your steak knife as you go. Experiment with the types of animal protein, cuts of meat, and seasonings you use, and remember to rotate through different greens to maximize the health benefits. If you feel the greens are bitter, add up to 2 tablespoons of vinegar, lime juice, or lemon juice. The bitterness is the alkalinity of the food, so a bit of acidic liquid will often mellow that out.

ANY VARIETY OF meat and greens will work well together using this recipe. Zebby is particularly fond of salmon and cooked greens, while Zach really likes steak and has come to enjoy his nearly as rare as I eat mine. Jackie and I consider heart to be like a very fine filet mignon. It's a terrific source of ubiquinone, or coenzyme Q10. (Eating brain is another more potent source, but few are doing this now.) We get bison hearts from our local butcher and they are marvelous. Ideally, we have heart once a week. My great-grandmother knew that heart, liver, and kidneys were a vital part of family nutrition. I like to make enough meat to have leftovers for a quick and easy breakfast.

HERE ARE THE basic proportions:

1 tablespoon coconut oil

Your favorite seasonings to taste (experiment!): garlic (add with greens), ginger, fresh or dried herbs (basil, rosemary, thyme, etc.), dried spices (cumin, curry powder, chili powder, turmeric, paprika, even cinnamon)

1–2 tablespoons vinegar and/or citrus juice: apple cider vinegar, balsamic vinegar, lemon juice, lime juice, red wine vinegar

1 teaspoon organic kelp powder, like Starwest Botanicals organic
  kelp powder (optional)

1 teaspoon iodized sea salt

1–2 pounds meat or fish: nitrate-free bacon (cooked before the
  main protein source, with excess fat drained from pan), ham,
  steak, chicken, turkey, pork, salmon, lamb, heart, liver

6–7½ cups greens and other vegetables: broccoli, collard greens,
  kale, mustard greens, spinach, turnip greens, plus cabbage,
  carrots, eggplant, mushrooms, onions

❖ Add coconut oil to a large skillet with cover over medium heat. Add seasonings, vinegar, kelp powder, and salt. Add meat or fish, and simmer until it
is cooked to your liking. Keep in mind that the more done the meat is, the
more tough it is likely to be. I like my meat rare, so I cook it for about 5 minutes. Add greens, and steam for another 1 to 2 minutes. Before serving, I slice
the meat into thin slices. If it is too raw for some at the table, put the slices
back in the skillet for another minute to make them well-done.

Algerian Chicken/Algerian Vegetarian

SERVES 4

My DAUGHTER AND I enjoy an Algerian restaurant in Elkader, Iowa, and decided we needed to add Algerian flair to our repertoire. It does take a bit
longer than basic skillet meals, but it is delicious! This is a flexible recipe that
you can make vegetarian if you wish. It can be enjoyed at the Wahls Diet
(served over quinoa with red pepper), Wahls Paleo (served over cauliflower
rice, spaghetti squash, winter squash, yams, or sautéed cabbage), or Wahls
Paleo Plus levels (replace the green beans with asparagus).

4 cloves garlic

1½ pounds chicken, with skin on (You can use breasts, legs, or
  thighs. Omit for vegetarian version.)

1 14.5-ounce can chopped tomatoes

2 cups sliced leeks

1 cup Bone Broth (page 440; use vegetable broth or water
    if vegetarian)

1 medium-size banana pepper, sliced

1 medium-size carrot, sliced

1 tablespoon coconut oil

2 teaspoons ground turmeric

1 teaspoon ground cinnamon

1 teaspoon ground cumin

1 teaspoon organic kelp powder, such as Starwest Botanicals
    organic kelp (optional)

½ teaspoon iodized sea salt

4 cups green beans (Wahls Diet/Wahls Paleo) or 4 cups asparagus
    (Wahls Paleo Plus)

2 cups chopped cilantro, with stems separated from leaves

❖ Mince garlic and let sit for 15 minutes prior to use to allow sulfur to stabilize. Add garlic, chicken, tomatoes, leeks, Bone Broth, pepper, carrot, coconut oil, spices, kelp powder, and salt to large skillet over medium heat. Simmer for 15 minutes. Add green beans or asparagus and chopped cilantro stems to the skillet and simmer for another 5 minutes. Stir in chopped cilantro leaves just prior to serving.

Rosemary Chicken

SERVES 8

ROSEMARY AND CHICKEN go together beautifully. Rosemary is an easy herb to grow in your garden or container garden.

6 cloves garlic

2 teaspoons chopped fresh rosemary

2 pounds cut-up chicken thighs, skin on (or any cut
    of chicken)

1 *medium eggplant, sliced*

1 *pound mushrooms, sliced*

2 *large carrots, sliced*

2 *tablespoons distilled vinegar*

1 *tablespoon coconut oil*

½ *teaspoon organic kelp powder, such as Starwest Botanicals*
   organic kelp (optional)

½ *teaspoon iodized sea salt*

❖ Mince garlic and let stand for 15 minutes. Put rosemary under the skin of the chicken. Place garlic, chicken, eggplant, mushrooms, carrots, vinegar, coconut oil, kelp powder, and salt in a skillet. Simmer for 20 minutes. Serve.

Liver, Onions, and Mushrooms

SERVES 4

THIS RECIPE IS adapted from my great-grandmother's cookbook *Compendium of Cookery and Reliable Recipes and Book of Knowledge*, which has a chapter devoted to the use of organ meats, liver, heart, brain, sweetbread (thymus), and kidney. Chicken liver is milder than the other livers, so it is a good place to start. You can also make this in the oven, baking at 250°F for 1 to 2 hours, which is my favorite way to prepare liver. In that recipe, one lays the bacon pieces between the liver slices, which rest on top of the onions and mushrooms. We intentionally make enough to use the leftovers to make liver pâté, which I have for breakfast.

½ *pound bacon (nitrate-free)*

½ *pound mushrooms, sliced*

1 *teaspoon organic kelp powder, such as Starwest Botanicals*
   organic kelp (optional)

1 *pound onions, chopped*

⅔ *pound lamb liver or chicken livers (must be organic)*

1 *tablespoon balsamic vinegar*

½ *teaspoon iodized sea salt*

❖ In a large skillet, fry the bacon. Pour off all the fat. Add mushrooms, kelp, and onions, and cook for 3 to 5 minutes over medium-low heat. Take the onion and mushrooms out of the skillet and set aside. Add livers, vinegar, and salt. Cook over medium heat for 1 to 2 minutes and then flip and cook another 1 to 2 minutes. Do not overcook. Make sure to leave the livers medium-rare because overcooking will make them tough. You can use any liver in this recipe, though lamb liver is our current favorite.

Liver Pâté

SERVES 2

WHILE LIVER PÂTÉ is not a skillet meal in the traditional sense, I put it here, because each time I make liver and onions I intentionally make enough to make a batch of pâté. I use this liver pâté as my morning protein after having liver and onions. We particularly enjoy it with turnip, rutabaga, radish, or kohlrabi slices. Celery is also good.

> Liver, onions, and mushrooms
> ¼ cup olive oil, coconut oil, or ghee
> ¼ cup balsamic vinegar (or Bragg apple cider vinegar)

❖ Take your leftover liver, onions, and mushrooms—about half of the preceding recipe—and add it to a food processor with oil and vinegar. Process on high until smooth. If it seems too thick, add more water or vinegar to make a runny pudding consistency. Store in the refrigerator.

Wahls Pizza

SERVES 1

GIVING UP PIZZA was difficult for my family. While it is possible to find gluten-free pizzas, it is more challenging to find pizzas that are both gluten-free and dairy-free. Zebby and Jackie often have pizza while I stick to Wahls Paleo Plus. Here is an example of how you can use gluten-free tortillas as a crust to build your own pizza. Add a bunch of vegetables, your meat of choice, and a dairy-free cheese such as Daiya (daiyafoods.com), and you are set. Serve with a large salad and you have comfort food to make the transition a little easier for you and your family. Be sure to read the ingredient labels of the gluten-free products to know that they are gluten-, dairy-, and (ideally) egg-free, too.

2 6-inch corn tortillas (or gluten-free flour tortillas)
¼ cup pizza sauce (look for sauce without sugar or gluten)
¼ pound ground beef, browned
¼ cup chopped sweet red peppers
¼ cup chopped onions
¼ cup sliced black olives
¼ cup spinach
1 clove garlic, minced
6 ounces soy-based or nut-based imitation cheese (you can find
    nondairy cheese substitutes in health food stores and regular
    grocery stores)

❖ Place the tortillas on a large cookie sheet. Place the pizza sauce and beef on the tortilla. Add the peppers, onions, olives, spinach, and garlic to each tortilla. Top with the gluten-free, dairy-free cheese alternative. Bake at 375°F, or until the cheese melts, about 5 to 10 minutes. Alternatively, you can broil the pizzas in a toaster oven or put the tortilla in a large covered skillet and cook on the stove over medium heat until the cheese melts, usually 2 to 3 minutes. Carefully slide the pizzas out of the oven, toaster oven, or skillet, and serve.

Note:

The amounts in this recipe are for two 6-inch corn tortillas, but if you decide to make your own version on a larger gluten-free pizza crust or gluten-free tortilla to share, add more ingredients according to your taste. It is important to use the optimum amounts of Daiya on pizza for the best performance. These are the amounts I have found work best:

❖ 10-inch gluten-free tortilla = 4 ounces; 12-inch = 5–6 ounces; 14-inch = 8 ounces; 16-inch = 10 ounces; 18-inch = 12 ounces.

❖ If you like the convenience of frozen pizza, Daiya also makes a frozen dairy-free, gluten-free pizza now.

Rawmesan

MAKES 16 SERVINGS

THIS IS A vegan recipe that tastes much like Parmesan cheese. (Of course, you don't have to be vegan to enjoy it on your Wahls Pizza or cooked veggies.)

½ cup nutritional yeast
½ cup ground walnuts
½ teaspoon iodized sea salt

❖ Combine ingredients in a food processor and process in short pulses until the mixture resembles Parmesan cheese.

Cheez Sauce

MAKES ABOUT 1½ CUPS SAUCE

This "cheezy" sauce can stand in for cheese in any appropriate recipe. The nutritional yeast adds more minerals and B vitamins. Add turmeric and or paprika to give it a pleasing yellowish hue. You can increase or decrease the water to adjust to your desired level of thickness.

⅓ cup sesame butter
¼ cup nutritional yeast
2 teaspoons onion powder
½ teaspoon sea salt
1 teaspoon paprika (optional)
½ teaspoon turmeric (optional)

1 tablespoon lemon juice
⅔ cup water

❖ Cream together sesame butter, nutritional yeast, onion powder, sea salt, optional paprika and/or turmeric, and lemon juice. Gradually stir in the water using a whisk until smooth. Alternatively, place the all the ingredients in a food processor and pulse until smooth.

Almond Dipping Sauce
MAKES ABOUT 2 CUPS

WE JUST DISCOVERED this sauce this summer. It is a lovely dip with raw vegetables, and it is also excellent over grilled meats. You can add fresh green herbs to make additional variations—we have experimented with cilantro, savory, oregano, and rosemary from our garden, and all have been quite tasty. You can make a beet version by adding half a cup of grated raw or chopped boiled/roasted beets—it's a beautiful magenta-colored dip and also delicious. The nutritional yeast adds minerals and B vitamins. Don't skip soaking the almonds (page 211)—just six hours begins the sprouting process that will reduce the lectin content of the nuts. This reduces the inflammatory reaction for those who are sensitive to lectins in nuts, legumes, and nightshades.

½ cup soaked/sprouted almonds
½ cup olive oil
½ cup water, plus more as needed
¼ cup nutritional yeast
¼ cup lemon juice
4 cloves garlic, minced
1 to 2 tablespoons fresh minced garden herbs (optional—cilantro, basil, oregano, savory, and thyme have all been delicious) or ½ cup ground raw or chopped cooked beet (optional, to make this into beet dip)
1 tablespoon coconut liquid aminos
½ tablespoon salt

❖ Place all of the ingredients in the food processor and pulse. Add additional water 2 tablespoons at a time, pulsing after each addition until achieving the desired texture of the sauce.

SOUPS

Bone Broth

MAKES VARYING AMOUNTS, DEPENDING
ON HOW MUCH WATER YOU USE

BONE BROTH WILL keep in the refrigerator for three days, in sealed airtight glass jars, or in the freezer for three months. The more bones you have in the pot, the longer you should let it steam and simmer to increase the collagen and minerals in the broth. Knucklebones and chicken feet add a lot of gelatin and collagen. My goal is to have 1 to 2 cups a day, especially during the winter.

Water (filtered or reverse osmosis water), enough to fill the pot or
  Crock-Pot
1 onion, chopped
3–4 cloves garlic
2–4 tablespoons cider vinegar (1 tablespoon per quart of water
  added is a good place to start)
1 teaspoon kelp powder or 1 tablespoon dulse flakes (optional)
½ teaspoon black pepper
½ teaspoon iodized sea salt
Bones (knucklebones are particularly good)
4 chicken feet (optional but recommended)
Any vegetables in your fridge that are getting a little bit limp

❖ Heat the water to steaming or a light simmer and add the rest of the ingredients. Simmer anywhere from 4 hours to 2 days. If any foamy materials come to the top of the pot, skim them off and discard. After you turn off the heat, allow to cool. Strain out the vegetables and bones.

THE POWER OF BONE BROTH

People spend a lot of money on expensive joint supplements for arthritis. These include substances like glucosamine, chondroitin sulfate, and methylsulfonylmethane (or MSM, another sulfur-containing compound). People also spend a lot of money on hyaluronic acid joint injections. I prefer a more natural approach: Get all these joint-strengthening, bone-building substances and more by making your own bone broth and drinking it every day. Bones with cartilage and tendons attached have more glucosamine to help benefit bones and joints even more. Those with a lot of marrow have more DHA fat, which, as I mentioned earlier, is really good for you, too!

Bone Broth–Avocado Soup

MAKES ABOUT 2½ CUPS

THIS WILL MAKE a lovely thick creamy soup. If it is too thick, simply add more broth or water.

 2 cups Bone Broth (page 440)
 ⅓ can full-fat coconut milk
 1 avocado, pitted and peeled
 2 cloves garlic, crushed
 1 teaspoon grated fresh gingerroot

❖ Mix all the ingredients. Blend in a high-powered blender until smooth. You may wish to heat again, although this soup is equally wonderful cold.

Bone Broth–Carrot Soup

SERVES 1

1 cup Bone Broth (page 440)
⅓ can full-fat coconut milk (or 2 to 3 tablespoons extra virgin olive oil)

½ cup cooked or raw carrots

1 teaspoon minced fresh gingerroot

½ teaspoon ground turmeric

❖ Bring the Bone Broth to a simmer over medium heat. Stir in remaining ingredients. Puree in a Vitamix or other high-speed blender.

Bone Broth–Cauliflower Turmeric Soup

SERVES 1

1 cup Bone Broth (page 440)

⅓ can full-fat coconut milk (or 2 to 3 tablespoons extra virgin olive oil)

½ cup cauliflower florets (cooked or raw)

1 clove garlic, minced

½ teaspoon ground turmeric

❖ Bring the Bone Broth to a simmer over medium heat. Stir in remaining ingredients. Puree in a Vitamix or other high-speed blender.

Bone Broth–Pepper Soup

SERVES 1

1 cup Bone Broth (page 440)

½ cup chopped red peppers

⅓ can (or more) full-fat coconut milk (or 2 to 3 tablespoons extra virgin olive oil)

❖ Bring the Bone Broth to a simmer over medium heat. Add remaining ingredients, and then blend in a Vitamix or other high-speed blender.

Coconut Milk–Fish Soup

SERVES 4

THIS IS A family favorite. It's very easy to adjust this to any combination of seafood, or even poultry.

> *6 cups Bone Broth (page 440)*
> *1 13.5-ounce can full-fat coconut milk*
> *1 teaspoon organic kelp powder, such as Starwest Botanicals*
>   *organic kelp (optional)*
> *½ teaspoon iodized sea salt*
> *5 cups chopped bok choy*
> *3 cups chopped broccoli*
> *1 medium carrot, sliced*
> *½ pound shiitake mushrooms, sliced*
> *1 tablespoon thinly sliced gingerroot*
> *1½ pounds Chinook salmon*
> *2 tablespoons lime juice*

❖ In large kettle, combine broth, coconut milk, kelp powder, salt, vegetables, and ginger. Add additional water if you want more broth in the soup. Bring to a simmer. Add salmon and lime juice. Bring soup to a boil. Turn off heat. Let kettle sit for 10 minutes and serve.

Seafood-Tomato Soup

SERVES 4

THIS SOUP IS marvelous and the saffron is a wonderful addition. We alternate between this and the Coconut Milk–Fish Soup. Both are very big hits with both Zach and Zebby. Neither takes long to make.

> *4 cups Bone Broth (page 440)*
> *1 18-ounce bottle clam juice*

1 14.5-ounce can chopped tomatoes

4 cloves garlic

1 cup chopped sweet red pepper

1 cup chopped sweet yellow pepper

1 leek, sliced

1 teaspoon organic kelp powder, such as Starwest Botanicals
     organic kelp (optional)

½ teaspoon iodized sea salt (or to taste)

⅛ teaspoon saffron

½ pound scallops

½ pound shrimp

❖ Place broth, clam juice, tomatoes, garlic, vegetables, kelp powder, salt, and saffron in a large pot over medium heat. Simmer 5 minutes. Add scallops and shrimp to the pot. Bring to boil. Turn heat off, let sit 5 to 10 minutes, then serve.

Kale Sausage Soup/Vegetarian Kale Soup

SERVES 4

THIS RECIPE IS particularly good for winter meals. Zach enjoys it with kale and sausage, but any type of leafy green will work well. You can also use any variety of sausage you like or omit it entirely to make the recipe vegetarian.

8 cups Bone Broth (page 440; or vegetable broth, if vegetarian)

4 cups chopped kale

2 cups chopped sweet potato

1 cup chopped onion

1 medium banana pepper, sliced

1 teaspoon organic kelp powder, such as Starwest Botanicals
     organic kelp (optional)

½ teaspoon iodized sea salt

4 bratwursts (If vegetarian, omit or substitute 2 cups
     black-eyed peas, canned, or soaked then cooked

from dried, or cooked in a pressure cooker to best
decrease the lectins/phytates.)
1 13.5-ounce can full-fat coconut milk

❖ Add broth, vegetables, kelp powder, and salt to a Crock-Pot or soup pot. Add brats and simmer for at least 30 minutes, or add black-eyed peas, which will be tender in 30 minutes if they were soaked first. Fish out the sausages, slice them, and add them back to the soup. Add coconut milk, stir, and serve.

Red Chili with Beans
SERVES 4

YOU CAN USE Louisiana hot sauce or other pepper sauce on the table to make your chili as hot as you like. Jackie prefers a milder chili, but Zebby and I like it hot. Zebby probably has the hottest taste preference of us all. The heat from the hot sauce is capsaicin, which has been a traditional treatment for chronic nerve pain. If you soak the beans overnight and sprout them, the cooking time is shortened, plus you will have reduced the lectins and phytates (or cook in a pressure cooker on high).

8 cups Bone Broth (page 440)
1 pound ground bison meat
1 cup chopped onion
1 15-ounce can black beans, drained
2 6-ounce cans tomato paste
1 medium carrot, sliced
1 jalapeño pepper, minced
1 teaspoon chili powder
1 teaspoon organic kelp powder, such as Starwest Botanicals
    organic kelp (optional)
½ teaspoon iodized sea salt

❖ Put all ingredients in kettle. Simmer 30 minutes.

Seafood Stew

SERVES 4

THIS STEW IS great with oysters or scallops, and it can be varied to fit the Wahls Protocol level you've selected. For the Wahls Paleo version, double the amount of seafood and keep the rest of the recipe the same. For Wahls Paleo Plus, use 1 pound of seafood but omit the butternut squash.

> 1 13.5-ounce can full-fat coconut milk
> 2 cups chicken broth (or Bone Broth, page 440, or store-bought broth)
> 1 pound mushrooms, sliced
> 1 large onion, chopped
> 2 cups cubed butternut squash (omit on Wahls Paleo Plus)
> 1 teaspoon organic kelp powder, such as Starwest Botanicals organic kelp (optional)
> ½ teaspoon iodized sea salt
> 1 pound oysters or scallops (use 2 pounds for Wahls Paleo)
> 2 cups chopped cauliflower
> 1 cup minced fresh cilantro

❖ Place coconut milk, broth, mushrooms, onion, squash, kelp powder, and salt in a pot. Heat to simmering until squash is nearly tender, 5 to 10 minutes. Add oysters or scallops and cauliflower, bring back to a gentle simmer, and turn the heat off. Let stew sit for 10 minutes. Stir in the cilantro and serve. Add coarse ground pepper to each bowl as you like.

SALADS

I OFTEN RECOMMEND HAVING a salad, but nutritional content can vary drastically depending on which vegetables, fruits, nuts, seeds, fat sources, and meats you choose. In general, I recommend piling your plate with fresh raw leafy greens of all types, chopping other vegetables you have, and adding them (cucumber, carrots, radishes, bell peppers, mushrooms, green onions, or whatever you like, but try to include sulfur-rich vegetables to balance the greens), drizzling with a cold-pressed olive oil and a splash of fresh lemon juice or vinegar, and adding some animal protein like steak, chicken, or fish.

Salmon or Chicken Salad

SERVES 3

You can use these meat salads as a spread, side dish, or salad accent. If using salmon, find a can of wild sockeye salmon that contains the bones. By keeping the bones in the salad, you will markedly increase your calcium intake. Serve with gluten-free crackers or bread. My daughter is very fond of having this with a collard green as a wrap. You can steam the collard green for a minute to soften it before using it in place of flatbread. If you prefer, warm the salad slightly on the stove before eating. This is an easy meal that you can make from pantry foods.

> 1 14.7-ounce can salmon, drained, or 4 medium skinless cooked
>   chicken breasts (about 13 ounces)
> ½ small onion, minced
> 1 clove garlic, minced
> ¼ cup minced celery
> ¼ cup chopped parsley
> 2 tablespoons gluten-free peanut sauce
> ⅓ teaspoon organic kelp powder, such as Starwest Botanicals
>   organic kelp (optional)
> ¼ teaspoon iodized sea salt

❖ Put the salmon in a bowl and mash the bones. If using chicken, chop the breasts into bite-size pieces. Place salmon or chicken and onion, garlic, celery, parsley, peanut sauce, kelp powder, and salt in a food processor and pulse until the mixture reaches your desired texture. You can also chop and mix by hand.

Parsley Onion Sumac Salad

MY DAUGHTER SERVED this when she was making a fancy meal that featured lamb liver (see the Bacon-Wrapped Lamb Liver recipe on page 428). It has since become one of our favorite salads! This is terrific nutrition for your mitochondria, your detox pathways, and your brain. And it is delicious. The parsley is a lovely green color and the pomegranate seeds are a great addition if they are available. Powdered sumac is available at Middle Eastern grocery stores. It is a dark purple, tart, and full of polyphenols. If you can't find sumac, you can substitute a dark balsamic vinegar of your choice. We love sumac and have added it to chicken when we roast chicken (or lamb) with root vegetables.

> 1 large or 2 medium red onions
> 1 bunch of parsley
> ¼ cup extra virgin olive oil
> ¼ to ½ cup pomegranate seeds (optional)
> 1 to 2 tablespoons ground sumac
> Juice of one lemon or 1 tablespoon lime juice or balsamic vinegar
> 1 teaspoon sea salt

❖ Slice the onions thinly or chop into bite-size pieces. Chop the parsley leaves and mince the stems. (No need to throw the stems away!) Mix the parsley and onions together, add the remaining ingredients, and stir thoroughly. Let sit for at least 5 minutes and then serve.

SIDE DISHES

THESE ARE VEGETABLE dishes to have on the side. One of the things I discovered was that by adding bacon to a dish, it cut the bitterness and made vegetables much more appealing to Zach and Zebby. When we discovered gluten-free, nitrate-free bacon, we were all much happier.

Greens and Bacon

SERVES 3

ANY TYPE OF green will work well with this recipe.

  4 slices bacon, cut into bite-size pieces (nitrate-free)
  6 cups chopped greens (beet, mustard, or any other greens)
  3 cloves garlic, chopped
  1 tablespoon balsamic vinegar
  1 teaspoon organic kelp powder, such as Starwest Botanicals
     organic kelp (optional)
  ½ teaspoon iodized sea salt

❖ Fry bacon. Retain all fat. Add greens, garlic, vinegar, kelp powder, and salt to the pan. Cook until greens are wilted. Serve.

Garlic and Onion Green Beans

THIS IS A dish that one of our nannies introduced to our family. It was an immediate hit with both of our kids and it is delicious warm or cold. This recipe also works wonderfully well with sugar snap peas or asparagus standing in for the green beans.

  ¼ cup olive oil
  ¼ cup flax oil or hemp oil
  6 to 12 garlic cloves, minced
  ½ medium onion, minced
  1 pound fresh green beans, stems removed
  1 to 2 tablespoons minced herbs such as savory, thyme, oregano,
     or basil

❖ Combine the olive oil and flax or hemp oil. Add the garlic and onion to the oil mixture and let sit for at least 30 minutes. Steam the green beans for

3 minutes. After steaming, stir the garlic, onion, and oil mixture into the green beans. Serve the green beans warm or serve cool as a salad. Top with the herbs (optional).

Brussels Sprouts, Bacon, and Cranberries

SERVES 4

As a child, I did not care for Brussels sprouts, but now both Jackie and I are very fond of them. The trick here is not to overcook them, because they'll become bitter if you do. The cranberries are a lovely addition visually and taste-wise, and the almonds add a little more calcium to the meal. This is a quick and easy dish to prepare.

4 slices bacon (nitrate-free)
4 cups halved Brussels sprouts
1 cup whole fresh cranberries
¼ cup chopped onion
2 tablespoons balsamic vinegar
1 teaspoon organic kelp powder, such as Starwest Botanicals
    organic kelp (optional)
¼ cup raw almonds, chopped (soaked once you are doing Wahls
    Paleo or Wahls Paleo Plus)

❖ Fry bacon. Pour off half the fat (or retain all of the fat to increase your intake of healthy fats). Add Brussels sprouts, cranberries, onion, vinegar, and kelp powder to skillet. Cover and simmer for two minutes. Add the chopped almonds when you serve it.

Mashed Turnips

SERVES 4

1 pound turnips
½ cup nutritional yeast
¼ cup chopped chives
4 cloves garlic, minced
2 tablespoons coconut oil
1 teaspoon organic kelp powder, such as Starwest Botanicals
*   organic kelp (optional)*
¼ teaspoon iodized sea salt
¼ teaspoon ground black pepper

❖ Wash and cut up turnips into bite-size pieces. Place in a steamer basket and steam until tender, which will be 5 to 10 minutes, depending on how small you cut the pieces. When the turnips are tender, place in a bowl with the remaining ingredients and mash with a potato masher. (You can also pulse the mixture in a food processor until the desired texture is achieved.) Add more coarsely ground black pepper to individual servings if desired.

Sautéed Red Cabbage

SERVES 4

My mother was very fond of red cabbage, and introduced our family to eating it sautéed.

2 tablespoons coconut oil
4 cups chopped red cabbage
1½ tablespoons sliced fresh gingerroot
1 tablespoon balsamic vinegar

❖ Heat coconut oil in a skillet over medium heat. Add cabbage, ginger, and vinegar. Sauté for 2 to 4 minutes.

Quinoa and Red Peppers

SERVES 4

ZEBBY IS FOND of this recipe. We based it on a dish served at an Algerian restaurant in Elkader, Iowa.

1 cup quinoa
1½ cups water
1 cup chopped red pepper

❖ Soak quinoa for 10 minutes and rinse carefully to remove the skin (which has a bitter coating called saponin) or sprout by soaking 6 to 24 hours and then rinse. Return to pot, add the water, cover the pan, and simmer 10 minutes. Add chopped red pepper and simmer another 5 minutes. Remove from heat and let it sit in the pot for another 5 minutes. Fluff with a fork and serve. (Or you can cook using a pressure cooker on high, to reduce the lectins.)

Cauliflowerice

SERVES 4

1 medium cauliflower

❖ Cut cauliflower into pieces that will fit in through the food processor chute (unless you choose to grate it by hand). Place cauliflower in a steamer basket in large pot on the stove. Steam for 2 to 4 minutes. Put the grating blade in the food processor. Run the steamed cauliflower, including stems and leaves, through the food processor. This is a great substitute for rice. You could also put it through the processor to make mashed cauliflower, which can be eaten like mashed potatoes. This is a low-carbohydrate alternative to potatoes. It tastes great, goes with any dish that has a lovely sauce, and will not cause a rise in insulin levels.

Spaghetti Squash

SERVES 4

1 large spaghetti squash

❖ Poke holes in the squash to allow steam to escape. Bake in oven at 375°F for 1 hour or in a Crock-Pot on low for 10 hours. The squash is done when a carving fork can easily pierce the skin. Split the squash in half and scoop out and discard the seeds. Scrape out the squash, which will look like noodles, and serve.

Sweet Potato or Winter Squash

MAKES ½ TO 1 SWEET POTATO OR SQUASH
PER SERVING, DEPENDING ON SIZE

❖ Cut up and steam for 10 to 15 minutes or until a carving fork can easily pierce the skin. Place sweet potatoes or squash in a serving dish and serve.

Beet and Red Cabbage Mixture

SERVES 1

You can make this two ways. Use the freshly grated ginger or the cinnamon-cocoa combination, or you can omit the spices and simply have the beet–red cabbage mixture. The beets and cabbage are excellent for mitochondria and detoxification. Ginger, cinnamon, and cocoa are all powerhouse spices that add even more mitochondrial and detoxification support, which is why I started adding them to more of my foods.

¼ *cup beets, raw*
¼ *cup chopped red cabbage*
1 *tablespoon flaxseed oil or hemp oil or olive oil*
1 *tablespoon olive oil*

1 teaspoon ground cinnamon (optional)
¼ teaspoon unsweetened cocoa (optional) or 1 teaspoon grated
fresh gingerroot (instead of the cocoa-cinnamon combination)

❖ Combine all ingredients. Place in a food processor and pulse to your desired consistency.

Beet and Cranberry Mixture

SERVES 1

¼ cup beets, raw
¼ cup fresh whole cranberries
1½ tablespoons sliced or grated fresh gingerroot

❖ Combine all ingredients. Place in a food processor and pulse to desired consistency.

BEVERAGES

Bone Broth Tea

I LIKE TO COMBINE Bone Broth and coconut milk to make a warm drink for mornings, especially during the winter. The basis is a cup of hot Bone Broth and ⅓ of a can of full-fat coconut milk. Then I add spices (like turmeric) and some vegetables (like carrots or garlic). The Vitamix can handle anything, so I add vegetables raw or cooked and put the entire mixture on high until blended smooth. If it seems too thick, I add more broth until it reaches my desired thickness. Again, experiment with spices and your local in-season vegetables.

Turmeric Tea

SERVES 1

1 cup Bone Broth (page 440)
⅓ can (or more) full-fat coconut milk
½ tablespoon ground turmeric
1 clove garlic, peeled and crushed

❖ Bring the Bone Broth to a simmer over medium heat. Add remaining ingredients, then blend with an immersion blender, or in a Vitamix or other high-speed blender. (Be careful blending hot liquid. Cover tightly and start on low speed.)

Hot Cocoa

SERVES 1

OUR GREAT-GREAT-GRANDMOTHERS AND great-great-grandfathers knew to use spices to make foods seem sweeter. Spices that have a little heat, such as cinnamon, cloves, mint, and ginger, will help reduce the perceived bitterness of food and improve the relative sweetness. I make hot cocoa using just organic cocoa powder, cinnamon, coconut milk, and water. There is no sugar in the cocoa, but the cinnamon cuts the bitterness nicely. The longer you are away from sugar, the more your taste buds and taste sensibility will change. You will likely find your foods tasting sweeter, and you may find bitter tastes more appealing. If this chocolate seems too bitter for your taste, add a very ripe banana or some of the approved sweeteners, such as a teaspoon of honey. Stevia leaves are certainly fine, but once stevia is processed, I am not certain about the impact of the processing, so I do not use it.

¼ to 1 teaspoon unsweetened cocoa
½ to 1 teaspoon ground cinnamon
½ can full-fat coconut milk (or 2 cups any nut milk)

½ *cup water*
Optional: Make a mint cocoa by adding a few drops of oil of mint.

❖ Combine all ingredients in a blender and process until smooth. (Stirring alone will not produce a smooth cocoa.) Heat gently in a saucepan over medium heat on the stove.

FERMENTED FOODS

FERMENTED FOODS WERE a long tradition in most of our great-grandmothers' kitchens. They are not hard to make and add a lot of nutrition to your diet. Here are some easy recipes that I enjoy. Fermented foods are an acquired taste, so start slowly. Kombucha is the easiest. Then add other fermented foods as condiments to your meals.

Kombucha Tea

MAKES 16 CUPS

KOMBUCHA IS A symbiotic culture of strains of *Saccharomyces* (including *Saccharomyces cerevisiae*) and bacteria, making it very helpful at reducing problems related to yeast overgrowth after antibiotic use. I like to have a glass of kombucha every day. You can purchase kombucha tea at the store, but for the freshest possible tea where you control the ingredients, make it yourself. To make a gallon of tea, you can either add tea bags to heated water or make sun tea. Either way, you must ensure that there is no chlorine in your water or you'll kill the kombucha "mother," or SCOBY, which is responsible for fermenting the tea. I always use reverse osmosis water, but if you don't have that type of filter, you can also let the water sit uncovered for 24 hours or boil it for 5 minutes to get rid of the chlorine. The metals from your pans may also disrupt the kombucha, so you should use a nonreactive container such as a one-gallon glass jar to make the tea. Make sure to wash all of your containers with hot, soapy water before starting. You can order kombucha mothers through the Internet (find both mothers and supplies at Kombucha Kamp, kombuchakamp.com), or if you are lucky, you can get a mother from a friend.

I DRINK KOMBUCHA TEA regularly; however, there have been a couple of reported cases of people becoming ill from too much acid in their bloodstreams attributed to drinking kombucha. If you have any kidney or liver disease or diabetes, you are at a higher risk to have problems with kombucha. Start with drinking just ¼ cup when you first begin, just to confirm that you have no problems with it. Then you can increase to ½ cup and then a full cup or more each day.

1 gallon black tea, green tea, rooibos tea, or yerba maté
1 cup white granulated sugar
1 mother

❖ Add the sugar while the tea is still warm and stir until dissolved. After the tea has cooled to room temperature, remove the tea bags. Pour the tea into a gallon jar that holds the mother or SCOBY. Place a mesh bag over the jar and cover the jar with a towel to let the mixture breathe. Store the mixture at room temperature in a well-ventilated area without light for 7 to 10 days, though fermentation time can vary. You can check whether it's done by taste or by using a pH strip to see if its pH is between 2.6 and 4.0. Discard any kombucha that smells rancid or looks to be contaminated with mold or insects. A well-fermented batch will be cloudy and fizzy with stringy brown pieces from the SCOBY. Pour the kombucha into quart jars, seal them, let them sit on the counter for another day, then place them in the refrigerator. Consume within the month. Leave 1 to 2 cups of tea with the mother and put the mother back in the refrigerator to reuse. You can make a fresh batch of kombucha every other weekend, but kombucha that has been fermented too long turns into usable vinegar. Because of its acidity, the tea should not be prepared or stored in lead-glazed ceramic or lead crystal containers, as toxic elements can leach into the tea.

Beet Kvass

SERVES 3

EASTERN EUROPE HAS a long history of fermenting foods, including root vegetables. The fermentation process increases the production of vitamins and enzymes, and it helps put the correct health-promoting bacteria back in your bowels. Beets are traditionally an excellent support for your detoxification enzymes, and fermented beets offer even more support to the detoxification process. I like to alternate between drinking kombucha and beet kvass, and I dilute the beet kvass with an equal amount of water when I drink it. It is very important to use organic beets for the kvass and water that has absolutely no chlorine. You also need a starter from some fermented beets or a single probiotic capsule, like an acidophilus capsule you can buy at your grocery store or pharmacy, with the supplements. Open the capsule and dump it into the mix. Get one with as large a number of different species as possible. (The one I use has fifteen different strains of health-promoting bacteria in it.)

> 1 cup coarsely sliced or chopped beets
> 1 tablespoon grated gingerroot
> 1 tablespoon grated orange zest
> 1 tablespoon iodized sea salt
> 1 probiotic capsule
> 2½ cups water

❖ Clean a canning jar and lid carefully in hot soapy water. Rinse well. Place beet pieces in the jar, sprinkling ginger, orange zest, and salt as you go. Open the probiotic capsule and sprinkle the contents on beets to introduce the helpful bacteria. Fill with water. Place a jar with a diameter smaller than the opening of the canning jar on the beets to keep them submerged. After 2 to 3 days, the fermentation should be sufficient, and the jar can be sealed and placed in the refrigerator. Drain the liquid and drink it. (You can also eat the beets or discard them, but they are good in smoothies or salads.)

CHOOSING A PROBIOTIC CAPSULE

Saccharomyces boulardii is a probiotic that is very closely related to *Saccharomyces cerevisiae*, which is used to make nutritional and brewer's yeast. They both outcompete *Candida albicans* and are quite effective at reducing symptoms related to *Candida*/fungal overgrowth. For those who have taken repeated courses of antibiotics throughout their lifetime, particularly at an early age, adding *S. boulardii* via probiotic supplementation can be helpful. Look for varieties that include this beneficial yeast. You can use it in any of the fermentation recipes in this chapter, or take it with water before meals. I have people start with one capsule per day. The following day, I increase to a capsule twice per day. Next, I advise two capsules in the morning and then one in the evening. Finally, we move to two capsules twice a day. In some cases, I have the person go up to 3 capsules twice a day. If the *Candida* die-off leads to headaches, fatigue, or malaise as the *S. boulardii* is introduced, that confirms that the *Candida albicans* is probably present, overgrown, and contributing to that person's symptoms.

Sauerkraut and Fermented Vegetables

THIS IS A very easy fermented food recipe and was a staple for American settlers. Both my grandmothers would have made fermented root vegetables and pickles regularly. (All vegetables need to be organic.)

1 small organic cabbage
Organic carrots, garlic, and/or onions, to taste
Gingerroot, to taste
Hot peppers, chopped or whole, to taste
1 tablespoon sea salt
1 probiotic capsule

❖ Clean a wide-mouth canning jar and lid carefully in hot soapy water. Rinse carefully. Wash the cabbage and vegetables. The goal is to have 80 percent or more grated cabbage in the mixture. Grate the cabbage and carrots. Grate the ginger. Place the cabbage in the jar, sprinkling ginger, hot peppers, other root vegetables (to taste), and salt as you go. Pack the vegetables into the canning jar with a spoon. Open the probiotic capsule and sprinkle on the cabbage. Place a jar with a diameter smaller than the opening of the canning jar on the cabbage to submerge it below the brine. Place the jar in another container to catch any brine that overflows during the fermentation process, and store in a cool, dark place. Check the jar periodically to remove any unsubmerged pieces of vegetables or mold that has appeared. If the level of brine is below the top of the vegetables, add additional salted water until the vegetables are completely submerged (2 teaspoons salt to 1 cup filtered water). Remember, tap water has chlorine and will kill the friendly bacteria. After a week, the fermentation should be sufficient and the jar can be sealed and placed in the refrigerator. Fermentation time can vary; if desired, the vegetables can be fermented longer until the desired taste and texture have been achieved.

DESSERTS

You do get to have some treats. Your taste buds will adjust and you will discover new flavors in your foods. These are some wonderful desserts using dried fruit, fresh berries, and spices to accent and sweeten the dish.

Fruit Pudding
SERVES 2

In this recipe, the spices enhance the fruit's natural sweetness. After you've gone two weeks without sugar, your cravings for sweets will fade.

> 1 cup full-fat coconut milk (or any nut milk)
> 1 cup any berries, or combination of berries (such as blackberries, blueberries, raspberries, and strawberries)

1 *medium Hass avocado, peeled, pitted, and chopped*
1 *teaspoon ground cardamom*
1 *teaspoon ground cinnamon*

❖ Heat coconut milk or nut milk until it is steaming. Add hot coconut milk, berries, avocado, and spices to a Vitamix and blend for 3 minutes. (Be careful blending hot liquids—cover tightly and start on low speed.) Pour into a bowl and refrigerate.

Raspberry-Flaxseed Pudding

ONCE YOU GET to Wahls Paleo, the flaxseeds should be soaked for 2 to 6 hours before use to eliminate phytates and lectins. This will make them softer and easier to blend, so you won't have to grind the seeds separately. If you're not on Wahls Paleo or Wahls Paleo Plus, grind the flaxseeds immediately before use in a coffee grinder. That way the omega-3 fatty acids won't have broken down. You may increase or decrease the flaxseed to make the pudding your desired level of firmness. Fresh berries and a tablespoon of full-fat coconut milk make a lovely garnish for serving.

¼ *cup flaxseeds*
1 *cup full-fat coconut milk (or any nut milk)*
1 *cup raspberries*
1 *teaspoon ground cardamom*
1 *teaspoon ground cinnamon*

❖ Grind flaxseeds just prior to use (Wahls Diet) or soak seeds for 2 to 6 hours prior to use (Wahls Paleo and Wahls Paleo Plus). Heat the coconut milk (or nut milk) until it is steaming. Place ground flaxseeds or whole soaked flaxseeds, hot coconut milk, raspberries, and spices in a Vitamix or other high-speed blender, cover, and blend for 1 to 3 minutes. Pour into a bowl and refrigerate.

Mitochondria Support Pudding

LIKE THE MITOCHONDRIA Support Smoothie (page 426), this pudding supports the mitochondrial membranes that keep your mitochondria healthy and young, thanks to the phosphatidylcholine (PC). This pudding is rich in PC, so I make it most mornings and have it most evenings. It feeds my mitochondria and it feeds my microbiome. Honestly, I make the pudding more than I make the smoothie—I consider it one of my most powerful anti-aging strategies. (See the Resources for good sources for PC. The PC supplement is expensive but it is an excellent anti-aging, mitochondria-boosting, and brain repair strategy. Even my daughter agrees that in this recipe, it is delicious.) For best results, make a few hours before you'd like to enjoy it. I make mine in the morning and eat it in the evening.

2 cups water

1 teaspoon to 1 tablespoon PC (or up to 2 tablespoons as you adjust to it)

1 tablespoon organic hemp oil

¼ to ½ teaspoons organic extra virgin cod-liver oil

½ to 1 cup fresh or frozen berries (optional)

1 to 3 tablespoons inulin powder

1 to 2 tablespoons organic cocoa powder

1 tablespoon ground cinnamon

¼ to ½ inch coarsely chopped or sliced gingerroot (optional)

1 teaspoon powdered lion's mane mushroom (optional)

1 teaspoon powdered medicinal mushroom (e.g., turkey tail, reishi, chaga, or other medicinal mushroom blend)

1 teaspoon matcha green tea powder (organic)

1 probiotic capsule containing lactobacillus and bifidobacteria species

3 tablespoons (more or less, depending on how thick you like your pudding) organic chia seeds

Optional enhancements:

Fresh organic berries or chopped stone fruit (peaches, plums, or apricots)
Grated dark chocolate bar or cacao nibs
Coconut cream (skim off the solids from the top of your can of coconut milk and whip until fluffy)

❖ Blend the water, PC, hemp oil, and cod-liver oil in a high-speed blender for 1 to 3 minutes (it should look like cream). Add the berries, inulin, cocoa powder, cinnamon, ginger, mushrooms, and matcha and blend on high until everything looks thoroughly combined. Open the probiotic capsule and sprinkle onto the mixture. Add the chia seeds and gently stir into the mixture. Let this sit on the counter to begin the germination process for the seeds and the fermentation process for the bacteria, for at least 30 minutes or up to overnight. The pudding may not look thick at first, but the chia will expand and thicken over the next 30 to 60 minutes; as the bacteria ferments, it will also contribute to thickening the pudding. Experiment to find the amount of chia seed that achieves the desired texture. If the PC flavor is too strong, add more cocoa. If the cocoa is too bitter, add more cinnamon and ginger. Put it in a fancy glass or goblet and you have an elegant dessert for your family and friends.

Note:

Don't skip the long blending time for the water and oils. This is required to make liposomes, which are a form of fat more easily absorbed into the bloodstream and brain.

Wahls Fudge
MAKES 20 SERVINGS

WE USE THIS recipe when people are losing too much weight. We have people eat as much fudge as they need to maintain a healthy weight. This is a marvelous sweet treat with raisins, but you can use any dried fruit, like plums, dates, or cherries. The coconut oil keeps the carbohydrates from entering your bloodstream too quickly. This is an excellent dessert that will hopefully help you to adjust to a new way of eating. For those who are following Paleo Plus and reducing carbohydrate intake, omit the raisins, though you will have to cut back considerably on cocoa to keep the fudge from being too bitter. (Start with ¼ teaspoon.) If you are still losing too much weight, you may need to increase the carbs, even if you're on Paleo Plus. If so, add raisins and don't be concerned about whether you are in ketosis.

> 1 *cup coconut oil or ghee*
> 1 *cup raisins*
> 1 *cup walnuts (soaked once you are doing Wahls Paleo)*
> 1 *medium Hass avocado, peeled and pitted*
> ½ *cup dried unsweetened coconut*
> 1–2 *teaspoons ground cinnamon*
> 1 *teaspoon unsweetened cocoa powder*

❖ Put everything in a food processor and blend on high until smooth. Press mixture into an 8-inch square glass baking dish and place in the refrigerator. Keep refrigerated.

Appendix A

THE WAHLS PROTOCOL
COMPLETE FOOD LISTS

THE FIRST STEP we give our study subjects is to go through their homes and eating environments and remove all of the prohibited foods. Donate them to a food bank, give them to a neighbor, or toss them—whatever seems appropriate to you. Completing that step dramatically increases the probability of success. To help you do this, I am starting with the list of prohibited foods for the Wahls Diet, and then I'll tell you what you would be removing for Wahls Paleo and Wahls Paleo Plus. After that, I'll provide a table summarizing the three plans, followed by the list of foods you can eat by category.

PROHIBITED FOODS

All gluten-containing foods

1. Wheat, rye, malt, most commercial oats, and all products made from these:
   - Bread; most baked goods, like muffins, cookies, cake, rolls, biscuits, and croissants; most pasta; most crackers; flour tortillas; and any breakfast cereal containing wheat or other gluten grains
   - Many packaged foods contain wheat or other gluten-containing grains, so check the label! Foods that contain gluten but aren't obviously made of wheat include soy sauce (tamari is okay), seitan, and many brands of veggie "meats," like veggie burgers, veggie hot dogs, and veggie "chicken." Words to look for include: brominated flour, durum flour, enriched flour, farina, flour, graham flour, phosphate flour, plain flour, self-rising flour, semolina, white flour, teff, einkorn, emmer, Kamut, and spelt

2. Barley
  - Barley, including pearl barley, like the kind you might put in soup
  - All beer that isn't specifically labeled gluten-free
  - Cider and other fermented beverages (Note: Distilled non-grain-based alcohol, such as vodka or gin, is gluten-free, and some fermented ciders are gluten-free, but check the label. Most wine is also gluten-free.)
  - Malt products (malt syrup, malt extract, malt flavoring, malted beverages, and malted milk)

All dairy products

- All cow, sheep, and goat milks
- All products made from those milks, like cheese, yogurt, cream, and ice cream
- All products containing milk proteins, such as baked goods, pudding, and snacks containing cheese
- Many packaged foods contain milk or milk components, such as casein and whey, so check the label.

Other foods to avoid

- Chicken and duck eggs, omega-3 eggs, and all foods containing eggs
- Nonorganic soy products
- Processed meats—like hot dogs, bologna, and salami—that contain gluten or nitrates
- All oils other than the permitted oils listed in the following pages. Do not consume corn, soybean, canola, or grape-seed oils. Also, do not consume any trans fats, hydrogenated or partially hydrogenated oils, or any type of margarine.
- All foods sweetened with sugar, high-fructose corn syrup, or other refined sweeteners, including artificial sweeteners. This includes:
  - Desserts and snacks sweetened with sugar
  - Regular or diet soda
  - Sweetened juice drinks
  - Sports drinks
  - Fruit canned or frozen with added sugar or artificial sweetener

- Any drink or foods made with sugar, high-fructose corn syrup, or artificial sweetener
- Any foods made with monosodium glutamate (MSG)
- Do not microwave any food you intend to eat!
- With Wahls Paleo, reduce your intake of gluten-free grains, legumes, and potatoes to two servings a week, and remove soy milk completely.
- At the Wahls Paleo Plus level, remove all grains, legumes, peanuts, and soy.

WAHLS PROTOCOL FOOD RULES

That last section was about what you can't eat, but this section is what you *can* eat! Here are the general food rules for the three diet plans. After the summary, I provide a table comparing the three diets and then the list of foodstuffs contained in each of the various food categories. Make sure to vary the foods within each group that you consume each day.

Wahls Diet

- Remove all prohibited foods from your diet, as specified previously.
- Eat 9 cups of vegetables and fruit (3 cups greens, 3 cups sulfur-rich, 3 cups color).
- You may reduce your 9 cups in proportion to one another if it is making you feel uncomfortably full or giving you digestive trouble; in other words, if you reduce your intake to 6 cups, you should get 2 cups from each category. Or eat up to 12 cups!
- Eat high-quality protein, preferably animal, as desired (6 to 12 ounces daily according to gender and size). Gluten-free, nitrate-free processed meats are acceptable.
- Vegetarians are encouraged to soak, and preferably sprout, the grains and legumes consumed. (See chapter 6, "Wahls Paleo," for more information on the difference between the two.)
- Eating organic is encouraged.
- Limit gluten-free grain products to one per day.
- Limit sweeteners to 1 teaspoon.

- Avoid all artificial sweeteners.
- Avoid vegetable oils high in omega-6 fatty acids, like corn, soybean, canola, grape-seed, and palm kernel oils.
- Avoid hydrogenated fats.
- If constipated, use flaxseed or chia seed as needed to have soft bowel movements daily.
- Eat to satiety.

The food groups added in Wahls Paleo (soaked nuts and seeds, seaweed, organ meats, and fermented foods) are also permitted if desired in the Wahls Diet.

Wahls Paleo

- Continue eating 9 cups of vegetables and fruit and being gluten-, dairy-, and egg-free, as in the Wahls Diet.
- Increase protein to 9 to 21 ounces of meat daily, with 12 ounces of organ meat and 16 ounces of high omega-3 fish each week.
- Reduce all gluten-free grain products, potatoes, and legumes to two servings per week (soaked if consumed).
- Add seaweed and algae daily.
- Add lacto-fermented food daily.
- Add soaked nuts and seeds.
- Avoid soy and rice milk.
- Switch to coconut milk and soaked nut milks.

Wahls Paleo Plus

- Continue eating vegetables and fruit, and being gluten-, dairy-, and egg-free, as in the Wahls Diet. Continue with the fermented foods, organ meats, soaked nuts and seeds, coconut milk, soaked nut milks, seaweed, and algae as in Wahls Paleo.
- You may reduce your 9 cups to 6 cups, but retain an even distribution between leafy green, color, and sulfur categories. Remove apples, pears, and bananas. Raw starchy colored vegetables may be consumed as part of the color allotment. Limit fruit to one cup per day, with a preference for

berries and low-carbohydrate fruits. Avoid all dried and canned fruit and fruit juices.

- Avoid all legumes, grains, and white potatoes.
- Reduce protein back down to 6 to 12 ounces according to size and gender.
- Increase fat to a can of full-fat coconut milk (about 14 ounces) or 4 to 5 tablespoons coconut oil per day. Have full-fat coconut milk or coconut oil with each meal.
- Reduce cooked starchy vegetables and starchy fruit to 2 servings per week eaten with coconut milk/fat and protein. If you are losing too much weight, you may gradually add starchy cooked vegetables back into your diet to determine which level is right for you.
- Eliminate legumes, including pea pods and green beans.
- Eliminate even gluten-free soy sauce (coconut aminos are a good substitute).
- Limit alcohol to special occasions because of the carb content.
- If not showing urine ketones, you may need to reduce your intake of starchy vegetables and fruits and/or increase your fat intake.
- Note: The transition to Wahls Paleo Plus should occur over several weeks to avoid problems with nausea, vomiting, or diarrhea with the shift to a fat-burning metabolism.

The following chart summarizes the food categories and the goal for each food group. Note the colors are broken down into high-carbohydrate and low-carbohydrate foods. Remember that Wahls Paleo Plus stresses low-carbohydrate colors and limits high-carbohydrate vegetables and fruits.

Food Category	Wahls Diet	Wahls Paleo	Wahls Paleo Plus
Fruits and Vegetables	Goal	Goal	Goal
Leafy greens (6 cups raw)	3 cups/day	3 cups/day	2–3 cups/day
Sulfur-rich (raw or cooked)	3 cups/day	3 cups/day	2–3 cups/day
Nonstarchy colorful (raw or cooked)	3 cups/day	3 cups/day	2–3 cups/day

Food Category	Wahls Diet	Wahls Paleo	Wahls Paleo Plus
Fruits and Vegetables	Goal	Goal	Goal
Starchy color (raw or cooked) as part of the 3 cups color category	As part of 3 cups of color	As part of 3 cups of color	Raw as part of 2–3 cups of color; cooked 2 servings/week maximum
Apple, pear, bananas	After 9 cups	After 9 cups	Avoid
Protein Sources			
Organ meats	As desired	12 ounces/week	12 ounces/week
Wild cold-water fish	As desired	16 ounces/week	16 ounces/week
Other meat, poultry, game	6–12 ounces/day	9–21 ounces/day	6–12 ounces/day
Beans, legumes, peas, lentils, peanuts	As desired	2 servings/week maximum	Avoid
Raw nuts and seeds	4 ounces/day maximum	Soaked, up to 4 ounces/day day maximum	Soaked, up to 4 ounces/day day maximum
Eggs	Avoid	Avoid	Avoid
Fats and Oils			
Flax, hemp, walnut	2 tablespoons/day maximum	2 tablespoons/day maximum	2 tablespoons/day maximum
Olive	As desired	As desired	As desired
Coconut (coconut oil, coconut butter)	As desired	As desired	4–6 tablespoons/day or more (or 1¾ cups full-fat coconut milk)
Animal fat (clarified butter, lard, bacon grease)	As desired	As desired	As desired
Milk and Milk Substitutes			
Full-fat coconut milk	As desired	As desired	1¾ cups/day (or 4–6 tablespoons coconut oil) or more
Rice (organic preferred)	As desired	Avoid	Avoid
Soy (organic only)	As desired	Avoid	Avoid
Nut and seed (almond, hazelnut, hemp)	As desired	Soaked, as desired	Soaked, as desired
Animal (cow, goat, sheep)	Avoid	Avoid	Avoid

Food Category	Wahls Diet	Wahls Paleo	Wahls Paleo Plus
Grains			
Gluten-free (rice, oat, quinoa, amaranth, buckwheat, corn)	1 serving/day maximum	2 servings/week maximum	Avoid
Gluten grains (wheat, rye, barley)	Avoid	Avoid	Avoid
Additional Items			
Seaweed	Permitted, up to 1 serving/day (serving = 2.5 ounces fresh or reconstituted, 1 teaspoon flakes, or ¼ teaspoon powder)	Up to 1 serving/day	Up to 1 serving/day
Dried algae (chlorella)	Up to 1 teaspoon chlorella	Up to 1 teaspoon/day	Up to 1 teaspoon/day
Nutritional yeast	1–2 tablespoons/day	1–2 tablespoons/day	1–2 tablespoons/day
Fermented nondairy, non-grain foods	As desired	1 or more servings/day	1 or more servings/day

COMPLETE FOOD LISTS FOR ALL LEVELS OF THE WAHLS PROTOCOL

Dark green leafy vegetables (3 cups cooked or 6 cups raw, daily)

(* = Vegetables high in calcium)

- Arugula*
- Beet greens
- Bok choy* and other Asian greens
- Chard, all colors
- Chicory
- Cilantro
- Collard greens*
- Dandelion greens*
- Endive
- Escarole
- Kale,* all types (curly, lacinato/dinosaur, red, etc.)
- Lettuce, all types of deep green, bright green, and red leaf (no iceberg)
- Mizuna
- Mustard greens*
- Parsley
- Radicchio
- Radish leaves
- Romaine lettuce
- Spinach*
- Tatsoi*
- Turnip greens*
- Watercress
- Wheatgrass

Colored vegetables and fruits (3 cups daily)

Even though they have white flesh, we allow zucchini and cucumbers because they are low in carbohydrates and their skins, which you should eat, are very high in antioxidants. Consume at least three different colors daily. Note: While on Wahls Paleo Plus, switch colors to the low-carbohydrate vegetables and fruits. Limit starchy produce to two servings per week eaten with 1 to 2 tablespoons of fat and protein. If not in nutritional ketosis, you may need to eliminate the higher-carbohydrate vegetables and fruits and/or increase coconut milk. Note: For the following lists, any food containing 30 grams of carbohydrates or more per cup qualifies it as a higher-carb choice.

Green

LOWER/MODERATE-CARBOHYDRATE

- Artichoke
- Asparagus
- Avocado
- Beans, green (avoid on Wahls Paleo Plus)
- Cabbage, green
- Celery
- Cucumber, with skin
- Grapes, green
- Green peas (avoid on Wahls Paleo Plus and Wahls Elimination)
- Honeydew melon
- Kiwi, green
- Limes
- Okra
- Olives, green
- Peppers, green (avoid for Wahls Elimination)
- Snow peas (avoid on Wahls Paleo Plus and Wahls Elimination)
- Sugar snap peas (avoid on Wahls Paleo Plus and Wahls Elimination)
- Zucchini with skin

HIGHER-CARBOHYDRATE

- Commercial juices (avoid on Wahls Paleo Plus)

Red

LOWER/MODERATE-CARBOHYDRATE

- Beets
- Blood oranges
- Cabbage, red
- Cherries
- Cranberries
- Currants, red
- Grapefruit, red
- Grapes, red
- Peppers, red (avoid for Wahls Elimination)
- Radicchio
- Raspberries, red
- Rhubarb
- Strawberries
- Tomatoes, red (avoid for Wahls Elimination)
- Watermelon

HIGHER-CARBOHYDRATE

- Commercial juices (avoid on Wahls Paleo Plus)
- Dried cranberries and other dried fruit (avoid on Wahls Paleo Plus)
- Pomegranate

Blue/Purple/Black

LOWER/MODERATE-CARBOHYDRATE

- Aronia berries
- Blackberries
- Blueberries
- Currants, black
- Eggplant (avoid for Wahls Elimination)
- Elderberries
- Grapes, black
- Grapes, purple
- Kale, purple
- Olives, black
- Plums
- Raspberries, black

HIGHER-CARBOHYDRATE

- Commercial juice (avoid on Wahls Paleo Plus)
- Dates (avoid on Wahls Paleo Plus)
- Dried currants (avoid on Wahls Paleo Plus)
- Figs, purple (avoid on Wahls Paleo Plus)
- Prunes (avoid on Wahls Paleo Plus)
- Raisins (avoid on Wahls Paleo Plus)

Yellow/Orange

LOWER/MODERATE-CARBOHYDRATE

- Apricots
- Carrots
- Grapefruit
- Kiwi, golden
- Lemon
- Mango
- Muskmelon
- Nectarines
- Oranges
- Papaya
- Peaches
- Peppers, orange and yellow (avoid for Wahls Elimination)
- Pineapple
- Pumpkin
- Squash, summer and winter
- Sweet potatoes
- Tangerines
- Tomatoes, yellow (avoid for Wahls Elimination)
- Yams

HIGHER-CARBOHYDRATE

- Acorn squash
- Commercial juice (avoid on Wahls Paleo Plus)

- Dried apricots, pineapple, or other dried fruit (avoid on Wahls Paleo Plus)
- Figs
- Sweet potatoes, cooked

Sulfur-rich vegetables (3 cups daily)

(* = Vegetables high in calcium)

- Arugula*
- Asparagus
- Bok choy*
- Broccoli
- Broccoli rabe (rapini)
- Brussels sprouts
- Cabbage
- Cauliflower
- Chives
- Collard greens*
- Daikon
- Garlic, all types (two cloves = 1 serving)
- Kale*
- Kohlrabi
- Leeks
- Mizuna
- Mushrooms
- Mustard greens
- Onions, red, yellow, and white
- Radishes
- Rutabagas
- Scallions
- Shallots
- Tatsoi
- Turnip greens*
- Turnips
- Watercress

Starchy fruits not included in the 9 cups (white flesh). Consume only after 9 cups are finished.

- Apples (avoid on Wahls Paleo Plus)
- Bananas (avoid on Wahls Paleo Plus)
- Pears (avoid on Wahls Paleo Plus)

Other white nonstarchy vegetables may be consumed after the 9 cups have been eaten.

- Bamboo shoots
- Cucumbers without skin
- Jicama
- Water chestnuts (canned)
- Zucchini without skin

Sea vegetables/algae (introduced with Wahls Paleo and Wahls Paleo Plus)

- Algae (serving = 1 teaspoon chlorella)
- Chlorella
- Seaweed (1 serving = 2.5 ounces fresh or reconstituted, 1 teaspoon flakes, or ¼ teaspoon powder)

Red

- Dulse
- Irish moss
- Nori

Brown

- Bladder wrack
- Kelp
- Kombu
- Wakame

Green

- Sea lettuce

Animal protein (strongly recommended in the Wahls Diet, mandatory for Wahls Paleo and Wahls Paleo Plus; prefer organic if possible, wild or grass-fed ideal)

- Beef
- Buffalo/bison
- Chicken
- Duck
- Elk
- Fish, all kinds (salmon, tuna, cod, sardines, mackerel, tilapia, sea bass, herring, etc.)
- Lamb
- Pork
- Processed meat with no gluten, nitrates, or monosodium glutamate
- Shellfish, all kinds (shrimp, crab, lobster, scallops, etc.)
- Turkey
- Veal
- Venison, rabbit, pheasant, quail, and other wild game

Organ meat (12 ounces per week; introduced with Wahls Paleo and continued in Wahls Paleo Plus)

- Brain
- Gizzard
- Heart
- Kidney
- Liver
- Sweetbreads
- Tongue
- Tripe

Omega-3-rich fish (16 ounces a week; encouraged in the Wahls Diet, mandatory with Wahls Paleo and Wahls Paleo Plus)

- Anchovies
- Clams
- Halibut
- Herring
- Mackerel
- Mussels
- Oysters
- Salmon
- Sardines
- Trout
- Tuna (fresh)

Dairy substitutes (organic preferred)

- Organic full-fat coconut milk, canned
- Organic unsweetened nut milk (like almond, hazelnut, or hemp milk; homemade soaked nut milk is strongly preferred for Wahls Paleo and Wahls Paleo Plus)
- Unsweetened coconut milk in a carton (for Wahls Diet and Wahls Paleo only, not for use on Wahls Paleo Plus. This is different from canned coconut milk, with much less fat and added fillers)
- Organic soy milk (avoid on Wahls Paleo and Wahls Paleo Plus)
- Yogurts and other products made from coconut milk, nut milks, or organic soy (Wahls Diet only), but watch the sugar content.

Nongluten grains and potatoes (eaten only after meeting your 9 cups goal: 1 serving per day on the Wahls Diet, 2 servings per week on Wahls Paleo, avoid on Wahls Paleo Plus and Wahls Elimination)

- Almond and other nut flours
- Amaranth
- Arrowroot
- Brown rice
- Buckwheat
- Chickpea flour
- Coconut flour
- Coconut meat, fresh or unsweetened dried (shredded or flaked)
- Corn
- Flaxseeds and flax meal
- Millet
- Quinoa
- Sago
- Sorghum
- Soy flour
- Tapioca
- White potatoes (Yukon gold or heirloom red or black potatoes)
- Wild rice

Legumes (2 servings per week maximum on Wahls Paleo, avoid on Wahls Paleo Plus and Wahls Elimination)

- Any dried beans (black, white, pinto, lima, peanuts, peanut butter, etc.)
- Lentils
- Pea pods and green beans

Nuts and seeds (for Wahls Paleo, Wahls Paleo Plus, and Wahls Elimination, all nuts and seeds and their butters should be sprouted)

    † = good source of fiber
    * = high in calcium

- Tree nuts (unless you are allergic to them, including almonds,* walnuts, hazelnuts, cashews, Brazil nuts, and pistachios), maximum 4 ounces of nuts and seeds per day
- Seeds (sunflower, pumpkin, sesame, flax,† and chia†)
- Peanuts (unless you are allergic to them; peanuts are technically a legume, so avoid on Wahls Paleo and Wahls Paleo Plus)
- Peas (green, split peas, black-eyed peas; avoid on Wahls Paleo Plus and Wahls Elimination)
- Tahini (sesame butter)
- Sunflower butter
- Almond butter

Cold-pressed oils (do not fry with or heat these oils)

- Avocado oil
- Flax oil
- Hemp oil
- Olive oil, extra virgin
- Nut oil (such as walnut or almond)

Cooking oils

- Clarified butter/ghee
- Coconut oil, extra virgin
- Rendered animal fats (e.g., lard, chicken fat, duck fat)
- Other oil/seed butters: Very occasional use of organic sesame oil. Coconut fat sources (use as desired on the Wahls Diet and Wahls Paleo, but highly

recommended on Wahls Paleo Plus; these are used to increase the intake of medium-chain triglycerides to assist in achieving nutritional ketosis)

Condiments/flavorings

- Brewer's yeast—though I prefer nutritional yeast because it has B_{12} added
- Coconut aminos (a soy-sauce-like condiment; one popular brand is Coconut Secret raw vegan aminos)
- Herbs/spices without added sugar or salt
- Horseradish
- Miso (brown rice and soy versions only, not barley or other miso containing gluten); avoid on Wahls Paleo and Wahls Paleo Plus (avoid on Wahls Elimination)
- Mustard
- Nutritional yeast (Make sure it is gluten-free; if it causes headaches or fatigue, add it to your "prohibited" list.)
- Pickles
- Sauerkraut
- Sea salt (iodized or regular)
- Tamari (Make sure it's gluten-free, preferably fermented instead of hydrolyzed (avoid for Wahls Elimination)
- Wasabi (The powder is gluten-free, but the paste may have gluten, so be sure to read the label.)

Sweeteners (limit to 1 teaspoon per day and avoid on Wahls Paleo Plus)

- Honey
- Real maple syrup, organic (Do not use "pancake syrup" or anything containing high-fructose corn syrup. Organic maple syrup is important—formaldehyde may have been added to nonorganic brands.)
- Molasses* (high in calcium)
- Sorghum
- Stevia leaves or extract
- Raw sugar, evaporated cane juice, or other relatively unrefined forms of cane sugar (I prefer that you choose one of the other sweeteners, if possible, and avoid sugar entirely. *Do not* consume white sugar.)

Fermented foods (introduced with Wahls Paleo and Wahls Paleo Plus; start with one serving per day for Paleo and two servings per day for Paleo Plus, though additional servings are fine. You can find these in the refrigerator section of grocery and natural food stores, or of course you can make them yourself using the recipes in this book.)

- ½ cup lacto-fermented almond, soy, and coconut milk cultures
- ½ cup kombucha tea
- ½ cup beet kvass
- ¼ cup kimchi
- ¼ cup lacto-fermented cabbage, sauerkraut, pickles, or other vegetables

Beverages

- Water
- Club soda
- Coffee
- Tea (black or green, white, red rooibos, oolong, matcha, herbal)
- Yerba maté
- Kombucha tea
- Unsweetened 100 percent fruit juice (Avoid on Wahls Paleo Plus; have smoothies blended with water and/or coconut milk instead.)
- 100 percent vegetable juice
- 100 percent vegetable/fruit juice unsweetened (Avoid fruit juice on Wahls Paleo Plus; have smoothies blended with water instead.)
- Alcohol (daily limit to no more than one drink for women and two for men—special occasions only on Wahls Paleo Plus):
  - Gluten-free beer
  - Non-grain-based alcohol (like potato vodka)
  - Wine

Appendix B
NUTRIENT COMPARISON TABLES

Wahls versus the average U.S. intake mean for females aged 50–59

The following table summarizes the nutrient comparison of the average U.S. dietary intake for a woman my age and the intake for the one-week menus of the Wahls Diet, Wahls Paleo, and Wahls Paleo Plus. The Wahls Elimination diet nutrient content was reported in *Nutrients* and was found to be low in calcium but was otherwise nutrient dense.[1] The nutrients with ** are the key thirty-one nutrients that we have identified as most important for brain health.[2] The additional micro- and macronutrients are provided to demonstrate how healthful the Wahls Diets are in comparison to the average U.S. diet.

I have also provided information about the macronutrient content, glycemic index, and glycemic load from the three weeks of menus we provided to show that all three Wahls diets are more nutrient-dense than the average American diet.

Key Brain Nutrient Comparison of the U.S., Wahls Diet, Wahls Paleo Diet, Wahls Paleo Plus Diets					
Nutrients	*U.S.**	*Wahls Diet*	*Wahls Paleo*	*Wahls Paleo Plus*	*Dietary Reference Intakes†*
Macronutrients and Dietary Fiber					
Energy, kcal	1,759	2,009	1,991	2,012	
Protein, g	70	107	158	84	46
Fat, g	66	80	80	152	
Carbohydrate, g	219	244	178	103	130
Dietary fiber, g	17	52	40	31	*21*
Protein, percent energy	16	20	32	16	
Fat, percent energy	33	34	35	65	
Carbohydrate, percent energy	50	46	33	19	

Nutrients	U.S.*	Wahls Diet	Wahls Paleo	Wahls Paleo Plus	Dietary Reference Intakes†
Macronutrients and Dietary Fiber					
Glycemic Index (≤55 is low; ≥70 is high)	n/a	52	53	38	
Glycemic Load (<80 is low; 100 is moderate)	n/a	100	74	28	
Cholesterol and Fatty Acids					
Cholesterol, mg**	228	165	567	351	
Trans-fatty acids, g**	2.06‡	0.46	0.62	0.38	
Palmitic acid 16:0, g**	11.36	9.41	10.82	16.47	
Linoleic acid 18:2, g**	13.51	15.94	10.99	11.08	11
Linolenic acid 18:3, g**	1.47	3.16	3.09	2.32	
Arachidonic acid 20:4, g**	0.12	0.10	0.50	0.33	
Eicosapentaenoic acid 20:5 (EPA), g**	0.03	0.27	0.37	0.40	
Docosahexaenoic acid 22:6 (DHA), g**	0.07	0.44	0.59	0.46	
Vitamins					
Retinol, mcg**	420	341	1,406	1,388	
Vitamin B_1 (thiamin), mg **	1.4	9.3	8.7	2.7	1.1
Vitamin B_2 (riboflavin), mg**	1.9	10.4	9.7	3.8	1.1
Vitamin B_3 (niacin), mg**	21.5	72.2	84.2	38.3	14††
Vitamin B_6 (pyridoxine), mg**	1.8	10.7	10.8	3.9	1.5
Vitamin B_9 (folic acid), mcg DFE**	487	947	1137	872	400
Vitamin B_{12} (cobalamin), mcg**	4.8	19.3	23.1	14.4	2.4
Vitamin C (ascorbic acid), mg**	99	440	561	337	75
Vitamin D, mcg**	4.6	12.8	8.8	10.1	15
Vitamin E (total alpha-tocopherol), mg**	8.2	24.5	18.4	16.7	15
Vitamin K, mcg**	152	1,346	1,384	1,120	90

Nutrients	U.S.*	Wahls Diet	Wahls Paleo	Wahls Paleo Plus	Dietary Reference Intakes†
Minerals					
Calcium, mg**	890	1,731	957	736	1,200
Phosphorus, mg**	1,202	1,771	1,986	1,438	700
Magnesium, mg**	283	635	501	448	320
Iron, mg**	13.1	21.5	27.4	21.8	8
Zinc, mg**	9.8	16.3	31.8	18.3	8
Copper, mg**	1.2	3.0	3.6	3.2	0.9
Selenium, mcg**	95.8	118.4	209.9	129.9	55
Minerals					
Sodium, mg	2,992	2,380	3,042	2,539	1,300
Potassium, mg	2,592	6,140	6,234	4,807	4,700
Carotenoids					
Beta-carotene, mcg**	3,097	27,190	31,223	21,494	
Alpha-carotene, mcg**	490	1,510	2,745	1,717	
Beta-cryptoxanthin, mcg**	98	1,195	493	1,033	
Lutein + Zeaxanthin, mcg**	2,428	37,460	23,273	31,327	
Lycopene, mcg**	4,238	10,832	2,917	1,362	

* Mean intake for females 50–59 years in the United States, 2009–2010. Premenopausal women and men will have slightly different average intakes. ars.usda.gov/SP2UserFiles/Place/12355000/pdf/0910/Table_1_NIN_ GEN_09.pdf and ars.usda.gov/SP2UserFiles/Place/12355000/pdf/0910/Table_5_EIN_GEN_09.pdf accessed June 7, 2013.

** Key Brain Nutrients

‡ Based on median intake (third quintile) of 6,183 women ≥45 years who participated in the Women's Health Study; Annals of Neurology 72 (2012): 124–34.

† Recommended Dietary Allowances and Adequate Intakes for females 51–70 years; usual intake at or above these levels have a low probability of inadequacy. Adequate Intake values are in italics. iom.edu/Activities/ Nutrition/SummaryDRIs/DRI-Tables.aspx

†† mg niacin equivalents

Appendix C
RESOURCES

This Resource Guide includes things that I either personally use in my every-day life or is a product or service I believe you would find useful in your health journey. Many of these companies sponsor my annual seminar (https://terry wahls.com/seminar/) so that we are able to include meals for attendees and make the ticket price more affordable. I also use affiliate links when available. This means I get a small amount of money if you purchase through my link. This helps support my work and my research and I am grateful for your support.

WAHLS RESOURCES

On the following pages find information for all the products and services mentioned in this book. Because resources are ever-changing, check my web-site, thewahlsprotocol.com/bonus, for the most up-to-date product and sup-plement recommendations.

Electrical therapy devices for NMES

The device I used to use, which was in this list in the first edition, is no longer available. I advise you to work with your therapist to find the right device for you.

COMPEX

compex.com

This product is made for athletes and is available over the counter. It will not be as high-powered as what your physical or occupational therapist would have access to.

NEUFIT

neu.fit

Neufit is a company out of Austin, Texas, that has an electrical therapy de-vice. You can do an initial consult with them for an evaluation and develop-ment of a home training program and a device to have at home to use for exercise and training in your rehabilitation program.

Functional electrical therapy cycles

Cycles that are powered by hand (ergonomic) or legs (bicycle) are augmented with electrical stimulation of muscles. This is another excellent training device with case examples of patients with multiple sclerosis and spinal cord injury who have benefited from using functional electrical stimulation to support the use of cycling exercise machines.

RESTORATIVE THERAPIES
restorative-therapies.com

MYOLYN
myolyn.com/

WALKAIDE
walkaide.com/en-US/Pages/default.aspx

BIONESS
bioness.com/Home.php

These devices use functional electrical stimulation, or FES. A sequential firing of the device helps the person contract muscles in the leg, pick up their toes, and flex their ankle upward as they swing their leg forward. Bioness also has devices to improve the function of the thigh muscles and improve hand function.

Whole-body vibration machines

slimvibes.com/compare.html

This site allows the consumer to compare several manufacturers and models. You will need to assemble the device once it is delivered to your home.

powerplate.com

Power Plate is a company that will deliver the device and set it up in your home.

Endless Pools

endlesspools.com

EMF Protection

EMF Analysis information and products

emfanalysis.com

rfreduce.com/mxdna2

SafeSleeve

safesleevecases.com

The EMF Safety Superstore

lessemf.com

Food and Supplement Resources
Emu Oil

WALKABOUT HEALTH PRODUCTS

walkabouthealthproducts.com

The emus that produce emu oil (manufactured by Walkabout Health Products) have been bred to have more vitamin K2MK4 (a useable sub-type of vitamin K2). I use this product routinely—it comes in capsule or liquid form. Most emu oil on the market is a waste product from birds that have not been cultivated for high K2MK4 content in their fat. I prefer to use the Walk-about emu oil for this reason.

Organ meat capsules

DR. RON'S ULTRA-PURE

drrons.com

If you can't get used to eating organ meat, you could consider capsules of dried organ meat. He also has a number of vitamin and other supplements.

PALEOVALLEY

paleovalley.com/store

This is another business offering organ meat capsules and other products from grass-fed animals. Their meat sticks are excellent.

Seaweed

Maine Coast Sea Vegetables

seaveg.com/shop

Phosphatidylcholine (PC)

BodyBio

bodybio.com

Most of the PC available online is soy-derived and is actually just lecithin. When you blend it with water, you will not be able to make liposomes (cream) because it is not actually a phospholipid. The phospholipid is a molecule that has a fat-soluble tail and a water-soluble head. When it is blended at very high speed with water, it will make tiny spheres with the head inside and the tails to the outside. These are liposomes. These liposomes will more easily enter the bloodstream and cross the blood-brain barrier to facilitate the repair of myelin.

PC is also helpful at improving the detoxification pathways. It is something I routinely use in my clinical practice for those with mental health issues or neurological issues. It is also helpful for those who have a high toxin burden due to heavy metals, solvents, pesticides, or biotoxins such as Lyme or mold from water-damaged buildings.

The PC that I have found that consistently makes liposome is the PC that can be purchased from BodyBio. They offer a variety of high-quality nutritional supplements and vitamins. This is the only place to order phosphatidylcholine that is capable of making liposomes when blended with water in a high-speed blender (such as a Vitamix). Liposomes are more readily absorbed than PC capsules, which is why I recommend making them into smoothies and pudding (pages 426 and 462).

PC is expensive, so I recommend using the coupon code Wahls-P for a discount.

Note: There is also intravenous PC that is egg-derived (and manufactured in Russia) and can be administered in an infusion center familiar with high-dose intravenous PC. Most people won't choose to do this, but it is an option you may want to investigate.

Labs and other nutrition, microbiome, and genetic testing companies

FUNCTIONAL MEDICINE TESTING

yourlabwork.com/wahlsprotocol/

This link will take you to a comprehensive listing of functional medicine tests you can order for yourself without a prescription from a doctor. This will allow you to get information on many tests your conventional doctor may not order for you. Insurance will not typically cover these tests, but many are relatively inexpensive. This is a powerful tool for taking control of your own health! For help interpreting your results, consult a functional medicine doctor (to find one, consult the search function on the IFM website at ifm.org/find-a-practitioner/).

GLUTEN DETECTIVE
glutendetective.com

This test detects whether you have been exposed to gluten.

EZ GLUTEN TEST
ezgluten.com

NIMA GLUTEN SENSOR
Nimasensor.com/gluten

Both of these tests detect the presence of gluten in food or beverages.

METAGENICS
metagenics.com

Metagenics is a nutrition company that was founded by Dr. Jeffrey Bland, a nutritional biochemist who based it on the principle of using nutrition to overcome the less effective enzymes a person has because of his or her particular DNA.

NUTRITION GENOME
nutritiongenome.com/consultations/

Nutrition Genome does DNA analysis and creates a review of the known DNA variants that impact nutrition pathways. You get a 50-page report that discusses the implications of your genetics and makes recommendations for dietary choices (e.g., high-fat diet or low-fat diet, risk of gluten sensitivity, need for higher dosing for specific vitamins, etc.).

GENOPALATE
genopalate.com

This company will test your DNA and give you dietary recommendations based on the results. If you already have results from another test (such as 23andMe), they will supplement and interpret your data for a lower fee.

EMBODYDNA
embodydna.com

This DNA test and results are specifically oriented toward weight loss.

ENTEROLAB
enterolab.com/default.aspx

This lab offers testing for sensitivities to a variety of foods, including gluten, dairy, and other foods such as soy and nightshades. It also offers genetic testing for the genes that put that person at a high risk for developing a severe type of food sensitivity reaction. A physician's prescription is not required for these tests. This is how I convinced my family to go gluten- and dairy-free.

Such labs offer a wide variety of nutritional and functional medicine assessments. They have information for patients and clinicians on their webpages and can assist the layperson with finding a health care practitioner who can oversee a functional medicine evaluation.

CELL SCIENCE SYSTEMS
cellsciencesystems.com/

This lab (among others) offers the ALCAT food sensitivity test.

NOW LEAP
nowleap.com/leap/

This is a food sensitivity test, but the focus is on the foods you can eat, rather than the foods you can't eat.

GREAT PLAINS LABORATORY, INC.
greatplainslaboratory.com

This company provides testing for physicians and for patients, for the organic metabolites (by-products) of our cellular metabolism. Tests can be done using blood (sometimes from a finger-stick blood sample you can collect at home), or from urine, stool, saliva, or hair, to better understand how your cells are conducting the chemistry of life, how you are managing your toxin burden, what your food sensitivities are, what your vitamin and nutrient status is, and what your genetic risks are. They do have an option to have one of their in-house physicians act as the ordering physician. Details for what is available can be found on their website.

GENOVA DIAGNOSTICS

gdx.net/

Genova Diagnostics provides extensive testing for underlying environmental, nutritional, and genetic factors contributing to health and disease. The tests must be ordered by a health care practitioner. They can assist patients in locating a practitioner with whom to work. Find details on their website.

CYREX LABS

cyrexlabs.com

This company is very helpful, with more advanced testing related specifically to autoimmunity. They also offer many other complex panels, but a physician will need to order the labs.

VIOME MICROBIOME

viome.com

This microbiome test provides you with a food list based on your results.

BIOHM HEALTH MICROBIOME TESTING

biohmhealth.com

This company offers comprehensive microbiome testing including Candida testing, and also offers probiotic and prebiotic supplements.

Self-Monitoring Technology

APPLE WATCH

apple.com

This smartwatch has a fitness tracker and a heart rate monitor.

FITBIT

fitbit.com

This is an easy-to-use fitness tracker and step counter.

HEARTMATH

heartmath.com

This device monitors your heart rate and gives you feedback for stress management purposes.

MUSE

choosemuse.com/

This EEG device translates your mental activity into weather sounds for feedback and meditation.

MELOMIND

melomind.com/

This device is for brain training and relaxation.

Kitchen Tools
High-performance blending machines

VITAMIX

Vitamix.com

Enter the code 06-004969 to get free standard shipping when ordering online. These will cost $200 to $600 depending on the features you choose. I waited until my blender died and got a Vitamix. After that, I wondered why I had waited so long. You can look for the refurbished models and save some money that way.

HEALTHMASTER

myhealthmaster.com

Montel Williams has the Health Master, another high-performance blending machine. I have not used it, however.

Food-processing machines

Cuisinart has several food processors that you can consider. We have used the Custom 14. cuisinart.com/products/food_processors.html

Dehydrators

Many virtual and brick-and-mortar sporting goods and camping supply stores will carry dehydrators. Prices will likely range from approximately $100 to $300 or more, depending on the features you choose.

- Open Country and Nesco are round dehydrators. You can get additional trays to make the dehydrator taller.
- Excalibur is a rectangular dehydrator that has nine trays.

Pressure Cooking

INSTANT POT

instantpot.com

This is the newest incarnation of the old-fashioned pressure cooker, made easier and safer. They are trendy, but they are also excellent for anyone on the Wahls Diet who wants to reduce the lectin content in grains, legumes, and nightshade vegetables via pressure cooking. It is also provides a fast way to make bone broth.

Other Health Tools

SAUNAS

saunaspace.com

Near-infrared incandescent light provides light and heat therapy that improves mitochondrial function and detoxification. SaunaSpace's single bulb units are helpful for those suffering from heat intolerance, but who would benefit fron sauna and light therapy.

MELATONIN ENHANCING

lowbluelights.com/index.asp?

LowBlueLights sells products to boost melatonin production naturally. This is done by limiting your exposure to light in the blue frequency range. Products will include amber-tinted glasses and amber lightbulbs.

MOLEKULE AIR PURIFIERS

molekule.com

Molekule has new technology that improves air quality, reducing particulates in the air including mold and animal dander. Many of my patients have found this to be remarkably helpful in reducing problems related to pet allergies and problems with water damage in a building that they cannot avoid.

Books
ELECTRICAL THERAPY TEXTBOOKS

- Greta Vrbová, Olga Hudlicka, and Kristen Schaefer Centofani, *Application of Muscle/Nerve Stimulation in Health and Disease (Advances in Muscle Research).* New York: Springer, 2008.
  - This is a reference book for the research on the use of electrical therapy to recover from injury and restore function, including the setting in of progressive brain and spinal cord disorders. It also includes a chapter that is written as a how-to for performing electrical stimulation for the lay individual.

GROWING YOUR OWN FOOD

- Mel Bartholomew. *All New Square Foot Gardening,* 3rd ed. Brentwood, TN: Cool Springs Press, 2018.
  - This book is an excellent resource for growing more of your own food with less work.

IMPACT OF CHRONIC MOLD AND OTHER BIOTOXIN-RELATED PROBLEMS

- Ritchie C. Shoemaker. *Surviving Mold: Life in the Era of Dangerous Buildings.* Baltimore, MD: Otter Bay Books, 2010.
  - The presence of mold in the internal environment of a building's ventilation, heating, and cooling systems can, in the genetically susceptible person, lead to chronic fatigue and numerous medical, neurological, and psychological symptoms.

ATHEROSCLEROSIS (BLOOD VESSEL HEALTH)

- Mark Houston. *What Your Doctor May Not Tell You About Heart Disease.* New York: Grand Central Life and Style, 2012.
  - Atherosclerosis (clogging of the arteries and veins) is very common in those with autoimmune problems.

Informational organizations about the subjects in this book

Local Harvest Inc. localharvest.org/csa/

This website is focused on organic and local foods. It will help you find a farmer who offers shares in a community-supported agriculture near you.

THE QUANTIFIED SELF

quantifiedself.com/

This organization is dedicated to the furthering of self-monitoring through technology.

THE VITAMIN D COUNCIL

vitamindcouncil.org

This website provides information about vitamin D deficiency, toxicity, health conditions related to vitamin D, and vitamin D supplementation for public and health professionals. You can also request a home test kit to obtain your vitamin D level without a doctor's order.

INSTITUTE FOR FUNCTIONAL MEDICINE

ifm.org

You can search the site for more information about functional medicine and use the "Find a Functional Medicine Practitioner" page to search for a provider.

ANCESTRAL HEALTH SOCIETY

ancestralhealth.org

The Ancestral Health Society fosters interdisciplinary collaboration among scientists, health care professionals, and laypersons to promote an evolutionary perspective on current health challenges. They have many fascinating materials for anyone interested in the concepts of ancestral health and how they can apply them today.

THE WAHLS RESEARCH FUND

terrywahls.com/about/the-wahls-research-fund/

We have dissolved the Wahls Foundation. Instead, we are utilizing the University of Iowa Foundation to fund the Wahls Research Fund. Having philanthropic support to collect the pilot data for use in our grants has been critical to the success of our research lab. For grants to be competitive, we need to have pilot data from 10 to 20 subjects to present as part of the grant proposal. My goal is to expand the number of disease states that we are investigating so that we can study how diet and lifestyle can be used to improve quality of life and reduce symptoms in other neurological diseases such as Parkinson's, amyotrophic lateral sclerosis (ALS), Alzheimer's, and other dementias; mental health conditions such as depression and anxiety; other autoimmune conditions such as rheumatoid arthritis and lupus; and other medical problems such as obesity, fatty liver disease, and diabetes. If you are interested in helping us collect pilot data for a disease state that is important to you and your family, please reach out and partner with us.

In addition, we have several studies in various stages of development. We have philanthropic support to collect some additional biospecimens as part of the Dietary Approaches to Treating MS Related Fatigue clinical trial and are conducting analysis for a study in newly diagnosed MS patients to compare therapeutic diet/lifestyle to usual care. If you wish to partner with us to help launch this study, please reach out.

We are always writing grants, submitting proposals, and looking for collaborators. Philanthropic support that allows us to collect pilot data for these studies is crucial because it allows us to make grant proposals much stronger. We have already received generous support and hope to secure more, so that we can build on these proposals, generate more pilot data, and submit more competitive grants to the National MS Society and the National Institutes of Health. Please contact Megan Rife (megan.rife@foriowa.org) at the University Center for Advancement to learn more about any of these research proposals.

Donations by check should be made payable to the University of Iowa Center for Advancement. Include The Wahls Research Fund on the memo line. Please mail checks to: University of Iowa Center for Advancement, PO Box 4550, Iowa City, IA 52244, USA.

ACKNOWLEDGMENTS

I GOT MY LIFE BACK. I wrote this book so that you can get yours back, too, and I wrote this revised edition so you can continue to advance and take advantage of the evolving knowledge, technologies, and support increasingly available to us all.

This book would not be possible without the love and support of my wife, Jackie, and our children, Zach and Zebby. They are my sustenance.

There are many others who have given me critical support and encouragement in this journey. It was a global village of named and unnamed who made this work possible. There are multiple parallel journeys: the memoir, my recovery, the research, the teaching, the public outreach. All have been necessary to give birth to this book. First, I needed to become ill and experience relentless decline and suffering, despite receiving the best care from the best institutions. Then the work on the memoir began, when I thought that all I could do was create a legacy for my children, for that time when I'd no longer be there, physically or cognitively. How lucky and glad I am to be with them still, in both capacities! Critical support came from the Patient Voices Project with the University of Iowa and the editors Paul Cassel and Kate Gleeson, who worked closely with me for over a year to shape my early storytelling. Kate Gleeson connected me with my literary agent, Lynn Franklin, who saw the possibilities in my work years ahead of everyone else. Without their early guidance and support, this work would never have blossomed.

My discovery and creation of the Wahls Protocol is of course critical to this book and could not have happened without my discovery of Dr. Ashton Embry. It was his organization, the Direct-MS charity of Canada, that encouraged the very first steps in my journey back to health. This could not have happened without Dr. Lael Stone, the physician who first directed me to look at Dr. Ashton Embry's work. Through Dr. Embry, I found Loren Cordain and then eventually the Ancestral Health movement. Next I discovered the role of neuromuscular electrical stimulation through Dr. Richard Shields's work and the Institute for Functional Medicine and their community of health professionals. I especially need to thank Drs. Jeff Bland, David Jones, Catherine Willner, Jay Lombardi, David Perlmutter, Mark Hyman, Michael Stone, Kristi Hughes, and Laurie Hoffman, their president. I have to thank my personal physicians, Drs. Lael Stone, E. Torage Shivapour, and Gwen Beck, for their willingness to work with me through the years.

In the development of the research program I have many to thank, and they include Drs. Paul Rothman, Warren Darling, Kathryn Chaloner, Linda Snetselaar, Susan Lutgendorf, Ergun Uc, E. Torage Shivapour, Garry Buettner, Jeff Murray, Zuhair Ballas, John Cowdery, Peter Cram, Nicole Nisly, and Cathy Swanson. I must specifically thank Babita Bisht, who was my first research assistant and was critical to our lab's success. I also have to thank the many undergraduate students who volunteered their time in the lab.

Big thanks to Cathy Chenard, the registered dietitian who worked in my research lab and provided critical support to the development of our study diets and the first edition of this manuscript, and to Tom Nelson, our graphic designer, who created the wonderful illustrations for this book.

My initial editor, Marisa Vigilante, has been invaluable from the beginning, nursing the early concepts for this book all the way to its current form. My current editor, Lucia Watson, has helped me see this book into the future.

I must also thank Jonathan Sabin, Leanne Ely, and JJ Virgin, who were key mentors as I developed my business so that I could create a website and begin spreading my message to a wider audience. Teaching the public began with an email to Theresa Carbrey, the person in charge of education at the local organic food co-op, pitching the idea of giving a lecture about how changing my diet led to improvement in my MS. Theresa agreed, and over the next several years I taught many courses for the co-op.

In 2011, Cliff Missen gave me the opportunity to give a presentation at the TEDx talk in November, and that was the beginning of a viral movement that has changed hundreds of thousands, if not millions of lives. At the time, I would never have suspected that would or could happen.

That same summer, Eve Adamson approached me as I stood in line to pick up that week's vegetables from my local CSA, suggested that we write a book together, and helped me rework my book proposal. When my TEDx talk went viral, I soon had a book contract for *The Wahls Protocol*. That meant, of course, that I now had to write while also working full-time in the clinic and doing my research. Fortunately for me, Eve is a tremendous writer with a vast amount of experience in crafting a how-to book for the public, and we have now partnered not only on the first edition of this book but also on the cookbook and on this revised edition. That was the beginning of a partnership that I hope will continue to produce many more books.

This brings me back to all of you, the public. Every day we receive countless messages through social media, emails, and phone calls from people whose lives have been helped by the Wahls Protocol. It is the global village that created the change in the research priorities for the NMSS. That led to a change in funding. More research about diet and lifestyle is happening because of your collective voice. It is this global village that will reclaim its health by teaching one another that we are in charge of the food we eat and the way we choose to live. With hearts filled with gratitude for having our lives back again, we teach, and the teaching spreads around the world.

NOTES

Preface to the Revised Edition

1. nationalmssociety.org/NationalMSSociety/media/MSNationalFiles/Documents/Diet-and -Multiple-Sclerosis-Bhargava-06-26-15.pdf

2. nationalmssociety.org/NationalMSSociety/media/MSNationalFiles/Documents/Diet-and -Multiple-Sclerosis-Bhargava-06-26-15.pdf.

3. Lee JE, Bisht B, Hall MJ, Rubenstein LM, Louison R, Klein DT, Wahls TL. A multimodal, nonpharmocologic intervention improves mood and cognitive function in people with multiple sclerosis. *Journal of the American College of Nutrition* 36 (2017): 150–68. doi.org/10.1080 /07315724.2016.1255160.

4. Irish AK, Erickson CM, Wahls TL, Snetselaar LG, Darling WG. Randomized control trial evaluation of a modified Paleolithic dietary intervention in the treatment of relapsing-remitting multiple sclerosis: a pilot study. *Degenerative Neurological and Neuromuscular Disease* 7 (2017): 1–18. doi: 10.2147/DNND.S116949; Bisht B, Darling WG, White EC, White KA, Shivapour ET, Zimmerman MB, Wahls TL. Effects of a multimodal intervention on gait and balance of subjects with progressive multiple sclerosis: a prospective longitudinal pilot study. *Degenerative Neurological and Neuromuscular Disease* 7 (2017): 79–93. doi: 10.2147 /DNND.S128872.

5. Maxwell KF, Wahls T, et al. "Lipid profile is associated with decreased fatigue in individuals with progressive multiple sclerosis following a diet-based intervention. Results from a pilot study." *PLoS One* 14, 6 (2019): e0218075.

6. 1)Wahls T, Scott MO, Alshare Z, Rubenstein L, Darling W, Carr L, Smith K, Chenard CA, LaRocca N, Snetselaar L. Dietary approaches to treat MS-related fatigue: comparing the modified Paleolithic (Wahls Elimination) and low saturated fat (Swank) diets on perceived fatigue in persons with relapsing-remitting multiple sclerosis: study protocol for a randomized controlled trial. *Trials* 19 (2018): 309. doi: 10.1186/s13063-018-2680-x; 2)Rezapour-Firouzi S, Arefhosseini SR, Mehdi F, Mehrangiz EM, Baradaran B, Sadeghihokmabad E, Mostafaei S, Fazlijou SM, Torbati MA, Sanaie S, Zamani F. Immunomodulatory and therapeutic effects of Hot-nature diet and co-supplemented hemp seed, evening primrose oils intervention in multiple sclerosis patients. *Complementary Therapies in Medicine* 21 (2013): 473–80. doi: 10.1016/j.ctim.2013.06.006; 3)Choi IY, Piccio L, Childress P, Bollman B, Ghosh A, Brandhorst S, Suarez J, Michalsen A, Cross AH, Morgan TE, Wei M, Paul F, Bock M, Longo VD. A diet mimicking fasting promotes regeneration and reduces autoimmunity and multiple sclerosis symptoms. *Cell Reports* 15 (2016): 2136–46. doi: 10.1016/j.celrep.2016.05.009; 4)Bisht B, Darling WG, Grossmann RE, Shivapour ET, Lutgendorf SK, Snetselaar LG, Hall MJ, Zimmerman MB, Wahls TL. A multimodal intervention for patients with secondary progressive multiple sclerosis: feasibility and effect on fatigue. *Journal of Alternative and Complementary Medicine* 20 (2014): 347–55. doi: 10.1089/acm.2013.0188; 5)Fellows Maxwell K, Wahls T, Browne RW,

Rubenstein L, Bisht B, Chenard CA, Snetselaar L, Weinstock-Guttman B, Ramanathan M. Lipid profile is associated with decreased fatigue in individuals with progressive multiple sclerosis following a diet-based intervention: Results from a pilot study. Public Library of Science One 14,6 (2019). doi: 10.1371/journal.pone.0218075. 6)Chenard CA, Rubenstein LM, Snetselaar LG, Wahls TL. Nutrient composition comparison between the low saturated fat swank diet for multiple sclerosis and healthy U.S.-style eating pattern. *Nutrients* 11,3 (2019): 616. doi: 10.3390/nu11030616; 7)Wahls TL, Chenard CA, Snetselaar LG. Review of two popular eating plans within the multiple sclerosis community: Low saturated fat and modified paleolithic. *Nutrients* 11,2 (2019): 352. doi: 10.3390/nu11020352; 8)Fellows Maxwell K, Wahls T, Browne RW, Rubenstein L, Bisht B, Chenard CA, Snetselaar L, Weinstock-Guttman B, Ramanathan M. Lipid profile is associated with decreased fatigue in individuals with progressive multiple sclerosis following a diet-based intervention: Results from a pilot study. *Public Library of Science One* 14,6 (2019). doi: 10.1371/journal.pone.0218075.

7. Chenard CA, Rubenstein LM, Snetselaar LG, Wahls TL. Nutrient composition comparison between the low saturated fat swank diet for multiple sclerosis and healthy U.S.-style eating pattern. *Nutrients* 11,3 (2019): 616. doi: 10.3390/nu11030616; Chenard CA, Rubenstein LM, Snetselaar LG, Wahls TL. *Nutrients* 11,3 (2019): 537. doi: 10.3390/nu11030537; Wahls TL, Chenard CA, Snetselaar LG. Review of two popular eating plans within the multiple sclerosis community: Low saturated fat and modified paleolithic. *Nutrients* 11,2 (2019): 352. doi: 10.3390/nu11020352; Fellows Maxwell K, Wahls T, Browne RW, Rubenstein L, Bisht B, Chenard CA, Snetselaar L, Weinstock-Guttman B, Ramanathan M. Lipid profile is associated with decreased fatigue in individuals with progressive multiple sclerosis following a diet-based intervention: Results from a pilot study. *Public Library of Science One* 14,6 (2019). doi: 10.1371/journal.pone.0218075.

Introduction

1. Cordain L. *The Paleo Diet: Lose Weight and Get Healthy by Eating the Foods You Were Designed to Eat.* New York: John Wiley & Sons, 2002.
2. Lin Y, Desbois A, Jiang S, Hou ST. Group B vitamins protect murine cerebellar granule cells from glutamate/NMDA toxicity. *Neuroreport* 15 (2004): 2241–44.
3. Beal MF. Bioenergetic approaches for neuroprotection in Parkinson's disease. *Annals of Neurology* 53, Suppl 3 (2003): S39–S47; Zhang W, Narayanan M, Friedlander RM. Additive neuroprotective effects of minocycline with creatine in a mouse model of ALS. *Annals of Neurology* 53 (2003): 267–70.
4. Bisht B; Darling WG; Grossmann RE; Shivapour ET; Lutgendorf SK; Snetselaar LG; Hall MJ; Zimmerman MB; Wahls TL. A multimodal intervention for patients with secondary progressive multiple sclerosis: feasibility and effect on fatigue. *Journal of Alternative and Complementary Medicine* 20 (2014).

Chapter 1

1. Willett WC. Balancing life-style and genomics research for disease prevention. *Science* 296 (2002): 695–98.
2. Alberts B, Johnson A, Lewis J, Raff M, Roberts K, Walter P. *Molecular Biology of the Cell*, 4th ed. New York: Garland Publishing, 2002.
3. Ibid.

4. Drug Influences on Nutrient Levels and Depletion. *Natural Medicines Comprehensive Database* (serial online) 2012; available from Therapeutic Research Faculty (accessed November 16, 2012).

5. Montagna P, Sacquegna T, Martinelli P et al. Mitochondrial abnormalities in migraine. Preliminary findings. *Headache* 28 (1988): 477–80; Stuart S, Griffiths LR. A possible role for mitochondrial dysfunction in migraine. *Molecular Genetics and Genomics* 287 (2012): 837–44; Welch KM, Ramadan NM. Mitochondria, magnesium and migraine. *Journal of the Neurological Sciences* 134 (1995): 9–14.

6. Pieczenik SR, Neustadt J. Mitochondrial dysfunction and molecular pathways of disease. *Experimental and Molecular Pathology* 83 (2007): 84–92.

7. Alberts et al. *Molecular Biology of the Cell.*

8. Ibid.

9. Ames BN, Liu J. Delaying the mitochondrial decay of aging with acetylcarnitine. *Annals of the New York Academy of Sciences* 1033 (2004): 108–16; Ames BN. Prevention of mutation, cancer, and other age-associated diseases by optimizing micronutrient intake. *Journal of Nucleic Acids* (2010): pii: 725071. doi: 10.4061/2010/725071.

10. Ames BN. Prevention of mutation.

11. Bowman GL, Silbert LC, Howieson D, et al. Nutrient biomarker patterns, cognitive function, and MRI measures of brain aging. *Neurology* 78 (2012): 241–49.

12. Ibid.

13. Bourre JM. Effects of nutrients (in food) on the structure and function of the nervous system: update on dietary requirements for brain. Part 2: macronutrients. *Journal of Nutrition, Health and Aging* 10 (2006): 386–99; Bourre JM. Effects of nutrients (in food) on the structure and function of the nervous system: update on dietary requirements for brain. Part 1: micronutrients. *Journal of Nutrition, Health and Aging* 10 (2006): 377–85.

14. Ames, Liu. Delaying the mitochondrial decay, 108–16.

15. Bourre. Effects of nutrients (in food), part 2: macronutrients, 386–99; Bourre. Effects of nutrients (in food): part 1: micronutrients, 377–85.

16. Mateljan G. *The World's Healthiest Foods.* Seattle: World's Healthiest Foods, 2006; Higden J, Drake V. *An Evidence-Based Approach to Dietary Phytochemicals* [serial online], 2012.

17. Ibid.; The World's Healthiest Foods, whfoods.com, updated March 24, 2013; The George Mateljan Foundation (accessed May 22, 2013); Ground Beef Calculator, ndb.nal.usda.gov/ndb/beef/show, updated January 13, 2012; Nutrient Data Laboratory United States Department of Agriculture (accessed March 5, 2013; online interactive database); Linus Pauling Institute Micronutrient Research for Optimum Health, Oregon State University, lpi.ore gonstate.edu/infocenter (accessed May 22, 2013).

18. Martone AM, Bianchi L, Abete P, Bellelli G, Bo M, Cherubini A, Corica F, Di Bari M, Maggio M, Manca GM, Marzetti E, Rizzo MR, Rossi A, Volpato S, Landi F. The incidence of sarcopenia among hospitalized older patients: Results from the Glisten study. *Journal of Cachexia, Sarcopenia and Muscle* 8 (2017): 907–914; Wall BT, Dirks ML, van Loon LJ. Skeletal muscle atrophy during short-term disuse: implications for age-related sarcopenia. *Ageing Research Reviews* 12 (2013): 898–906.

19. Glouzon BK, Barsalani R, Lagacé JC, Dionne IJ. Muscle mass and insulin sensitivity in postmenopausal women. *Climacteric* 18 (2015): 846–51.

20. Frankl V. *Man's Search for Meaning*, rev., updated ed. Boston: Beacon Press, 2006.

Chapter 2

1. Wucherpfennig KW. Structural basis of molecular mimicry. *Journal of Autoimmunity* 16 (2001): 293–302.

2. Członkowska A, Smoliński Ł, Litwin T. Severe disease exacerbations in patients with multiple sclerosis after discontinuing fingolimod. *Neurologia i Neurochirurgia Polska* 51 (2017): 156–62. doi: 10.1016/j.pjnns.2017.01.006; Fagius J, Feresiadou A, Larsson EM, Burman J. Discontinuation of disease modifying treatments in middle-aged multiple sclerosis patients. First line drugs vs natalizumab. *Multiple Sclerosis and Related Disorders* 12 (2017): 82–87. doi: 10.1016/j.msard.2017.01.009; Kister I, Spelman T, Alroughani R, Lechner-Scott J, Duquette P, Grand'Maison F, Slee M, Lugaresi A, Barnett M, Grammond P, Iuliano G, Hupperts R, Pucci E, Trojano M, Butzkueven H. Discontinuing disease-modifying therapy in MS after a prolonged relapse-free period: a propensity score-matched study. *Journal of Neurology, Neurosurgery, and Psychiatry* 87 (2016): 1133–7; Melesse DY, Marrie RA, Blanchard JF, Yu BN, Evans C. Persistence to disease-modifying therapies for multiple sclerosis in a Canadian cohort. *Patient Preference and Adherence* 11 (2017): 1093–1101. doi: 10.2147/PPA.S138263.

3. Ramagopalan SV, Sadovnick AD. Epidemiology of multiple sclerosis. *Neurologic Clinics* 29 (2011): 207–17.

4. Zamboni P, Menegatti E, Bartolomei I, et al. Intracranial venous haemodynamics in multiple sclerosis. *Current Neurovascular Research* 4 (2007): 252–58; Zamboni P, Galeotti R, Menegatti E, et al. Chronic cerebrospinal venous insufficiency in patients with multiple sclerosis. *Journal of Neurology, Neurosurgery, and Psychiatry* 80 (2009): 392–99.

5. Malagoni AM, Galeotti R, Menegatti E, et al. Is chronic fatigue the symptom of venous insufficiency associated with multiple sclerosis? A longitudinal pilot study. *International Angiology* 29 (2010): 176–82.

6. Mandato KD, Hegener PF, Siskin GP, et al. Safety of endovascular treatment of chronic cerebrospinal venous insufficiency: a report of 240 patients with multiple sclerosis. *Journal of Vascular and Interventional Radiology* 23 (2012): 55–59; Zamboni P, Galeotti R, Weinstock-Guttman B, Kennedy C, Salvi F, Zivadinov R. Venous angioplasty in patients with multiple sclerosis: results of a pilot study. *European Journal of Vascular and Endovascular Surgery* 43 (2012): 116–22.

7. Pelizzari L, Jakimovski D, Laganà MM, Bergsland N, Hagemeier J, Baselli G, Weinstock-Guttman B, Zivadinov R. Five-year longitudinal study of neck vessel cross-sectional area in multiple sclerosis. *American Journal of Neuroradiology* 39 (2018): 1703–09.

8. Marder E, Gupta P, Greenberg BM, et al. No cerebral or cervical venous insufficiency in US veterans with multiple sclerosis. *Archives of Neurology* 68 (2011): 1521–25.

9. Zamboni P, Tesio L, Galimberti S, Massacesi L, Salvi F, D'Alessando R, Cenni P, Galeotti R, Papini D, D'Amico R, Simi S, Valsecchi MG, Filippini G. Efficacy and safety of extracranial vein angioplasty in multiple sclerosis: a randomized clinical trial. *JAMA Neurology* 75 (2018): 35–43. doi: 10.1001/jamaneurol.2017.3825.

10. Blasi C. The autoimmune origin of atherosclerosis. *Atherosclerosis* 201 (2008): 17–32.

11. Virtanen JK, Rissanen TH, Voutilainen S, Tuomainen TP. Mercury as a risk factor for cardiovascular diseases. *Journal of Nutritional Biochemistry* 18 (2007): 75–85.

12. Blasi F, Tarsia P, Arosio C, Fagetti L, Allegra L. Epidemiology of *Chlamydia pneumoniae*. *Clinical Microbiology and Infection* 4 Suppl 4 (1998): S1–S6.

13. Dyslipidemia: Nutritional and Nutraceutical Functional Medicine Approach. Cardiometabolic Module, 2012 Annual International Symposium, Institute for Functional Medicine, Gig Harbor, Washington, June 1, 2012.

14. The New Era of Managing Cardiovascular Disease, Metabolic Dysfunctions and Obesity. Cardiometabolic Module, 2012 Annual International Symposium, Institute for Functional Medicine, Scottsdale, Arizona, May 31, 2012.

15. Fire in the Hole: The Metabolic Connecting Points Between Major Chronic Diseases. Cardiometabolic Module, 2012 Annual International Symposium, Institute for Functional Medicine, Scottsdale, Arizona, May 30, 2012.

16. Bland JS, Levin B, Costarella L, et al. *Clinical Nutrition: A Functional Approach*, 2nd ed. Gig Harbor, WA: Institute for Functional Medicine, 2004.

17. Fire in the Hole: The Metabolic Connecting Points Between Major Chronic Diseases. Cardiometabolic Module, 2012 Annual International Symposium, Institute for Functional Medicine, Scottsdale, Arizona, May 30, 2012.

18. Dean B. Understanding the role of inflammatory-related pathways in the pathophysiology and treatment of psychiatric disorders: evidence from human peripheral studies and CNS studies. *International Journal of Neuropsychopharmacology* 14 (2011): 997–1012; Suvisaari J, Loo BM, Saarni SE, et al. Inflammation in psychotic disorders: a population-based study. *Psychiatry Research* 189 (2011): 305–11.

19. Kaptoge S, Di Angelantonio E, Lowe G, et al. C-reactive protein concentration and risk of coronary heart disease, stroke, and mortality: an individual participant meta-analysis. *Lancet* 375 (2010): 132–40.

20. Lord RS, Bralley A. *Laboratory Evaluations for Integrative and Functional Medicine*, 2nd ed. Atlanta, GA: Metametrix Institute, 2008.

21. Ames BN. Prevention of mutation, cancer, and other age-associated diseases by optimizing micronutrient intake. *Journal of Nucleic Acids* (2010): pii: 725071. doi: 10.4061/2010/725071; Ames BN, Liu J. Delaying the mitochondrial decay of aging with acetylcarnitine. *Annals of the New York Academy of Sciences* 1033 (2004): 108–16; Ames BN. Optimal micronutrients delay mitochondrial decay and age-associated diseases. *Mechanisms of Ageing and Development* 131 (2010): 473–79.

22. Dyslipidemia: Nutritional and Nutraceutical Functional Medicine Approach. Cardiometabolic Module, 2012 Annual International Symposium, Institute for Functional Medicine, Gig Harbor, Washington, June 1, 2012; The New Era of Managing Cardiovascular Disease, Metabolic Dysunctions and Obesity. Cardiometabolic Module, 2012 Annual International Symposium, Institute for Functional Medicine, Scottsdale, Arizona, May 31, 2012; Fire in the Hole: The Metabolic Connecting Points Between Major Chronic Diseases. Cardiometabolic Module, 2012 Annual International Symposium, Institute for Functional Medicine, Scottsdale, Arizona, May 30, 2012.

23. Ibid.

Chapter 3

1. Koizumi M, Ito H, Kaneko Y, Motohashi Y. Effect of having a sense of purpose in life on the risk of death from cardiovascular diseases. *Journal of Epidemiology* 18 (2008): 191–96.

2. Ventegodt S, Andersen NJ, Merrick J. The life mission theory II. The structure of the life purpose and the ego. *Scientific World Journal* 3 (2003): 1277–85.

3. Emmons R, McCullough E. *The Psychology of Gratitude*. New York: Oxford University Press, 2004.

Chapter 4

1. Cordain L, Eaton SB, Sebastian A, Mann N, Lindeberg S, Watkins BA, O'Keefe JH et al., eds. Origins and evolution of the Western diet: health implications for the 21st century. *American Journal of Clinical Nutrition* 81:2 (2005): 341–45; Cordain L, Eaton SB, Miller JB, Mann N, Hill K. The paradoxical nature of hunter-gatherer diets: meat-based, yet non-atherogenic. *European Journal of Clinical Nutrition* 56, Suppl 1 (2002): S42–S52; Cordain L, Eades MR, Eades MD. Hyperinsulinemic diseases of civilization: more than just Syndrome X. *Comparative Biochemistry and Physiology Part A: Molecular & Integrative Physiology* 36 (2003): 95–112; Eaton SB, Konner M, Shostak M. Stone agers in the fast lane: chronic degenerative diseases in evolutionary perspective. *American Journal of Medicine* 84 (1988): 739–49.

2. Miller D. *Farmacology: Total Health from the Ground Up*, reprint ed. New York: William Morrow Paperbacks, 2014.

3. Wahls T, Scott MO, Alshare Z, Rubenstein L, Darling W, Carr L, Smith K, Chenard CA, LaRocca N, Snetselaar L. Dietary approaches to treat MS-related fatigue: comparing the modified Paleolithic (Wahls Elimination) and low saturated fat (Swank) diets on perceived fatigue in persons with relapsing-remitting multiple sclerosis: study protocol for a randomized controlled trial. *Trials* 19 (2018): 309. doi: 10.1186/s13063-018-2680-x.

4. Gurven M, Kaplan H. Longevity among hunter-gatherers: a cross-cultural examination. *Population and Development Review* 33 (2007): 321–65.

5. Mummert A, Esche E, Robinson J, Armelagos GJ. Stature and robusticity during the agricultural transition: evidence from the bioarchaeological record. *Economics & Human Biology* 9 (2011): 284-301; Sajantila A. Major historical dietary changes are reflected in the dental microbiome of ancient skeletons. *Investigative Genetics* 4 (2013): 10.

6. Gurven M, Kaplan H. Longevity among hunter-gatherers, 321–65; Mummert A, Esche E, Robinson J, Armelagos GJ. Stature and robusticity during the agricultural transition: evidence from the bioarchaeological record. *Economics & Human Biology* 9 (2011): 284-301.

7. Sajantila A. Major historical dietary changes are reflected in the dental microbiome of ancient skeletons. *Investig Genet* 4 (2013): 10; Egger G. Health, "illth," and economic growth: medicine, environment, and economics at the crossroads. *American Journal of Preventive Medicine* 37 (2009): 78–83.

8. Obesity and Overweight (updated May 13, 2012), Centers for Disease Control and Prevention, cdc.gov/nchs/fastats/overwt.htm (accessed August 18, 2013).

9. Frassetto LA, Schloetter M, Mietus-Synder M, Morris RC, Jr., Sebastian A. Metabolic and physiologic improvements from consuming a paleolithic, hunter-gatherer type diet. *European Journal of Clinical Nutrition* 63 (2009): 947–55; Osterdahl M, Kocturk T, Koochek A, Wandell PE. Effects of a short-term intervention with a paleolithic diet in healthy volunteers. *European Journal of Clinical Nutrition* 62 (2008): 682–85.

10. Jonsson T, Granfeldt Y, Ahren B, et al. Beneficial effects of a Paleolithic diet on cardiovascular risk factors in type 2 diabetes: a randomized cross-over pilot study. *Cardiovascular Diabetology* 8 (2009): 35.

11. Fasano A. Leaky gut and autoimmune diseases. *Clinical Reviews in Allergy & Immunology* 42 (2012): 71–78; Guandalini S, Newland C. Differentiating food allergies from food intolerances. *Current Gastroenterology Reports* 13 (2011): 426–34.

12. Sedaghat F, Jessri M, Behrooz M, Mirghotbi M, Rashidkhani B. Mediterranean diet adherence and risk of multiple sclerosis: a case-control study. *Asia Pacific Journal of Clinical Nutrition* 25 (2016): 377–84. doi: 10.6133/apjcn.2016.25.2.12.

13. Sanfilippo, D. *Practical Paleo: A Customized Approach to Health and a Whole-Foods Lifestyle*, updated, expanded ed. Auberry, CA: Victory Belt Publishing, 2016.

14. Calton, M, Calton J. *Naked Calories: The Caltons' Simple 3-Step Plan to Micronutrient Sufficiency*. Cleveland, OH: Changing Lives Press, 2013.

15. Treem WR. Emerging concepts in celiac disease. *Current Opinion in Pediatrics* 16 (2004): 552–59.

16. Pruimboom L, de Punder K. The opioid effects of gluten exorphins: asymptomatic celiac disease. Journal of *Health, Population and Nutrition* 33 (2015): 24. doi: 10.1186/s41043-015 -0032-y.

17. Fallon S, Enig MG. *Nourishing Traditions*, revised 2nd ed. Brandywine, MD: New Trends Publishing, 2000.

18. Kvehaugen AS, Tveiten D, Farup PG. Is perceived intolerance to milk and wheat associated with the corresponding IgG and IgA food antibodies? A cross sectional study in subjects with morbid obesity and gastrointestinal symptoms. *BMC Gastroenterology* 18, 1(2018):22.

19. Shakoor Z, AlFaifl A, AlAmro B, AlTawil LN, AlOhaly RY. Prevalence of IgG-mediated food intolerance among patients with allergic symptoms. *Annals of Saudi Medicine* 36 (2016): 386–90; Guo H, Jiang T, Wang J, Chang Y, Guo H, Zhang W. The value of eliminating foods according to food-specific immunoglobulin G antibodies in irritable bowel syndrome with diarrhoea. *Journal of International Medical Research* 40 (2012): 204–10; Drisko J, Bischoff B, Hall M, McCallum R. Treating irritable bowel syndrome with a food elimination diet followed by food challenge and probiotics. *Journal of the American College of Nutrition* 25 (2006): 514–22; Karakula-Juchnowicz H, Gałecka M, Rog J, Bartnicka A, Łukaszewicz Z, Krukow P, Morylowska-Topolska J, Skonieczna-Zydecka K, Krajka T, Jonak K, Juchnowicz D. The food-specific serum IgG reactivity in major depressive disorder patients, irritable bowel syndrome patients and healthy controls. *Nutrients* 10 (2018): pii: E548; Neuendorf R, Corn J, Hanes D, Bradley R. Impact of food immunoglobulin G-based elimination diet on subsequent food immunoglobulin G and quality of life in overweight/obese adults. *Journal of Alternative and Complementary Medicine* 25 (2019): 241–48.

20. Coca, AF. *The Pulse Test*, 5th ed. New York: St. Martin's Press, 1996.

Chapter 5

1. Moriya M, Nakatsuji Y, Okuno T, Hamasaki T, Sawada M, Sakoda S. Vitamin K2 ameliorates experimental autoimmune encephalomyelitis in Lewis rats. *Journal of Neuroimmunology* 170 (2005): 11–20.

2. Ferland G. Vitamin K and the nervous system: an overview of its actions. *Advances in Nutrition* 3 (2012): 204–12; Ferland G. Vitamin K, an emerging nutrient in brain function. *Biofactors* 38 (2012): 151–57.

3. Watzl B. Anti-inflammatory effects of plant-based foods and of their constituents. *International Journal for Vitamin and Nutrition Research* 78 (2008): 293–98; Shukitt-Hale B, Lau FC, Joseph JA. Berry fruit supplementation and the aging brain. *Journal of Agricultural and Food Chemistry* 56 (2008): 636–41; Joseph J, Cole G, Head E, Ingram D. Nutrition, brain aging, and neurodegeneration. *Journal of Neuroscience* 29 (2009): 12:795–801; Holt EM, Steffen LM, Moran A, et al. Fruit and vegetable consumption and its relation to markers of inflammation and oxidative stress in adolescents. *Journal of the American Dietetic Association* 109 (2009): 414–21.

4. Webb AJ, Patel N, Loukogeorgakis S, et al. Acute blood pressure lowering, vasoprotective, and antiplatelet properties of dietary nitrate via bioconversion to nitrite. *Hypertension* 51 (2008): 784–90.

5. Frostegård J. Arteriosclerosis in patients with autoimmune disorders. *Arteriosclerosis, Thrombosis, and Vascular Biology* 9 (2005): 1776–85.

6. Guerrero-Beltran CE, Calderon-Oliver M, Pedraza-Chaverri J, Chirino YI. Protective effect of sulforaphane against oxidative stress: recent advances. *Experimental and Toxicologic Pathology* 64 (2012): 503–508; Morihara N, Sumioka I, Moriguchi T, Uda N, Kyo E. Aged garlic extract enhances production of nitric oxide. *Life Sciences* 71 (2002): 509–17; Noyan-Ashraf MH, Sadeghinejad Z, Juurlink BH. Dietary approach to decrease aging-related CNS inflammation. *Nutritional Neuroscience* 8 (2005): 101–10; Ping Z, Liu W, Kang Z et al. Sulforaphane protects brains against hypoxic-ischemic injury through induction of Nrf2-dependent phase 2 enzyme. *Brain Research* 1343 (2010): 178–85; Thakur AK, Chatterjee SS, Kumar V. Beneficial effects of Brassica juncea on cognitive functions in rats. *Pharmaceutical Biology* 51 (2013): 1304–10; Holt EM, Steffen LM, Moran A, et al. Fruit and vegetable consumption and its relation to markers of inflammation and oxidative stress in adolescents. *Journal of the American Dietetic Association* 109 (2009): 414–21; Vasanthi HR, Mukherjee S, Das DK. Potential health benefits of broccoli: a chemico-biological overview. *Mini-Reviews in Medicinal Chemistry* 9 (2009): 749–59; Wierinckx A, Breve J, Mercier D, Schultzberg M, Drukarch B, Van Dam AM. Detoxication enzyme inducers modify cytokine production in rat mixed glial cells. *Journal of Neuroimmunology* 166 (2005): 132–43.

7. Guerrero-Beltran CE, Calderon-Oliver M, Pedraza-Chaverri J, Chirino YI. Protective effect of sulforaphane against oxidative stress, 503–508; Latte KP, Appel KE, Lampen A. Health benefits and possible risks of broccoli: an overview. *Food and Chemical Toxicology* 49 (2011): 3287–3309; Vasanthi HR, Mukherjee S, Das DK. Potential health benefits of broccoli, 749–59; Williams MJ, Sutherland WH, McCormick MP, Yeoman DJ, de Jong SA. Aged garlic extract improves endothelial function in men with coronary artery disease. *Phytotherapy Research* 19 (2005): 314–19.

8. Borek C. Garlic reduces dementia and heart-disease risk. *Journal of Nutrition* 136 (2006): 810S–812S; Chauhan NB. Multiplicity of garlic health effects and Alzheimer's disease. *Journal of Nutrition, Health and Aging* 9 (2005): 421–32.

9. Borek C. Antioxidant health effects of aged garlic extract. *Journal of Nutrition* 131 (2001): 1010S–1015S; Borek C. Garlic reduces dementia, 810S–812S; Williams MJ, Sutherland WH, McCormick MP, Yeoman DJ, de Jong SA. Aged garlic extract improves endothelial function, 314–19.

10. Akramiene D, Kondrotas A, Didziapetriene J, Kevelaitis E. Effects of betaglucans on the immune system. *Medicina* (Kaunas, Lithuania) 43 (2007): 597–606.

11. Lull C, Wichers HJ, Savelkoul HF. Antiinflammatory and immunomodulating properties of fungal metabolites. *Mediators of Inflammation* 2005(2): 63–80; Borek C. Antioxidant health effects, 1010S–1015S; Akramiene D, Kondrotas A, Didziapetriene J, Kevelaitis E. Effects of beta-glucans on the immune system. *Medicina* (Kaunas, Lithuania) 43 (2007): 597–606.

12. Chatrou ML, Winckers K, Hackeng TM, Reutelingsperger CP, Schurgers LJ. Vascular calcification: the price to pay for anticoagulation therapy with vitamin K-antagonists. *Blood Reviews* 26 (2012): 155–66; Shea MK, Holden RM. Vitamin K status and vascular calcification: evidence from observational and clinical studies. *Advances in Nutrition* 3 (2012): 158–65.

13. Huebner FR, Lieberman KW, Rubino RP, Wall JS. Demonstration of high opioid-like activity in isolated peptides from wheat gluten hydrolysates. *Peptides* 5 (1984): 1139–47; Teschemacher H, Koch G. Opioids in the milk. *Endocrine Regulations* 25 (1991): 147–50.

14. Gearhardt AN, Davis C, Kuschner R, Brownell KD. The addiction potential of hyperpalatable foods. *Current Drug Abuse Reviews* 4 (2011): 140–45.

15. *Textbook of Functional Medicine*. Gig Harbor, WA: Institute for Functional Medicine, 2010; Brown AC. Gluten sensitivity: problems of an emerging condition separate from celiac disease. *Expert Review of Gastroenterology & Hepatology* 6 (2012): 43–55; Cascella NG, Kryszak D, Bhatti B et al. Prevalence of celiac disease and gluten sensitivity in the United States clinical antipsychotic trials of intervention effectiveness study population. *Schizophrenia Bulletin* 37 (2011): 94–100; da Silva Neves MM, Gonzalez-Garcia MB, Nouws HP, Delerue-Matos C, Santos-Silva A, Costa-Garcia A. Celiac disease diagnosis and gluten-free food analytical control. *Analytical and Bioanalytical Chemistry* 397 (2010): 1743–53; Hadjivassiliou M, Grunewald RA, Lawden M, Davies-Jones GA, Powell T, Smith CM. Headache and CNS white matter abnormalities associated with gluten sensitivity. *Neurology* 56 (2001): 385–88; Hadjivassiliou M, Sanders DS, Grunewald RA, Woodroofe N, Boscolo S, Aeschlimann D. Gluten sensitivity: from gut to brain. *Lancet Neurology* 9 (2010): 318–30; Humbert P, Pelletier F, Dreno B, Puzenat E, Aubin F. Gluten intolerance and skin diseases. *European Journal of Dermatology* 16 (2006): 4–11; Jackson JR, Eaton WW, Cascella NG, Fasano A, Kelly DL. Neurologic and psychiatric manifestations of celiac disease and gluten sensitivity. *Psychiatric Quarterly* 83 (2012): 91–102; Valentino R, Savastano S, Maglio M, et al. Markers of potential coeliac disease in patients with Hashimoto's thyroiditis. *European Journal of Endocrinology* 146 (2002): 479–83; Vereckei E, Szodoray P, Poor G, Kiss E. Genetic and immunological processes in the pathomechanism of gluten-sensitive enteropathy and associated metabolic bone disorders. *Autoimmunity Reviews* 10 (2011): 336–40.

16. *Textbook of Functional Medicine*. Gig Harbor, WA: Institute for Functional Medicine, 2010.

Chapter 6

1. Konijeti GG, Kim N, Lewis JD, Groven S, Chandrasekaran A, Grandhe S, Diamant C, Singh E, Oliveira G, Wang X, Molparia B, Torkamani A. Efficacy of the autoimmune protocol diet for inflammatory bowel disease. *Inflammatory Bowel Diseases* 23 (2017): 2054–60. doi: 10.1097/MIB.0000000000001221.

2. Afifi L, Danesh MJ, Lee KM, Beroukhim K, Farahnik B, Ahn RS, Yan D, Singh RK, Nakamura M, Koo J, Liao W. Dietary behaviors in psoriasis: patient-reported outcomes from a U.S. national survey. *Dermatology and Therapy* 7 (2017): 227–42. doi: 10.1007/s13555-017-0183-4.

3. Otten J, Stomby A, Waling M, Isaksson A, Söderström I, Ryberg M, Svensson M, Hauksson J, Olsson T. A heterogeneous response of liver and skeletal muscle fat to the combination of a Paleolithic diet and exercise in obese individuals with type 2 diabetes: a randomised controlled trial. *Diabetologia* 61 (2018): 1548–59. doi: 10.1007/s00125-018-4618-y; Otten J, Mellberg C, Ryberg M, Sandberg S, Kullberg J, Lindahl B, Larsson C, Hauksson J, Olsson T. Strong and persistent effect on liver fat with a Paleolithic diet during a two-year intervention. *International Journal of Obesity* (London) 40 (2016): 747–53. doi: 10.1038/ijo.2016.4.

4. Manheimer EW, van Zuuren EJ, Fedorowicz Z, Pijl H. Paleolithic nutrition for metabolic syndrome: systematic review and meta-analysis. *American Journal of Clinical Nutrition* 102

(2015): 922–32. doi.org/10.3945/ajcn.115.113613; Boers I, Muskiet FA, Berkelaar E, Schut E, Penders R, Hoenderdos K, Wichers HJ, Jong MC. Favourable effects of consuming a Palaeolithic-type diet on characteristics of the metabolic syndrome: a randomized controlled pilot-study. Lipids in Health and Disease 13 (2014): 160. doi: 10.1186/1476-511X-13-160.

5. Otten J, Stomby A, Waling M, Isaksson A, Tellström A, Lundlin-Olsson L, Brage S, Ryberg M, Svensson M, Olsson T. Benefits of a Paleolithic diet with and without supervised exercise on fat mass, insulin sensitivity, and glycemic control: a randomized controlled trial in individuals with type 2 diabetes. *Diabetes/Metabolism Research and Reviews* 33 (2017). doi: 10.1002/dmrr.2828.

6. Genoni A, Lyons-Wall P, Lo J, Devine A. Cardiovascular, metabolic effects and dietary composition of ad-libitum Paleolithic vs. Australian Guide to Healthy Eating diets: a 4-week randomized trial. 8 (2016): pii: E314. doi: 10.3390/nu8050314.

7. Miller GJ, Field RA, Riley ML. Lipids in wild ruminant animals and steers. *Journal of Food Quality* 9 (1986): 331–41.

8. The New Era of Managing Cardiovascular Disease, Metabolic Dysfunctions and Obesity. Cardiometabolic Module, 2012 Annual International Symposium, Institute for Functional Medicine, Scottsdale, Arizona, May 31, 2012.

9. Simopoulos AP. Human requirement for N-3 polyunsaturated fatty acids. *Poultry Science* 79 (2000): 961–70.

10. Simopoulos AP. The importance of the omega-6/omega-3 fatty acid ratio in cardiovascular disease and other chronic diseases. *Experimental Biology and Medicine* 233 (2008): 674–88; Simopoulos AP. Importance of the omega-6/omega-3 balance in health and disease: evolutionary aspects of diet. *World Review of Nutrition and Dietetics* 102 (2011): 10–21.

11. Simopoulos AP. The importance of the omega-6/omega-3 fatty acid ratio, 674–88.

12. Deal CL, Moskowitz RW. Nutraceuticals as therapeutic agents in osteoarthritis. The role of glucosamine, chondroitin sulfate, and collagen hydrolysate. *Rheumatic Disease Clinics of North America* 25 (1999): 379–95.

13. Replace and Replenish: Treatment of Digestive Dysfunction. Advance Practice Module: Restoring Gastrointestinal Equilibrium: Practical Applications for Understanding, Assessing and Treating GI Dysfunction. Conference, Institute for Functional Medicine, Scottsdale, Arizona, December 9, 2011.

14. Young GS, Conquer JA, Thomas R. Effect of randomized supplementation with high dose olive, flax or fish oil on serum phospholipid fatty acid levels in adults with attention deficit hyperactivity disorder. *Reproduction Nutrition Development* 45 (2005): 549–58.

15. Tripoli E, Giammanco M, Tabacchi G, Di Majo D, Giammanco S, La Guardia M. The phenolic compounds of olive oil: structure, biological activity and beneficial effects on human health. *Nutrition Research Reviews* 18 (2005): 98–112.

16. Muskiet FAJ. Fat Detection, Taste, Texture, and Post Ingestive Effects, Chapter 2, 19–79, in Pathophysiology and Evolutionary Aspects of Dietary Fats and Long-Chain Polyunsaturated Fatty Acids Across the Life Cycle. Boca Raton, FL: CRC Press, 2009; Kavanagh K, Jones KL, Sawyer J, et al. Trans fat diet induces abdominal obesity and changes in insulin sensitivity in monkeys. *Obesity* (Silver Spring) 15 (2007): 1675–84.

17. Bowman GL, Silbert LC, Howieson D, Dodge HH, Traber MG, Frei B, Kaye JA, Shannon J, Quinn JF. Nutrient biomarker patterns, cognitive function, and MRI measures of brain aging. *Neurology* 78 (2012): 241–49.

18. Ibid.

19. Urbano G, Lopez-Jurado M, Aranda P, Vidal-Valverde C, Tenorio E, Porres J. The role of phytic acid in legumes: antinutrient or beneficial function? *Journal of Physiology and Biochemistry* 56 (2000): 283–94.

20. Cordain L, Toohey L, Smith MJ, Hickey MS. Modulation of immune function by dietary lectins in rheumatoid arthritis. *British Journal of Nutrition* 83 (2000): 207–17.

21. Flavin DF. The effects of soybean trypsin inhibitors on the pancreas of animals and man: a review. *Veterinary and Human Toxicology* 24 (1982): 25–28.

22. Mensah P, Tomkins A. Household-level technologies to improve the availability and preparation of adequate and safe complementary foods. *Food and Nutrition Bulletin* 24 (2003): 104–25.

23. Gasnier C, Dumont C, Benachour N, Clair E, Chagnon MC, Seralini GE. Glyphosate-based herbicides are toxic and endocrine disruptors in human cell lines. *Toxicology* 262 (2009): 184–91; Richard S, Moslemi S, Sipahutar H, Benachour N, Seralini GE. Differential effects of glyphosate and roundup on human placental cells and aromatase. *Environmental Health Perspectives* 113 (2005): 716–20.

24. Samsel A, Seneff S. Glyphosate's suppression of cytochrome p450 enzymes and amino acid biosynthesis by the gut microbiome: pathways to modern diseases. *Entropy* (2013) 15: 1416–63.

25. McEvoy M. Organic 101: Can GMOs Be Used in Organic Products? (updated May 13, 2013), United States Department of Agriculture, blogs.usda.gov/2013/05/17/organic-101-can-gmos-be-used-in-organic-products (accessed July 21, 2013).

26. Cordain L, Toohey L, Smith MJ, Hickey MS. Modulation of immune function by dietary lectins, 207–17.

27. Berk Z. Technology of production of edible flours and protein products from soybeans, 1992. Rome: Food and Agriculture Organization of the United Nations (updated July 8, 2012); fao.org/docrep/t0532e/t0532e00.htm (accessed June 15, 2013).

28. Tang G. Bioconversion of dietary provitamin A carotenoids to vitamin A in humans. *American Journal of Clinical Nutrition* 91 (2010): 1468S–1473S.

29. Carmel R. Nutritional vitamin-B12 deficiency. Possible contributory role of subtle vitamin-B12 malabsorption. *Annals of Internal Medicine* 88 (1978): 647–49; Dastur DK, Santhadevi N, Quadros EV, et al. Interrelationships between the B-vitamins in B12-deficiency neuromyelopathy. A possible malabsorptionmalnutrition syndrome. *American Journal of Clinical Nutrition* 28 (1975): 1255–70.

30. Blumenschine RJ, Cavallo JA. Scavenging and human evolution. *Sci Am* 267 (1992): 90–96.

31. Cooksley VG. *Seaweed: Nature's Secret to Balancing Your Metabolism, Fighting Disease, and Revitalizing Body & Soul.* New York: Stewart, Tabori & Chang, 2007.

32. Brownstein D. *Iodine: Why You Need It, Why You Can't Live Without It,* 3rd ed. West Bloomfield, IN: Medical Alternative Press, 2004.

33. Becker G, Osterloh K, Schafer S, et al. Influence of fucoidan on the intestinal absorption of iron, cobalt, manganese and zinc in rats. *Digestion* 21 (1981): 6–12; Tanaka Y, Waldron-Edward D, Skoryna SC. Studies on inhibition of intestinal absorption of radioactive strontium. VII. Relationship of biological activity to chemical composition of alginates obtained from North American seaweeds. *Canadian Medical Association Journal* 99 (1968): 169–75.

34. Damonte EB, Matulewicz MC, Cerezo AS. Sulfated seaweed polysaccharides as antiviral agents. *Current Medicinal Chemistry* 11 (2004): 2399–2419.

35. Price WA. *Nutrition and Physical Degeneration*, 8th ed. Lemon Grove, CA: Price Pottinger Nutrition, 2008; Fallon S, Enig MG. *Nourishing Traditions: The Cookbook that Challenges Politically Correct Nutrition and the Diet Dictocrats*, rev. 2nd ed. Washington, DC: New Trends, 2007.

36. Fallon S, Enig MG. *Nourishing Traditions*.

37. Ibid.

38. Ibid.

39. Howell E. *Enzyme Nutrition*. Garden City Park, NY: Avery Publishing Group, 1995.

40. Abbott A. Scientists bust myth that our bodies have more bacteria than human cells. *Nature*, January 8, 2016. nature.com/news/scientists-bust-myth-that-our-bodies-have-more-bacteria-than-human-cells-1.19136.

41. ncbi.nlm.nih.gov/pmc/articles/PMC4393509/

42. Kirby TO, Ochoa-Reparaz J. The Gut Microbiome in Multiple Sclerosis: A Potential Therapeutic Avenue. *Medical Sciences* 6, 3(2018):69. doi: 10.3390/medsci6030069.

43. Holmes E, Li JV, Marchesi JR, Nicholson JK. Gut microbiota composition and activity in relation to host metabolic phenotype and disease risk. *Cell Metabolism* 16 (2012): 559–64; Moschen AR, Wieser V, Tilg H. Dietary factors: major regulators of the gut's microbiota. *Gut and Liver* 6 (2012): 411–16.

44. Ghelardi E, Celandroni F, Salvetti S, Guevye SA, Lupetti A, Senesi S. Survival and persistence of Bacillus clausii in the human gastrointestinal tract following oral administration as spore-based probiotic formulation. *Journal of Applied Microbiology* 119, 2 (2015):552-9; Taverniti V, Koirala R, Dalla VA, Gargari G, Leonardis E, Arioli S, Guglielmetti S. Effect of Cell Concentration on the Persistence in the Human Intestine of Four Probiotic Strains Administered Through a Multispecies Formulation. *Nutrients* 11, 2(2019):E285.

45. Benito-Leon J, Pisa D, Alonso R, Calleja P, Diaz-Sanchez M, Carrasco L. Association between multiple sclerosis and Candida species: evidence from a case-control study. *European Journal of Clinical Microbiology & Infectious Diseases* 29 (2010): 1139–45.

46. *Neuroprotection: A Functional Medicine Approach for Common and Uncommon Neurologic Syndromes*. Institute for Functional Medicine, San Diego, California, February 11–13, 2005 (conference and continuing education module, including DVDs).

47. *Textbook of Functional Medicine*. Gig Harbor, Washington: Institute for Functional Medicine, 2010; *Clinical Nutrition: A Functional Approach*, 2nd ed. Levin JS, Levin B, Costarella L, et al. Gig Harbor, Washington: Institute for Functional Medicine, 2004.

Chapter 7

1. Guelpa G. La lutte contre l'épilepsie par la désintoxication et par la rééducation alimentaire. *Medico-Chirurgical Review* 78 (1911): 8–13.

2. Rogawski MA, Löscher W, Rho JM. Mechanisms of action of antiseizure drugs and the ketogenic diet. *Cold Spring Harbor Perspectives in Medicine* 6 (2016): pii: a022780. doi: 10.1101/cshperspect.a022780; Lutas A, Yellen G. The ketogenic diet: metabolic influences on brain excitability and epilepsy. *Trends in Neuroscience* 36 (2013): 32–40. doi: 10.1016/j.tins.2012.11.005; Zhang Y, Xu J, Zhang K, Yang W, Li B. The anticonvulsant effects of ketogenic diet on epileptic seizures and potential mechanisms. *Current Neuropharmacology* 16 (2018): 66–70. doi: 10.2174/1570159X15666170517153509.

3. Zhang Y, Xu J, Zhang K, Yang W, Li B. The anticonvulsant effects of ketogenic diet, 66–70.

4. Wilder RM. High fat diets in epilepsy. *Mayo Clinical Bulletin* 2 (1921): 308.

5. Peterman MG. The ketogenic diet in epilepsy. *Journal of the American Medical Association* 84 (1925): 1979–83.

6. Huttenlocher PR, Wilbourn AJ, Signore JM. Medium-chain triglycerides as a therapy for intractable childhood epilepsy. *Neurology* 21 (1971): 1097–1103.

7. Balietti M, Casoli T, Di Stefano G, Giorgetti B, Aicardi G, Fattoretti P. Ketogenic diets: an historical antiepileptic therapy with promising potentialities for the aging brain. *Ageing Research Reviews* 9 (2010): 273–79; Maalouf M, Rho JM, Mattson MP. The neuroprotective properties of calorie restriction, the ketogenic diet, and ketone bodies. *Brain Research Reviews* 59 (2009): 293–315; Milder J, Patel M. Modulation of oxidative stress and mitochondrial function by the ketogenic diet. *Epilepsy Research* 100 (2012): 295–303; Rho JM, Stafstrom CE. The ketogenic diet: what has science taught us? *Epilepsy Research* 100 (2012): 210–17; Stafstrom CE, Rho JM. The ketogenic diet as a treatment paradigm for diverse neurological disorders. *Frontiers in Pharmacology* 3 (2012): 59; Zhao Z, Lange DJ, Voustianiouk A, et al. A ketogenic diet as a potential novel therapeutic intervention in amyotrophic lateral sclerosis. *BMC Neuroscience* 7 (2006): 29.

8. Seyfried T. *Cancer as a Metabolic Disease: On the Origin, Management, and Prevention of Cancer.* New York: John Wiley & Sons, 2012.

9. *Neuroprotection: A Functional Medicine Approach for Common and Uncommon Neurologic Syndromes.* Institute for Functional Medicine, San Diego, California, February 11–13, 2005 (conference and continuing education module, including DVDs).

10. Fontan-Lozano A, Lopez-Lluch G, Delgado-Garcia JM, Navas P, Carrion AM. Molecular bases of caloric restriction regulation of neuronal synaptic plasticity. *Molecular Neurobiology* 38 (2008): 167–77.

Chapter 8

1. Carson R. *Silent Spring.* New York: Houghton Mifflin Harcourt, 1962.

2. Toxicity: Mechanisms of Toxic Insult and Recognizable Patterns. Detoxification Advanced Practice Module Detox: Understanding Biotransformation and Recognizing Toxicity, Evaluation and Treatment in the Functional Medicine Model, Institute for Functional Medicine, 2011 conference, Phoenix, Arizona, December 9, 2011.

3. Cox PA, Metcalf JS. Traditional food items in Ogimi, Okinawa: L-serine content and the potential for neuroprotection. *Current Nutrition Reports* 6 (2017): 24–31. doi: 10.1007/s13668-017-0191-0.

4. Cox PA, Davis DA, Mash DC, Metcalf JS, Banack SA. Dietary exposure to an environmental toxin triggers neurofibrillary tangles and amyloid deposits in the brain. *Proceedings of the Royal Society: Biological Sciences* 283 (2016): pii: 20152397. doi: 10.1098/rspb.2015.2397.

5. Roy-Lachapelle A, Solliec M, Bouchard MF, Sauvé S. Detection of cyanotoxins in algae dietary supplements. *Toxins* (Basel) 9 (2017): pii: E76. doi: 10.3390/toxins9030076.

6. Toxicity: Mechanisms of Toxic Insult and Recognizable Patterns. Detoxification Advanced Practice Module Detox: Understanding Biotransformation and Recognizing Toxicity, Evaluation and Treatment in the Functional Medicine Model, Institute for Functional Medicine, 2011 conference, Phoenix, Arizona, December 9, 2011.

7. Choi, AL, Sun G, Zhang Y, Grandjean P. Developmental fluoride neurotoxicity: a systematic review and meta-analysis. *Environmental Health Perspectives* 120 (2012): 1362–68.

8. who.int/peh-emf/about/WhatisEMF/en/index1.html

Chapter 9

1. Velikonja O, Curic K, Ozura A, Jazbec SS. Influence of sports climbing and yoga on spasticity, cognitive function, mood and fatigue in patients with multiple sclerosis. *Clinical Neurology and Neurosurgery* 112 (2010): 597–601.

2. Dalgas U, Stenager E, Jakobsen J, et al. Resistance training improves muscle strength and functional capacity in multiple sclerosis. *Neurology* 73 (2009): 1478–84; Dalgas U, Stenager E, Jakobsen J, et al. Fatigue, mood and quality of life improve in MS patients after progressive resistance training. *Multiple Sclerosis* 16 (2010): 480–90.

3. Kileff J, Ashburn A. A pilot study of the effect of aerobic exercise on people with moderate disability multiple sclerosis. *Clinical Rehabilitation* 19 (2005): 165–69.

4. Campbell E, Coulter EH, Paul L. High intensity interval training for people with multiple sclerosis: A systematic review. *Multiple Sclerosis and Related Disorders* 24 (2018): 55–63.

5. Carro E, Trejo JL, Busiguina S, Torres-Aleman I. Circulating insulin-like growth factor I mediates the protective effects of physical exercise against brain insults of different etiology and anatomy. *Journal of Neuroscience* 21 (2001): 5678–84; Carro E, Trejo JL, Nunez A, Torres-Aleman I. Brain repair and neuroprotection by serum insulin-like growth factor I. *Molecular Neurobiology* 27 (2003): 153–62; Cotman CW, Berchtold NC, Christie LA. Exercise builds brain health: key roles of growth factor cascades and inflammation. *Trends in Neurosciences* 30 (2007): 464–72; White LJ, Castellano V. Exercise and brain health: implications for multiple sclerosis. Part II: immune factors and stress hormones. *Sports Medicine* 38 (2008): 179–86.

6. de la Cerda P, Cervello E, Cocca A, Viciana J. Effect of an aerobic training program as complementary therapy in patients with moderate depression. *Perceptual and Motor Skills* 112 (2011): 761–69.

7. White LJ, Castellano V. Exercise and brain health, 179–86; Cotman CW, Berchtold NC, Christie LA. Exercise builds brain health, 464–72.

8. Rojas Vega S, Knicker A, Hollmann W, Bloch W, Struder HK. Effect of resistance exercise on serum levels of growth factors in humans. *Hormone and Metabolic Research* 42 (2010): 982–86.

9. Velikonja O, Curic K, Ozura A, Jazbec SS. Influence of sports climbing and yoga, 597–601.

10. Pilutti LA, Paulseth JE, Dove C, Jiang S, Rathbone MP, Hicks AL. Exercise training in progressive multiple sclerosis: a comparison of recumbent stepping and body weight-supported treadmill training. *International Journal of MS Care* 18 (2016): 221–29; Łyp M, Stanisławska I, Witek B, Olszewska-Żaczek E, Czarny-Działak M, Kaczor R. Robot-assisted body-weight-supported treadmill training in gait impairment in multiple sclerosis patients: a pilot study. *Advances in Experimental Medicine and Biology* 1070 (2018): 111–15. doi: 10.1007/5584 _2018_158.

11. Parker-Pope, T. Can't do the 7-Minute Workout? Neither can I. *New York Times*, June 5, 2018. nytimes.com/2018/06/05/well/move/05EASIER-7MINUTE.html

12. Gorgey AS, Mather KJ, Cupp HR, Gater DR. Effects of resistance training on adiposity and metabolism after spinal cord injury. *Medicine & Science in Sports & Exercise* 44 (2012): 165–74.

13. Lai CC, Tu YK, Wang TG, Huang YT, Chien KL. Effects of resistance training, endurance training, and whole-body vibration on lean body mass, muscle strength and physical performance in older people: a systematic review and network meta-analysis. *Age and Ageing* 47, 3 (2018):367–73.

14. Goudarzian M, Ghavi S, Shariat A, Shirvani H, Rahimi M. Effects of whole body vibration training and mental training on mobility, neuromuscular performance, and muscle strength

in older men. *Journal of Exercise Rehabilitation* 13 (2017): 573–80. doi: 10.12965/jer.1735024.512; Ko MC, Wu LS, Lee S, Wang CC, Lee PF, Tseng CY, Ho CC. Whole-body vibration training improves balance control and sit-to-stand performance among middle-aged and older adults: a pilot randomized controlled trial. *European Review of Aging and Physical Activity* 14 (2017): 11. doi: 10.1186/s11556-017-0180-8.

15. Wong A, Figueroa A. Effects of whole-body vibration on heart rate variability: acute responses and training adaptations. *Clinical Physiological and Functional Imaging* 39, 2 (2019): 115–21. doi: 10.1111/cpf.12524.

16. Ki-Hong K, Hyang-Beum L. The effects of whole body vibration exercise intervention on electroencephalogram activation and cognitive function in women with senile dementia. *Journal of Exercise Rehabilitation* 14, 4(2018):586-91. doi:10.12965/jer.1836230.115,

17. Pessoa MF, Muniz de Souza HC, Vasconcelos da Silva AP, dos antos Clemente R, Cunha Brandao D, Dornelas de Andrade A. Acute Whole Body Vibration Decreases the Glucose Levels in Elderly Diabetic Women. *Rehabilitation Research and Practice* 2018, Article ID 3820615, 7 pages, doi.org/10.1155/2018/3820615.

18. Sitja-Rabert M, Rigau D, Fort Vanmeerghaeghe A, Romero-Rodriguez D, Bonastre Subirana M, Bonfill X. Efficacy of whole body vibration exercise in older people: a systematic review. *Disability and Rehabilitation* 34 (2012): 883–93.

19. Zhou J, Pang L, Chen N, Wang Z, Wang C, Hai Y, Lyu M, Lai H, Lin F. Whole-body vibration training—better care for COPD patients: a systematic review and meta-analysis. *International Journal of Chronic Obstructive Pulmonary Disease* 13 (2018): 3243–254. doi: 10.2147/COPD.S176229. eCollection 2018; Neves CDC, Lacerda ACR, Lage VKS, Soares AA, Chaves MGA, Lima LP, Silva TJ, Vieira ÉLM, Teixeira AL, Leite HR, Matos MA. Whole body vibration training increases physical measures and quality of life without altering inflammatory-oxidative biomarkers in patients with moderate COPD. *Journal of Applied Physiology* 125 (2018): 520–28. doi: 10.1152/japplphysiol.01037.2017.

20. Yang F, Finlayson M, Bethoux F, Su X, Dillon L, Maldonado HM. Effects of controlled whole-body vibration training in improving fall risk factors among individuals with multiple sclerosis: a pilot study. *Disability and Rehabilitation* 40 (2018): 553–60. doi: 10.1080/09638288.2016.

21. Park YJ, Park SW, Lee HS. Comparison of the effectiveness of whole body vibration in stroke patients: a meta-analysis. *Biomedical Research International* 2018 (2018): 5083634. doi: 10.1155/2018/5083634. ncbi.nlm.nih.gov/pubmed/29114533.

22. Arena R, Pinkstaff S, Wheeler E, Peberdy MA, Guazzi M, Myers J. Neuromuscular electrical stimulation and inspiratory muscle training as potential adjunctive rehabilitation options for patients with heart failure. *Journal of Cardiopulmonary Rehabilitation and Prevention* 30 (2010): 209–23; Quittan M, Wiesinger GF, Sturm B, et al. Improvement of thigh muscles by neuromuscular electrical stimulation in patients with refractory heart failure: a single-blind, randomized, controlled trial. *American Journal of Physical Medicine & Rehabilitation* 80 (2001): 206–14.

23. Sillen MJ, Speksnijder CM, Eterman RM, Janssen PP, Wagers SS, Wouters EF, Uszko-Lencer NH, Spruit MA. Effects of neuromuscular electrical stimulation of muscles of ambulation in patients with chronic heart failure or COPD: a systematic review of the English-language literature. *Chest* 136 (2009): 44–61. doi: 10.1378/chest.08-2481.

24. Talbot LA, Gaines JM, Ling SM, Metter EJ. A home-based protocol of electrical muscle stimulation for quadriceps muscle strength in older adults with osteoarthritis of the knee. *Journal of Rheumatology* 30 (2003): 1571–78; Palmieri-Smith RM, Thomas AC, Karvonen-Gutierrez

C, Sowers M. A clinical trial of neuromuscular electrical stimulation in improving quadriceps muscle strength and activation among women with mild and moderate osteoarthritis. *Physical Therapy* 90 (2010): 1441–52; Gaines JM, Metter EJ, Talbot LA. The effect of neuromuscular electrical stimulation on arthritis knee pain in older adults with osteoarthritis of the knee. *Applied Nursing Research* 17 (2004): 201–6.

25. Piva SR, Goodnite EA, Azuma K, et al. Neuromuscular electrical stimulation and volitional exercise for individuals with rheumatoid arthritis: a multiple-patient case report. *Physical Therapy* 87 (2007): 1064–77.

26. Santos M, Zahner LH, McKiernan BJ, Mahnken JD, Quaney B. Neuromuscular electrical stimulation improves severe hand dysfunction for individuals with chronic stroke: a pilot study. *Journal of Neurologic Physical Therapy* 30 (2006): 175–83; Sullivan JE, Hedman LD. A home program of sensory and neuromuscular electrical stimulation with upper-limb task practice in a patient 5 years after a stroke. *Physical Therapy* 84 (2004): 1045–54.

27. Stackhouse SK, Binder-Macleod SA, Stackhouse CA, McCarthy JJ, Prosser LA, Lee SC. Neuromuscular electrical stimulation versus volitional isometric strength training in children with spastic diplegic cerebral palsy: a preliminary study. *Neurorehabilitation and Neural Repair* 21 (2007): 475–85; Carmick J. Clinical use of neuromuscular electrical stimulation for children with cerebral palsy, Part 1, 505–13; Carmick J. Clinical use of neuromuscular electrical stimulation for children with cerebral palsy, Part 2: Upper extremity. *Physical Therapy* 73 (1993): 514–22; Scheker LR, Chesher SP, Ramirez S. Neuromuscular electrical stimulation, 226–32.

28. Courtney AM, Castro-Borrero W, Davis SL, Frohman TC, Frohman EM. Functional treatments in multiple sclerosis. *Current Opinion in Neurology* 24 (2011): 250–54; McClurg D, Ashe RG, Marshall K, Lowe-Strong AS. Comparison of pelvic floor muscle training, electromyography biofeedback, and neuromuscular electrical stimulation for bladder dysfunction in people with multiple sclerosis: a randomized pilot study. *Neurourology and Urodynamics* 25 (2006): 337–48.

29. Wahls TL, Reese D, Kaplan D, Darling WG. Rehabilitation with neuromuscular electrical stimulation leads to functional gains in patients with secondary progressive and primary progressive multiple sclerosis: a case series report. *Journal of Alternative and Complementary Medicine* 16 (2010): 1343–49.

30. Burridge J, Taylor P, Hagan S, Swain I. Experience of clinical use of the Odstock dropped foot stimulator. *Artificial Organs* 21 (1997): 254–60; Taylor PN, Burridge JH, Dunkerley AL, et al. Clinical use of the Odstock dropped foot stimulator: its effect on the speed and effort of walking. *Archives of Physical Medicine and Rehabilitation* 80 (1999): 1577–83.

31. Davis GM, Hamzaid NA, Fomusek C. Cardiorespiratory, metabolic, and biomechanical responses during functional electrical stimulation leg exercise: health and fitness benefits. *Artificial Organs* 32 (2008): 625–29. doi: 10.1111/j.1525-1594.2008.00622.x; Dolbow DR, Gorgey AS. Effects of use and disuse on non-paralyzed and paralyzed skeletal muscles. *Aging and Disease* 7 (2016): 68–80. doi: 10.14336/AD.2015.0826.

32. Szecsi J, Schlick C, Schiller M, Pollmann W, Koenig N, Straube A. Functional electrical stimulation-assisted cycling of patients with multiple sclerosis: biomechanical and functional outcome: a pilot study. *Journal of Rehabilitation Medicine* 41 (2009): 674–80; Ratchford JN, Shore W, Hammond ER, et al. A pilot study of functional electrical stimulation cycling in progressive multiple sclerosis. *NeuroRehabilitation* 27 (2010): 121–28.

33. Edwards T, Moti RW, Sebastião E, Pilutti LA. Pilot randomized controlled trial of functional electrical stimulation cycling exercise in people with multiple sclerosis with mobility disabil-

ity. *Multiple Sclerosis and Related Disorders* 26 (2018): 103–11. doi: 10.1016/j.msard .2018.08.020; Edwards T, Moti RW, Pilutti. Cardiorespiratory demand of acute voluntary cycling with functional electrical stimulation in individuals with multiple sclerosis with severe mobility impairment. *Applied Physiology, Nutrition, and Metabolism* 43 (2018): 71–76. oi: 10.1139/apnm-2017-0397; Backus D, Burdett B, Hawkins L, Manella C, McCully KK, Sweatman M. Outcomes after functional electrical stimulation cycle training in individuals with multiple sclerosis who are nonambulatory. *International Journal of MS Care* 19 (2017): 113–21. doi: 10.7224/1537-2073.2015-036; Reynolds MA, McCully K, Burdett B, Manella C, Hawkins L, Backus D. Pilot study: evaluation of the effect of functional electrical stimulation cycling on muscle metabolism in nonambulatory people with multiple sclerosis. *Archives of Physical Medicine and Rehabilitation* 96 (2015): 627–32. doi: 10.1016/j.apmr.2014.10.010; Hammond ER, Recio AC, Sadowsky CL, Becker D. Functional electrical stimulation as a component of activity-based restorative therapy may preserve function in persons with multiple sclerosis. *Journal of Spinal Cord Medicine* 38 (2015): 68–75. doi: 10.1179/2045772314Y.0000000238.

Chapter 10

1. Smolders J. Vitamin D and multiple sclerosis: correlation, causality, and controversy. *Autoimmune Diseases* 2011 (2011): 629538; Mowry EM. Vitamin D: evidence for its role as a prognostic factor in multiple sclerosis. *Journal of the Neurological Sciences* 311 (2011): 19–22.
2. Yang CY, Leung PS, Adamopoulos IE, Gershwin ME. The implication of vitamin D and autoimmunity: a comprehensive review. *Clinical Reviews in Allergy & Immunology* 45 (2013):- 217–26; Pludowski P, Holick MF, Pilz S, et al. Vitamin D effects on musculoskeletal health, immunity, autoimmunity, cardiovascular disease, cancer, fertility, pregnancy, dementia and mortality: a review of recent evidence. *Autoimmunity Reviews* 12 (2013): 976–89.
3. Milliken SV, Wassall H, Lewis BJ, et al. Effects of ultraviolet light on human serum 25-hydroxyvitamin D and systemic immune function. *Journal of Allergy and Clinical Immunology* 129 (2012): 1554–61.
4. Faridar A, Eskandari G, Sahraian MA, Minagar A, Azimi A. Vitamin D and multiple sclerosis: a critical review and recommendations on treatment. *Acta Neurologica Belgica* 112 (2012): 327–33.
5. Kumar A, Singh RB, Saxena M, et al. Effect of carni Q-gel (ubiquinol and carnitine) on cytokines in patients with heart failure in the Tishcon study. *Acta Cardiologica* 62 (2007): 349–54; Sacher HL, Sacher ML, Landau SW, et al. The clinical and hemodynamic effects of coenzyme Q10 in congestive cardiomyopathy. *American Journal of Therapeutics* 4 (1997): 66–72; Singh RB, Niaz MA, Rastogi V, Rastogi SS. Coenzyme Q in cardiovascular disease. *Journal of the Association of Physicians of India* 46 (1998): 299–306; Kumar A, Singh RB, Saxena M, et al. Effect of carni Q-gel (ubiquinol and carnitine) on cytokines in patients with heart failure in the Tishcon study. *Acta Cardiologica* 62 (2007): 349–54.
6. Muller T, Buttner T, Gholipour AF, Kuhn W. Coenzyme Q10 supplementation provides mild symptomatic benefit in patients with Parkinson's disease. *Neuroscience Letters* 341 (2003): 201–4.
7. Brewer GJ. Copper excess, zinc deficiency, and cognition loss in Alzheimer's disease. *Biofactors* 38 (2012): 107–13; Loef M, von Stillfried, N, Walach H. Zinc diet and Alzheimer's disease: a systematic review. *Nutritional Neuroscience* 15 (2012): 2–12.
8. Ziegler D, Low PA, Litchy WJ, et al. Efficacy and safety of antioxidant treatment with alpha-lipoic acid over 4 years in diabetic polyneuropathy: the NATHAN 1 trial. *Diabetes Care* 34 (2011): 2054–60.

9. Muller T, Buttner T, Gholipour AF, Kuhn W. Coenzyme Q10 supplementation provides mild symptomatic benefit in patients with Parkinson's disease. *Neuroscience Letters* 341 (2003): 201–4.

10. Spain R, Powers K, Murchison C, Heriza E, Winges K, Yaday V, Cameron M, Kim E, Horak F, Simon J, Bourdette D. Lipoic acid in secondary progressive MS: A randomized controlled pilot trial. *Neurology Neuroimmunology & Neuroinflammation* 4, 5(2017):e374.

11. Liu J. The effects and mechanisms of mitochondrial nutrient alpha-lipoic acid on improving age-associated mitochondrial and cognitive dysfunction: an overview. *Neurochemical Research* 33 (2008): 194–203; Milgram NW, Araujo JA, Hagen TM, Treadwell BV, Ames BN. Acetyl-L-carnitine and alpha-lipoic acid supplementation of aged beagle dogs improves learning in two landmark discrimination tests. *FASEB Journal* 21 (2007): 3756–62.

12. Kumar A, Singh RB, Saxena M, et al. Effect of carni Q-gel (ubiquinol and carnitine) on cytokines in patients with heart failure in the Tishcon study. *Acta Cardiologica* 62 (2007): 349–54; Sacher HL, Sacher ML, Landau SW, et al. The clinical and hemodynamic effects of coenzyme Q10, 66–72; Singh RB, Niaz MA, Rastogi V, Rastogi SS. Coenzyme Q in cardiovascular disease, 299–306.

13. Pallas M, Verdaguer E, Tajes M, Gutierrez-Cuesta J, Camins A. Modulation of sirtuins: new targets for antiageing. *Recent Patents on CNS Drug Discovery* 3 (2008): 61–69.

14. James D, Devaraj S, Bellur P, Lakkanna S, Vicini J, Boddupalli S. Novel concepts of broccoli sulforaphanes and disease: induction of phase II antioxidant and detoxification enzymes by enhanced-glucoraphanin broccoli. *Nutrition Reviews* 70 (2012): 654–65; Applying Oral Chelation. Advanced Practice Module Detox: Understanding Biotransformation and Recognizing Toxicity, Evaluation and Treatment in the Functional Medicine Model, Institute for Functional Medicine, 2011 conference, Phoenix, Arizona, December 10, 2011.

15. Larijani VN, Ahmadi N, Zeb I, Khan F, Flores F, Budoff M. Beneficial effects of aged garlic extract and coenzyme Q10 on vascular elasticity and endothelial function: The FAITH randomized clinical trial. *Nutrition* 29 (2012): 71–75. Weiss N, Papatheodorou L, Morihara N, Hilge R, Ide N. Aged garlic extract restores nitric oxide bioavailability in cultured human endothelial cells even under conditions of homocysteine elevation. *Journal of Ethnopharmacology* 145 (2012): 162–67.

16. Jia K, Tong X, Wang R, Song X. The clinical effects of probiotics for inflammatory bowel disease: A meta-analysis. *Medicine (Baltimore)* 97, 51(2018):e13792.

17. Hayden MS, Ghosh S. Shared Principles in Nf-κB Signaling. *Cell* 132, 3(2008):344-62.

18. Kuboyama T, Tohda C, Komatsu K. Effects of Ashwagandha (roots of *Withania somnifera*) on neurodegenerative diseases. *Biological and Pharmaceutical Bulletin* 37 (2014): 892–97; Choudhary D, Bhattacharyya S, Bose S. Efficacy and safety of ashwagandha (*Withania somnifera* (L.) Dunal) root extract in improving memory and cognitive functions. *Journal of Dietary Supplements* 14 (2017): 599–612. doi: 10.1080/19390211.2017; Zhu LN, Mei X, Zhang ZG, Xie YP, Lang F. Curcumin intervention for cognitive function in different types of people: a systematic review and meta-analysis. *Phytotherapy Research* 33 (2019): 524–33. doi: 10.1002/ptr.6257; Saini N, Singh D, Sandhir R. Bacopa monnieri prevents colchicine-induced dementia by anti-inflammatory action. *Metabolic Brain Disease* 34 (2019): 505–18. doi: 10.1007/s11011-018-0332-1.

19. Scher JU, Abramson SB. Periodontal disease, *Porphyromonas gingivalis*, and rheumatoid arthritis: what triggers autoimmunity and clinical disease? *Arthritis Research & Therapy* 15 (2013): 122. doi.org/10.1186/ar4360.

20. Anderson JG, Taylor AG. Effects of healing touch in clinical practice: a systematic review of randomized clinical trials. *Journal of Holistic Nursing* 29 (2011): 221–28; Anderson JG, Taylor AG. Biofield therapies and cancer pain. *Clinical Journal of Oncology Nursing* 16 (2012): 43–48.

21. Rapaport MH, Schettler P, Bresee C. A preliminary study of the effects of repeated massage on hypothalamic-pituitary-adrenal and immune function in healthy individuals: a study of mechanisms of action and dosage. *Journal of Alternative and Complementary Medicine* 18 (2012): 789–97.

22. Hughes CM, Smyth S, Lowe-Strong AS. Reflexology for the treatment of pain in people with multiple sclerosis: a double-blind randomised sham-controlled clinical trial. *Multiple Sclerosis* 15 (2009): 1329–38.

23. Elster E. Eighty-one patients with multiple sclerosis and Parkinson's disease undergo upper cervical chiropractic care to correct vertebral subluxation: a retrospective analysis. *Journal of Vertebral Subluxation Research* 23 (2004): 1–9.

24. Foroughipour M, Bahrami Taghanaki HR, Saeidi M, Khazaei M, Sasannezhad P, Shoeibi A. Amantadine and the place of acupuncture in the treatment of fatigue in patients with multiple sclerosis: an observational study. *Acupuncture in Medicine* 31 (2013): 27–30.

25. Quispe-Cabanillas JG, Damasceno A, von Glehn F, et al. Impact of electroacupuncture on quality of life for patients with Relapsing-Remitting Multiple Sclerosis under treatment with immunomodulators: a randomized study. *BMC Complementary and Alternative Medicine* 12 (2012): 209.

26. Lappin MS, Lawrie FW, Richards TL, Kramer ED. Effects of a pulsed electromagnetic therapy on multiple sclerosis fatigue and quality of life: a double-blind, placebo controlled trial. *Alternative Therapies in Health and Medicine* 9 (2003): 38–48.

27. Piatkowski J, Kern S, Ziemssen T. Effect of BEMER magnetic field therapy on the level of fatigue in patients with multiple sclerosis: a randomized, double-blind controlled trial. *Journal of Alternative and Complementary Medicine* 15 (2009): 507–11; Ziemssen T, Piatkowski J, Haase R. Long-term effects of Bio-Electromagnetic-Energy Regulation therapy on fatigue in patients with multiple sclerosis. *Alternative Therapies in Health and Medicine* 17 (2011): 22–28.

28. Hashmi, JT, Huang Y-Y, Osmani BZ, Sharma SK, Naeser, MA, Hamblin MR. Role of low-level laser therapy in neurorehabilitation. *PM&R Journal* 2, Suppl 2 (2010): S292–S305. doi: 10.1016/j.pmrj.2010.10.013.

29. Rhee YH, Moon JH, Choi SH, Ahn JC. Low-Level Laser Therapy Promoted Aggressive Proliferation and Angiogenesis Through Decreasing of Transforming Growth Factor-beta1 and Increasing of Akt/Hypoxia Inducible Factor-1alpha in Anaplastic Thyroid Cancer. *Photomedicine and Laser Surgery* 34, 6(2016):229-35. But also note the positive results in this study: Hoefling DB, Chavantes MC, Juliano AG, Cerri GG, Knobel M, Yoshimura EM, Chammas MC. Low-level laser in treatment of patients with hypothyroidism induced by chronic autoimmune thyroiditis: a randomized, placebo-controlled clinical trial. *Lasers in Medical Science* 28, 3(2013):743-53.

30. Awasthi S, Peto R, Read S, Richards SM, Pande V, Bundy D, DEVTA team. Population deworming every 6 months with albendazole in 1 million pre-school children in North India: DEVTA, a cluster-randomised trial. *Lancet* 381 (2013): 1478–86. doi: 10.1016/S0140-6736(12)62126-6.

31. Liu C, Lu L, Zhang L, Luo R, Sylvia S, Medina A, Rozelle S, Smith DS, Chen Y, Zhu T. Effect of deworming on indices of health, cognition, and education among schoolchildren in Rural

China: a cluster-randomized controlled trial. *American Journal of Tropical Medicine and Hygiene* 96 (2017): 1478–89. doi: 10.4269/ajtmh.16-0354.

32. Szabo A. Psychedelics and Immunomodulation: Novel Approaches and Therapeutic Opportunities. *Frontiers in Immunology* 14, 6(2015):358.

33. Claflin SB, van der Mei IAF, Taylor BV. Complementary and alternative treatments of multiple sclerosis: a review of the evidence from 2001 to 2016. *Journal of Neurology, Neurosurgery & Psychiatry* 89 (2018): 34–41. doi.org/10.1136/jnnp-2016-314490.

34. Sharafaddinzadeh N, Moghtaderi A, Kashipazha D, Majdinasab N, Shalbafan B. The effect of low-dose naltrexone on quality of life of patients with multiple sclerosis: a randomized placebo-controlled trial. *Multiple Sclerosis* 16 (2010): 964–69. doi: 10.1177/1352458510366857; Ludwig MD, Zagon IS, McLaughlin PJ. Featured article: Serum [Met5]-enkephalin levels are reduced in multiple sclerosis and restored by low-dose naltrexone. *Experimental Biology and Medicine* (Maywood) 242 (2017): 1524–33. doi: 10.1177/1535370217724791.

35. Moore JJ, Massey JC, Ford CD, Khoo ML, Zaunders JJ, Hendrawan K, Barnett Y, Barnett MH, Kyle KA, Zivadinov R, Ma KC, Milliken ST, Sutton IJ, Ma DDF. Prospective phase II clinical trial of autologous haematopoietic stem cell transplant for treatment refractory multiple sclerosis. *Journal of Neurological and Neurosurgical Psychiatry* 90, 5(2019):514–21. doi: 10.1136/jnnp-2018-319446.

36. Mirshafiey A. Venom therapy in multiple sclerosis. *Neuropharmacology* 53 (2007): 353–61.

37. Zamboni P, Galeotti R, Weinstock-Guttman B, Kennedy C, Salvi F, Zivadinov R. Venous angioplasty in patients with multiple sclerosis, 116–22.

Chapter 11

1. Sabayan B, Foroughinia F, Mowla A, Borhanihaghighi A. Role of insulin metabolism disturbances in the development of Alzheimer's disease: mini review. *American Journal of Alzheimer's Disease & Other Dementias* 23 (2008): 192–99.

2. The New Era of Managing Cardiovascular Disease, Metabolic Dysfunctions and Obesity. Cardiometabolic Module, 2012 Annual International Symposium, Institute for Functional Medicine, Scottsdale, Arizona, May 31, 2012; Fire in the Hole: The Metabolic Connecting Points Between Major Chronic Diseases. Cardiometabolic Module, 2012 Annual International Symposium, Institute for Functional Medicine, Scottsdale, Arizona, May 30, 2012.

3. Richard A, Rohrmann S, Vandeleur CL, Schmid M, Barth J, Eichholzer M. Loneliness is adversely associated with physical and mental health and lifestyle factors: results from a Swiss national survey. *PLoS One* 12 (2017): e0181442. doi: 10.1371/journal.pone.01814422.

4. Hughes ME, Waite LJ, Hawkley LC, Cacioppo JT. A short scale for measuring loneliness in large surveys: results from two population-based studies. *Research on Aging* 26 (2004): 655–72.

5. Valtorta NK, Kanaan M, Gilbody S, Ronzi S, Hanratty B. Loneliness and social isolation as risk factors for coronary heart disease and stroke: systemic review and meta-analysis of longitudinal observational studies. *Heart* 102 (2016): 1009–16. doi: 10.1136/heartjnl-2015-308790.

6. Hyman M. *The Blood Sugar Solution.* New York: Little, Brown, 2012.

7. Rapaport MH, Schettler P, Bresee C. A preliminary study of the effects of repeated massage on hypothalamic-pituitary-adrenal and immune function in healthy individuals: a study of mechanisms of action and dosage. *Journal of Alternative and Complementary Medicine* 18 (2012): 789–97.

8. Bixler E. Sleep and society: an epidemiological perspective. *Sleep Medicine* 10, Suppl 1 (2009): S3–S6.

9. Bamer AM, Johnson KL, Amtmann D, Kraft GH. Prevalence of sleep problems in individuals with multiple sclerosis. *Multiple Sclerosis* 14 (2008): 1127–30; Manconi M, Ferini-Strambi L, Filippi M, et al. Multicenter case-control study on restless legs syndrome in multiple sclerosis: the REMS study. *Sleep* 31 (2008): 944–52; Moreira NC, Damasceno RS, Medeiros CA et al. Restless leg syndrome, sleep quality and fatigue in multiple sclerosis patients. *Brazilian Journal of Medical and Biological Research* 41 (2008): 932–37.

10. Khong TP, de Vries F, Goldenberg JS, Klungel OH, Robinson NJ, Ibáñez L, Petri H. Potential impact of benzodiazepine use on the rate of hip fractures in five large European countries and the United States. *Calcified Tissue International* 91 (2012): 24–31; Sylvestre MP, Abrahamowicz M, Capek R, Tamblyn R. Assessing the cumulative effects of exposure to selected benzodiazepines on the risk of fall-related injuries in the elderly. *International Psychogeriatrics* 24 (2012): 577–88.

Chapter 12

1. Alberts B, Johnson A, Lewis J, Raff M, Roberts K, Walter P. *Molecular Biology of the Cell*, 4th ed. New York: Garland Publishing, 2002.

2. *Textbook of Functional Medicine*. Gig Harbor, WA: Institute for Functional Medicine, 2010.

3. Philpott H, Nandurkar S, Royce SG, Thien F, Gibson PR. Allergy tests do not predict food triggers in adult patients with eosinophilic oesophagitis. A comprehensive prospective study using five modalities. *Alimentary Pharmacology & Therapeutics* 44 (2016): 223–33. doi: 10.1111/apt.13676; Hammond C, Lieberman JA. Unproven diagnostic tests for food allergy. *Immunology and Allergy Clinics of North America* 38 (2018): 153–63. doi: 10.1016 /j.iac.2017.09.011; Reddy K, Kearns M, Alvarez-Arango S, Carrillo-Martin I, Cuervo-Pardo N, Cuervo-Pardo L, Dimov V, Lang DM, Lopez-Alvarez S, Schroer B, Mohan K, Dula M, Zheng S, Kozinetz C, Gonzalez-Estrada A. YouTube and food allergy: an appraisal of the educational quality of information. *Pediatric Allergy, Immunology and Pulmonology* 29 (2018): 410–16. doi: 10.1111/pai.12885.

4. Shakoor Z, AlFaifi A, AlAmro B, AlTawil LN, AlOhaly RY. Prevalence of IgG-mediated food intolerance among patients with allergy symptoms. *Annals of Saudi Medicine* 36 (2016): 389–90; Kwiatkowski L, Mitchell J, Langland J. Resolution of allergic rhinitis and reactive bronchospasm with supplements and food-specific immunoglobulin G elimination: a case report. *Alternative Therapies in Health and Medicine* 22 (2016): 24–28; Vojdani A. Immune reactions to peanut proteins, agglutinins, and oleosins. *Alternative Therapies in Health and Medicine* 21 Suppl 1 (2015): 73–79; Guo H, Jiang T, Wang J, Chang Y, Guo H, Zhang W. The value of eliminating foods according to food-specific immunoglobulin G antibodies in irritable bowel syndrome with diarrhea. *Journal of International Medical Research* 40 (2012): 204–10.

5. Coca AF. *The Pulse Test*, 5th ed. New York: St. Martin's Press, 1996.

6. Morrison HI, Ellison LF, Taylor GW. Periodontal disease and risk of fatal coronary heart and cerebrovascular diseases. *Journal of Cardiovascular Risk* 6 (1999): 7–11; Seymour GJ, Ford PJ, Cullinan MP, Leishman S, Yamazaki K. Relationship between periodontal infections and systemic disease. *Clinical Microbiology and Infection* 13, Suppl 4 (2007): 3–10.

7. Chronic Infections and Neurological Disease: The Challenge of Emerging Infections in the 21st Century—Tolerance, Terrain, Susceptibility, 2011 International Annual Symposium Institute for Functional Medicine, Bellevue, Washington, April 30, 2011.

8. Ibid.; The Role of Chlamydophila in Autoimmune Disease. The Challenge of Emerging Infections in the 21st Century—Tolerance, Terrain, Susceptibility, 2011 International Annual Symposium Institute for Functional Medicine, Bellevue, Washington, April 30, 2011; Alam MZ, Alam Q, Kamal MA, Jiman-Fatani AA, Azhar EI, Khan MA, Haque A. Infectious agents and neurodegenerative diseases: Exploring the links. *Current Topics in Medicinal Chemistry* 17 (2017): 1390–99. doi: 10.2174/1568026617666170103164040.

Epilogue

1. De Luca F, Shoenfeld Y. The microbiome in autoimmune diseases. *Clinical & Experimental Immunology.* 195 (2019): 74–85. doi: 10.1111/cei.13158; Mowry EM, Glenn JD. The dynamics of the gut microbiome in multiple sclerosis. *Neurologic Clinics* 36 (2018): 185–206. doi: 10.1016 /j.ncl.2017.08.008; Chu F, Shi M, Lang Y, Shen D, Jin T, Zhu J, Cui L. Gut microbiota in multiple sclerosis and experimental autoimmune encephalomyelitis: current applications and future perspectives. *Mediators of Inflammation* 2018 (2018): 816817. doi: 10.1155/2018 8168717; Adamczyk-Sowa M, Medrek A, Madej P, Michlicka W, Dobrakowski P. Does the gut microbiota influence immunity and inflammation in multiple sclerosis pathophysiology? *Journal of Immunology Research* 2017 (2017): 7904821. doi: 10.1155/2017/7904821.

Appendix B

1. Chenard CA, Rubenstein LM, Snetselaar LG, Wahls TL. Nutrient Composition Comparison between a Modified Paleolithic Diet for Multiple Sclerosis and the Recommended Healthy U.S.-Style Eating Pattern. *Nutrients* 1, 11(2019): 3.
2. Wahls TL, Chenard CA, Snetselaar LG. Review of Two Popular Eating Plants within the Multiple Sclerosis Community: Low Saturated Fat and Modified Paleolithic. *Nutrients* 11, 2 (2019): E352.

INDEX

Note: Page numbers in *italics* refer to illustrations. Page numbers followed by a *t* refer to tables or boxed text.

and animal proteins, 189–191
and bone broth, 345, 441*t*
immune system's attack on, 58, 122–123
and sulfur-rich vegetables, 145, 328*t*
supplements for, 344–345
and Wahls Diet, 328*t*
and Wahls Elimination Diet, 122–123
journaling, 378. *See also* Wahls Diary
juicing, 152*t*

Kale Sausage Soup recipe, 444–445
Kaplan, Hilliard, 103
kefir, 218–219
kelp, 181, 204*t*, 205, 208, 274*t*, 275, 430–431, 476
ketogenic diets
about, 119*t*, 229, 231–233
and cancer, 231*t*, 232*t*
compared to Wahls Paleo Plus Diet, 229, 230–231*t*, 233
origin of, 230–231*t*
See also Wahls Paleo Plus Diet
ketones, 32, 121, 230*t*, 231–232, 249, 254
ketosis
about, 231–233
benefits, 232, 233
and cancer, 232*t*
and carbohydrate consumption, 120–121
and fasting, 252–253
and fats, 121, 249
and grains, legumes, and potatoes, 248
impact on mitochondria, 230*t*
lab tests guiding decisions on, 349
and low glycemic index foods, 234*t*
and monitoring blood ketones, 236–239, 249, 254
and protein consumption, 249
risks of long-term ketosis, 239–240*t*
and Wahls Elimination Diet, 125, 126
and Wahls Paleo Plus Diet, 121, 233, 249
and weight loss, 250*t*
without MCTs, 235*t*, 254
kidneys, consuming, 43*t*, 207
kidneys and kidney health
kidney stones, 182*t*
replacement of cells in, 389
testing function of, 345
and toxin elimination, 31, 269, 269, 272
kimchi, 119, 219, 480
kombucha tea, 119, 219, 220*t*, 456–457, 480

lab work, 345–350, 346–348*t*
lactose intolerance, 158*t*
L-carnitine, 32
lead, 71

leafy green vegetables
benefits, 138–140, 141*t*
and calcium, 182*t*, 236–238
and chloroplasts, 31*t*
choices in, 140, 472
and Coumadin, 156–157*t*
and eliminating food waste, 148*t*
goals/guidelines for, 469*t*
and ketosis, 236
and magnesium, 331
and managing digestive distress, 155
and Paleolithic nutrition, 100
recipes, 432–433, 446–448, 449
and rotating greens, 337
three cups of leafy green vegetables daily, 138–140
and vitamin D, 329
and vitamin K2, 329*t*
vitamins and minerals in, 138–140
leaky gut
about, 55–56
and autoimmune disease, 55–56, 114, 200
and bone broth, 190
and chronic stress, 365
and functional medicine, 10
impact of gluten and dairy on, 114
and lectin consumption, 122
and microbiome dysbiosis, 56, 57
and stomach acid of vegetarians, 200
and toxin exposure, 107
lectins, 122–123, 125–126, 165*t*, 195, 198, 211, 226
legumes
antinutrients found in, 112, 117, 165*t*, 195–196
carbohydrates in, 184
choices, 478
and digestive distress, 150*t*
and glyphosate (Roundup) exposure, 164*t*, 168
goals/guidelines for, 470*t*
and ketosis, 248
and microbiome, 106
and Paleolithic nutrition, 100, 103
preparation of, 125
as protein source, 186–187
reducing consumption of, 181
soaking and sprouting, 165*t*, 196, 211
and vegetarian diet, 165*t*, 195–196
and Wahls Diet, 112
and Wahls Paleo Diet, 117, 181, 183–184, 467
and Wahls Paleo Plus Diet, 120, 227, 248, 467
Lemtrada, 70*t*
liberation therapy, 361
light exposure and melatonin, 384–385
light therapy, 355–356
linoleic acid (LA), 187, 246, 246–247*t*
lipids levels, 121, 228, 333–334

ALSO BY TERRY WAHLS, M.D.

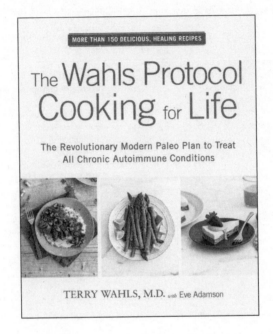

The cookbook companion to *The Wahls Protocol*,
featuring more than 150 delicious, nutritionally packed
recipes tailored to each level of the Wahls Paleo Diet.

terrywahls.com

AVERY